Clinical Handbook of Veterinary Medicine

Clinical Handbook of Veterinary Medicine

Edited by Peter Jones

SYRAWOOD
PUBLISHING HOUSE
New York

Published by Syrawood Publishing House,
750 Third Avenue, 9th Floor,
New York, NY 10017, USA
www.syrawoodpublishinghouse.com

Clinical Handbook of Veterinary Medicine
Edited by Peter Jones

International Standard Book Number: 978-1-68286-872-0 (Hardback)

Cataloging-in-Publication Data

Clinical handbook of veterinary medicine / edited by Peter Jones.
p. cm.
Includes bibliographical references and index.
ISBN 978-1-68286-872-0
1. Veterinary medicine. 2. Animals--Diseases. 3. Animals--Diseases--Treatment. 4. Animal health. I. Jones, Peter.
SF745 .C55 2020
636.089--dc23

Printed in China.

TABLE OF CONTENTS

PREFACE

Veterinary medicine is a medical specialty concerned with the diagnosis, prevention, control and treatment of conditions affecting the health of animals. The prevention and control of diseases that may be transmitted to other animals and humans is also under the scope of veterinary medicine. Medical and surgical procedures, such as caring for oral health, setting fractures and vaccinating are some of the responsibilities of a veterinarian. Vaccines have resulted in a dramatic decrease in companion animal diseases, such as feline distemper and canine distemper. Some of the specialties of veterinary medicine are dentistry, ophthalmology and dermatology. A number of instrumentation technologies used in veterinary medicine have a diagnostic or therapeutic functionality, such as echocardiography, endoscopy, laser lithotripsy, nuclear scintigraphy, ultrasonography, etc. This book elucidates the concepts and innovative models around prospective developments with respect to veterinary medicine. It presents researches and studies performed by experts across the globe. This book is a vital tool for all researching and studying this field.

This book has been the outcome of endless efforts put in by authors and researchers on various issues and topics within the field. The book is a comprehensive collection of significant researches that are addressed in a variety of chapters. It will surely enhance the knowledge of the field among readers across the globe.

It gives us an immense pleasure to thank our researchers and authors for their efforts to submit their piece of writing before the deadlines. Finally in the end, I would like to thank my family and colleagues who have been a great source of inspiration and support.

Editor

Construction of an *iss* deleted mutant strain from a native avian pathogenic *Escherichia coli* O78: K80 and in vitro serum resistance evaluation of mutant

Salari, S.[1], Zahraei Salehi, T.[1*], Nayeri Fasaei, B.[1], Karimi, V.[2]

[1] *Department of Microbiology, Faculty of Veterinary Medicine, University of Tehran, Tehran, Iran*

[2] *Department of Poultry Diseases, Faculty of Veterinary Medicine, University of Tehran, Tehran, Iran*

Key words:
iss, lambda red recombineering, Native APEC-O78 strain χ1378, serum resistance

Correspondence
Zahraei Salehi, T.
Department of Microbiology, Faculty of Veterinary Medicine, University of Tehran, Tehran, Iran

Email: tsalehi@ut.ac.ir

Abstract:

BACKGROUND: Colibacillosis, caused by different serotypes of avian pathogenic *Escherichia coli* (APEC), is one of the important diseases in poultry industry. The isolate O78 is the most prevalent serotype of APEC in Iran. One of the APEC virulence factors, increased serum survival (*iss*) gene, is related to serum resistance. The usual form of colibacillosis in avian is extraintestinal, and serum resistance is applied one way by APEC to reach internal organs; hence, it appears that the control of colibacillosis in poultry regarding the deletion of *iss* and the construction of a serum sensitive APEC strain is beneficial. Additionally, the knowledge about APEC serum resistance could be extended using mutant strains. **OBJECTIVES:** The present study was an attempt to generate an *iss* mutant strain from native APEC-O78 strain χ1378 and to study the level of serum resistance of native APEC-O78 strain χ1378 in comparison with its mutant (APEC-O78 strain χ1378Δ*iss*). **METHODS:** The lambda red recombinase system was utilized to delete *iss* gene in native APEC-O78 strain χ1378. This strain was first transformed with the plasmid pkD46 to introduce the lambda red recombinase system and then the PCR product with sequence homology to the *iss* gene and a kanamycin resistance marker was transformed into the APEC-O78 strain χ1378. Serum sensitivity of mutant and wild type strain was investigated by microtiter test. **RESULTS:** The generation of mutant was successful and the *iss* was replaced with kanamycin resistance cassette. Also, it was observed that the mutant was sensitive to serum. However, serum sensitivity of *iss* deleted mutant was not statistically different from its parents. **CONCLUSIONS:** Application of lambda red recombination could be a simple and useful technique for production of a precisely defined gene deletion. Also, there may be some genes that compensate the activity of *iss* gene.

Introduction

Colibacillosis is still considered the most important bacterial disease affecting the poultry industry (Barnes et al., 2008; Derakhshandeh et al., 2009; Kariyawasam et al., 2006; Kariyawasam and Nolan, 2009). This disease occurs by many serotypes of Avian Pathogenic *Escherichia coli* (APEC), such as O1, O2, and O78 (La Ragoine et al., 2000; Mellata et al., 2003; Nayeri Fasaei et al., 2009; Stordeur et al., 2004; Vandekerchove et al., 2004; Zahraei Salehi et al., 2004); however, it is usually the result of serotype

O78 in Iran (Zahraei Salehi et al., 2004). Clinical form of colibacillosis in avian, in contrast with mammalian colibasillosis, is extraintestinal, while intestinal form is more prevalent in mammals (Barnes and Gross, 2005; Gross, 1994). The use of prevalent pathogenic serotypes, in each country, is advisable to prepare vaccines and to control the vaccination strategies (Zahraei Salehi et al., 2004). Therefore, to this time, researches about the native APEC-O78 strain χ1378, along with other methods of colibacillosis control such as the use of antibiotics, farm sanitation, and other management practices, could be helpful. Farm sanitation and management practices are arduous and expensive, and also the cost involved in the treatment, undesirable side effects, appearance of apparent transferable antibiotic resistance, and public concerns over the use of antibiotics limit the use of antibiotics (Derakhshandeh et al., 2009; Gomis et al., 2003; La Ragione et al., 2001; La Ragione et al., 2004). Therefore, control of the disease through vaccination, especially with live attenuated vaccines, is thought to be a logical and desirable approach (Zahraei Salehi et al., 2004). It is worthwhile to consider native and frequent strains for studies of control and vaccine approaches (Zahraei Salehi et al., 2004). Live *E. coli* vaccine has been found to induce a more marked level of immunity (Kwaga et al., 1994). It is known that a properly delivered live bacterial vaccine will be more effective since all of the relevant antigens will be present to stimulate both cellular immunity and humoral immunity at the appropriate site, while these antigens may be absent or altered in killed bacteria. Also, the preparations of subunit vaccines are not cost effective (Kwaga et al., 1994). Many different live attenuated vaccines have been used to control colibacillosis; however, there is no vaccine currently available that is economical, functional in farms, and also effective against different strains of APEC (Derakhshandeh et al., 2009; Nolan et al., 2003; Nolan et al., 1992; Vidotto et al., 1990). One approach to develop attenuation and vaccination can be achieved through inactivation of one or more virulence factors (Nayeri Fasaei et al., 2009). In addition, identification and characterization of virulence factors in APEC, as a spectacular research area, could be done by construction of different mutants (Sharan et al., 2009). The role of different virulence factors related to serum resistance in mammalian *E. coli* and avian *E. coli* has been investigated; however, the knowledge about the serum resistance mechanism of APEC-O78 is ill-defined (Mellata et al., 2003). Increased serum survival (*iss*) gene, as a conserved virulence gene, has a role related to serum resistance and frequently occurs in avian *E. coli*, especially in avian pathogenic *E. coli* (Skyberg et al., 2008). Also, *iss* is located in different serotypes of APEC (Derakhshandeh et al., 2009). In addition, the ability of APEC to resist the host protective effects of serum plays a significant role in the development of APEC in body fluids and internal organs (Mellata et al., 2003). Since there is no report about the mechanism of serum resistance in native APEC-O78 strain χ1378, it seems worthwhile to delete *iss* and investigate the contribution of *iss* gene to serum resistance to have a better understanding of how to control colibacillosis.

Materials and Methodes

A. Construction of native APEC-O78 strain χ1378 Δ*iss*: The bacterial strains used in this study were routinely cultured on Luria-Bertani (LB) agar and broth, containing the appropriate antibiotics. The primers used in this study are listed in table 1. Deletion of *iss* gene was carried out in a virulent wild native strain of APEC-O78 χ1378, isolated from a chicken with systemic colibacillosis in Iran, as described previously (Datsenko and Wanner, 2000; Derakhshandeh et al., 2009; Horne et al., 2000; Lynne et al., 2007b; Nayeri Fasaei et al., 2009; Skyberg et al., 2008). Briefly, after serotyping of native APEC-O78 strain χ1378 (MAST serotyping kit; MAST Group Ltd, Merseyside, UK), the presence of *iss* gene (760bp) was detected by PCR using *iss* upper (F) and *iss* lower (R) primers. Then, *iss* gene was sequenced in APEC-O78 strain χ1378 (Derakhshandeh et al., 2009). The PCR was carried out on a total volume of 25 µL containing 1x PCR buffer, 1.6 mM MgCl2, 0.2 mM dNTPs, 0.5 µM of each primer, 1.25 U of Taq DNA polymerase and 10 µg of template DNA (PCR Set System, Sinaclon, Tehran, Iran). The amplification program was used at 94°C for 5 min, 30 cycles of 94°C for 30 sec, 55°C for 30 sec, 72°C for 30 sec, and 72°C for 7 min (Techne Thermocylcer, TC-512). Temperature sensitive plasmid pKD46, encoding the lambda Red recombinase (Nature Technology

Corporation, England), was transformed into electro-component native APEC-O78 strain χ1378 by electroporation. Plasmids were purified using commercial kit (Plasmid Isolation Kit Minipreparation, MBST, Tehran, Iran). L-Arabinose was used for the induction of the Lambda Red genes expression at 10 mM final concentration (BBL, USA). Overnight bacterial cultures of native APEC-O78 strain χ1378 were diluted 1: 100 into 8 mL of fresh SOB medium (each liter containing 20 g tripton, 0.5 g yeast extract, and 1 mL of 0.25 M KCl) and incubated at 37°C, while shaking, until they reached an OD600nm of 0.6. Culture was then concentrated by centrifugation at 3200 ×g for 15 min at 4°C. From this step, everything was maintained on ice. After discarding the supernatant, cells were then re-suspended in 4, 2 and 1 mL of ice-cold 10% glycerol (Merck, Germany) and centrifuged at 3200, 17900 and 17900 ×g for 15, 2 and 2 min, respectively, at 4°C. After these 3 washing steps, the cells were suspended in 80 µL ice-cold 10% glycerol and used immediately in 40 µL aliquots for electroporation step. Electroporation was carried out using Gene Pulser® II Electroporation System and cold Gene Pulser® 0.2 Cm gap Cuvettes (Bio-Rad® Laboratories Inc., Richmond, CA) at 2.5 kV with 25 µF and 200 Ω by adding 50 ng of pKD46 to native APEC-O78 strain χ1378 electrocompetent cells. Also, a control reaction, without adding plasmid, was electro-porated. Immediately after electroporation, cells were resuspended in 1 mL of cold LB and incubated for 1.5 h at 30°C. Five hundred microliters of the mixture were plated on LB containing 100 µg/mL ampicillin, and the plates were incubated at 30°C overnight. Ampicillin-resistant, temperature-sensitive colonies were selected for transformation by kanamycin cassette flanked by 5' and 3' sequences of the *iss* gene. Primers for - mut - *iss* and rev - mut - *iss*, and pKD4 as template, were used to amplify the kanamycin cassette flanked by homolog regions of 3' and 5' end of *iss* gene (1.6 kb). High fidelity PCR amplification was conducted using 15 reactions of AccuPower™ HF PCR PreMix (BIONEER) containing 1 µL of pKD4 template, 1 µL of each primer (10 µM) and 17 µL of distilled water. PCR conditions were as follows: 94°C for 3 min, followed by 30 cycles of 94°C for 30 sec, 58°C for 30 sec, and 72°C for 30 sec min and then an extension period of 72°C for 7 min (Techne Thermocycler, TC-512). The PCR product was purified from the agarose gel by manufacture's protocol (Gene Jet Gel Extraction Kit, Fermantase), then confirmed by agarose gel. A single fresh colony of native APEC-O78 strain χ1378 containing pKD46 was placed into 5 mL of LB-ampicillin and shaken at 30 °C overnight. Subsequently, 500 µL of this culture was mixed with 50 mL SOB containing 100µg/mL ampicillin and L-arabinose was added to a final concentration of 10 µm. The mixture was incubated at 30 °C with shake. At an OD_{600nm} of 0.6, the cells were made electrocompetent following this protocol. Cells were concentrated by centrifugation at 3200 ×g for 15 min, 4°C. Then, 4 washing steps, at 4°C, carried out by 10, 5, and 2.5 mL of cold 10% glycerol and centrifugation at 3200 ×g for 15 min for each step. Then pellet were mixed with 250 µL of cold 10% glycerol. 100 µL of electrocompetent cells (APEC-O78 strain µL378 containing pKD46) were mixed with 300 ng of purified PCR product and this mixture was electroporated as described above and then was spread on LB agar plates containing 50 µg/mL kanamycin. After kanamycin selection, the expected deletions in mutants were verified by PCR protocol targeting the new antibiotic resistance cassette junction fragment (1.8kb) through the use of the *iss* upper (F) and *iss* lower (R) primers on the kanamycin resistant colonies. The PCR reaction was performed in 25 µL reaction volume containing 2.5 µL of 10X PCR buffer, 1.6 mM of MgCl2, 0.2 mM of deoxynucleoside triphosphates, 0.5 mM of each of the upstream and downstream primers (10 pmol), 1.25 U of Taq DNA polymerase and 50 ng of DNA template (PCR Set System, Sinaclon, Tehran, Iran). PCR amplification involved 30 cycles of denaturation at 94°C for 30 sec, annealing at 55°C for 30 sec, and elongation at 72°C for 30 sec in a thermocycler (Techne Thermocylcer, TC-512). The reaction mixture was held at 94°C for 5 min before and 72°C for 7 min after the reaction.

B. In vitro serum resistance assay of native APEC-O78 strain χ1378 and its mutant by microtiter method: Tow hours culture of APEC-O78 strain χ1378, APEC-O78 strain χ1378Δ*iss*, and serum sensitive DH5α (control), grown in 3 mL Peptone Glucose (PG) broth (Difco), were adjusted to 0.5 McFarland standard (0.5 mL of 0.048 M BaCl2 (1.17% w/v BaCl2.2H2O) to 99.5 mL of 0.18 M

H2SO4 (1% v/v)). Then, 10-fold serial dilutions of each culture have been prepared and 100 μL of 10-3 dilution (104 CFU), verified by viable count was dispensed into flat-bottomed 96-well microtiter plates and mixed with 100 μL of 50% chicken serum diluted in phosphate-buffered saline. The experiment was repeated using PG broth instead of serum. Also, as medium control, 100 μL of serum mixed with 100 μL PG broth also included. Plates were incubated at 37°C and the growth was monitored using a microplate reader set at 490 nm (Stat fax-2100, UK) every 30 min for 4 hr. The experiment was repeated three times. The results are the average of three experiments. A one-way ANOVA was used to test the null hypothesis of equal mean growth rates among the strains. A post hoc test, Fisher LSD, was used to identify differences between strains with P-value 0.05 (Lee et al., 1991; Lynne et al., 2007a; Wooley et al., 1991).

Results

The *iss* gene was deleted in native APEC-O78 strain χ1378 to generate a mutant (APEC-O78 strain χ1378Δ*iss*) as described by Datsenko and Wanner (Datsenko and Wanner, 2000). At first, by PCR, with specific primers for *iss* in native APEC-O78 strain χ1378, the 760 bp PCR product was detected (Figure 1) and sequenced. The sequence was submitted to GenBank by Derakhshandeh et al. (2009) with the assigned accession number FJ416147. Then, the pKD46 electroporated to electrocompetent native APEC-O78 strain χ1378, and this strain was ampicillin resistante and sensitive to temperature higher than 30°C. The process of native APEC-O78 strain χ1378Δ*iss* construction is shown in Figure1. This figure shows 1.6 kb purified PCR product of the kanamycine cassette flanked with *iss* homology. Also, there are different sizes of band with the PCR protocol targeting the new antibiotic resistance cassette junction fragment in wild-type and mutant strain after the replacement of kananamycin cassette (Figure 1). The resistance of three strains to serum, native APEC-O78 strain χ1378 (wild), native APEC-O78 strain χ1378Δ*iss* (mutant), and DH5α (serum sensitive) were investigated using microtiter test. The results show that the growth of wild type, mutant strain, and DH5α were not statistically different in PG broth ($p<0.05$; Figure 2). DH5α grew significantly lower in chicken serum than it did in wild type and mutant strain (Figure 3; $p<0.05$). Also, in comparison with wild type, the growth of mutant in chicken serum decreased; however, it was not significant (Figure 3; $p<0.05$).

Discussion

Colibacillosis, an *Escherichia coli* infection, is a major problem for the poultry industry (Barnes et al., 2008; Derakhshandeh et al., 2009; Kariyawasam et al., 2006; Kariyawasam and Nolan, 2009). O1, O2, and O78 serotypes of APEC are the major etiological agent for colibacillosis in poultry (Vidotto et al., 1990); however, in Iran the majority of colibacillosis is related to O78 serotype (Zahraei Salehi et al., 2004). Prevention and control of colibacillosis by vaccination is one of the inquiries of researchers, and the use of native strain is advised in vaccine preparation (Zahraei Salehi et al., 2004). The present study investigated native APEC serotype O78. The pathogenesis of avian *E. coli* is different from mammalian *E. coli*, since in mammals intestinal form is more prevalent while the extraintestinal form occurs more in avian (Nolan et al., 2003). In addition, serum resistance is at least one of the mechanisms used by APEC to reach internal organs of chickens (Mellata et al., 2003). With regard to the act of *iss* gene, which increased serum resistance, it seems that deletion of *iss* from native APEC-O78 strain χ1378 could be profitable in controlling colibacillosis. On the other hand, there have been few investigations about the mechanism of serum resistance in APEC-O78 (Mellata et al., 2003). In the present study, the *iss* gene was deleted from native APEC-O78 strain χ1378 by lambda red recombineering (Datsenko and Wanner, 2000). *iss* gene was replaced with kanamycin cassette by homologous recombination due to red recombinase enzymes, produced by pKD46; as a result, the mutant strain was kanamaycin resistant and also the PCR result shows 1.8 kb of the PCR product. This confirms the deletion of *iss* from native APEC-O78 strain χ1378. Lynne et al. (2007) deleted *iss* from APEC-O2 by pSKY5000 (Lynne et al., 2007b), while in the present study pKD46 was used. The lambda Red recombinase was expressed by pSKY5000 rather than pKD46. pSKY5000 is a

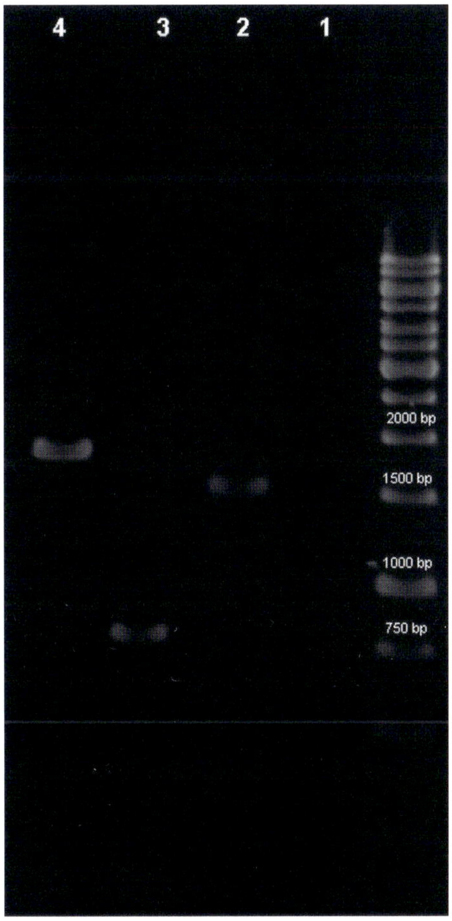

Figure 1. PCR results for mutant screening, Lane 1: 1 Kb marker; Lane 2 & 3: PCR results by for-mut-*iss* and rev-mut *iss* primers (no band in wild type, 1.6 kb in mutant); Lane 4 & 5: PCR results by *iss* upper and *iss* lower primers (760 bp in wild type, 1.8 kb in mutant).

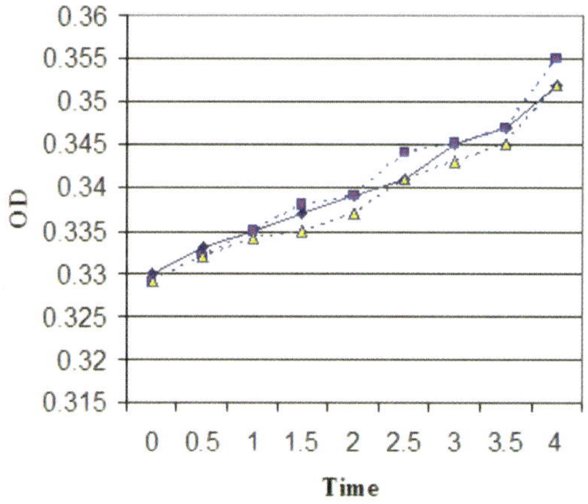

Figure 2. The growth rate of APEC-O78 strain χ1378, APEC-O78 strain χ1378Δ*iss* and DH5α in PG broth at different times. APEC-O78 strain χ 1378 DH5α APEC-O78 strain χ 1378 Δ *iss*

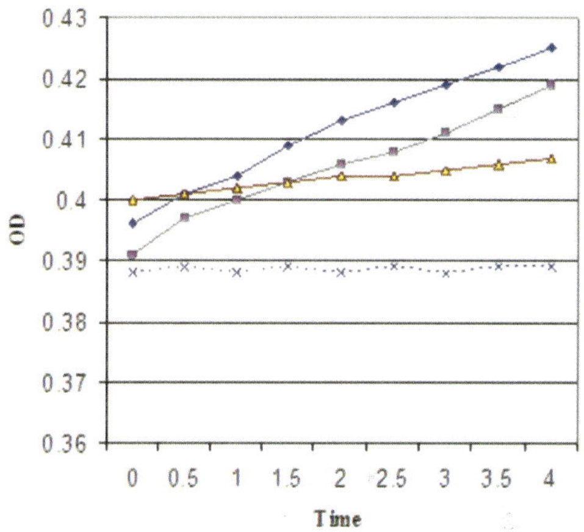

Figure 3. The growth rate of APEC-O78 strain χ1378, APEC-O78 strain χ1378Δ*iss* and DH5α (sensitive to serum) in chicken serum at different times. APEC-O78 strain χ 1378 DH5α APEC-O78 strain χ 1378 Δ *iss* Control

chloramphenicol resistant derivative of pKD46. Our results show that the method of mutagenesis, used in the present study, may be more comfortable than the suicide vector. The findings of Heiat et al. (2012), Nayeri et al. (2009) and Zare et al. (2008), that deleted different genes from different strains, confirmed this subject (Heiat et al., 2012; Nayeri Fasaei et al., 2009; Zare et al., 2008). This process is not difficult or expensive. In methods that use suicide vectors, there are two recombination steps (Herring et al., 2003). In addition, designing and construction of these vectors are labor intensive and depend on employment of several enzymes, while in the method used in our study, applied by little time and effort, and successfully, the mutant was generated by one step recombination. Moreover, in Datsenko and Wanner method, temperature sensitive helper plasmids could be easily eliminated by high temperature in mutant strain (Herring et al., 2003; Tischer et al., 2001). The mutant presented in this study could be examined in alternative or next researches, such as invivo evaluation of immunization, colonization, and invasion or used to construct multiple deletions. In the present study, the resistance of native APEC-O78 strain χ1378Δ*iss* to chicken serum, in comparison with wild type, was investigated by microtitr assay (Lynne et al., 2007a). Results demonstrated that there is no significant difference between mutant and wild type strain ($p<0.05$). Mellata et al. (2003) investigated the role of K1 capsule, P fimbriae, and O78 LPS in APEC in resistance to serum and demonstrated that the K1 capsule is probably required to prevent serum effect

Table 1. Primers used in this study.

Primers name	Sequences (5' to3')	Ref.
iss upper(F)	GTGGCGAAAACTAGTAAAACAGC	Derakhshandeh et al., 2009; Lynne et al., 2007a
iss lower(R)	CGCCTCGGGGTGGATAA	
for- mut- *iss*	TATTCATTTCCCATGATTCTGAGTACCTACCAAGTCTGAGTGTGTAGGCTGGAGCTGCTT	Lynne et al., 2007a
rev-mut- *iss*	AAAAACAACTGTAGGGAGCCCAGAAGTATATTAATGAACACATATGAATATCCTCCTTAG	

in particular strains, such as O1 and O2, but is not needed to protect O78. In addition, they showed that P fimbriae has not a significant role in serum resistance in O2 strain but maybe has a role in other serotypes and need to be investigated. Their study also implicated that in O1 strains, in addition to LPS, there may be other factors related to serum resistance. In their study, the presence of *iss* and *traT* were demonstrated in all mutant and wild type strains. Also, the mutant strains of APEC O78:K80 and APEC O2:K1 contained *iss* and *traT* genes but had lost the K1, or the O serotype was not protected against the bactericidal effect of serum. However, these mutant strains were more resistant than the control strains. The control strains were wild type and *iss* and *traT* negative (Mellata et al., 2003). Nolan et al. (2003) reported that *iss* might have a more important role in birds than mammals to produce virulence and resistance to serum. These differences may be due to the rout of initial entry and forms of clinical disease in these hosts (Nolan et al., 2003). Lynne et al. (2007) studied the contribution of *iss* and *bor* gene to *E. coli* serum resistance. They showed that *iss* contributes more to serum resistance than *bor* (Lynne et al., 2007a). Chuba and Colleagues reported that the effect of *iss* on serum resistance was not gene dosage dependent (Chuba et al., 1986). Skyberg et al. (2008) investigated the role of *iss*, *tsh*, *iutA*, *iroN*, *sitA* and *cvaB* genes in virulence of APEC-O2. They deleted these genes and mutants were compared to the wild type (APEC-O2) for lethality to chick embryos and growth in human urine. No significant differences between the mutants and the wild type were detected, and they reasoned that insensitivity of the virulence assays or other factor could have obscured changes in the virulence of the mutants (Skyberg et al., 2008). These finding showed that the serum resistance of native APEC-O78 strain χ 1378 is multifactorial. Moreover, the effects of single gene deletion might be obscured by some compensatory mechanism. Hence, deletion of more genes related to serum resistance is advisable to achieve serum sensitive native strain. Additionally, when differences in virulence between the mutants and the wild type were not detected, follow-up studies to determine if the genes are differentially expressed in native APEC-O78 strain χ1378 in serum is necessary (Skyberg et al., 2008). The mutant showed little, but not significant, growth in serum compared to the wild-type parent, showing that there are probably other genes to compensate the act of *iss*. Chuba et al. (1986) noted that *traT* gene, located on Col-V plasmid, like *iss* but less, was involved in serum resistance (Chuba et al., 1986). The finding of lynne et al. (2007) demonstrated that *iss* appears to play a major role in the serum resistance associated with pAPEC-O2-ColV (Lynne et al., 2007a). Chuba et al. (1989) showed that *iss* had significant homology to *bor* gene of lysogen bacteriophage lambda (Chuba et al., 1989). In our later work, *bor* gene in native APEC-O78 strain χ1378 have been identified and sequenced and 90% homology with *iss* has been observed (data have not published), therefore deletion of *bor* gene from native APEC-O78 strain χ1378Δ*iss* could be advisable. Our work added to the current understanding of serum resistance of native APEC-O78 strain χ1378. There are not so much data on virulent genes sequences of this bacterium, and the sequences of these genes are still unknown.

Aknowledgments

We are grateful to the Research Council of the University of Tehran and the Research Council of the Faculty of Veterinary Medicine of the University of Tehran for financial support of project no. 7504002/6/14. The authors are also grateful to the National Institute of Genetic Engineering and Biotechnology and also Mr. I. Ashrafi for their valuable collaboration.

References

1. Barnes, H.J., Gross, W.B. (2005) Colibacillosis. In: Diseases of Poultry. Calnek, B.W. (ed.). (10th ed.) Iowa State University press, Ames, IA, USA. p. 131-141.

2. Barnes, H.J., Nolan, L.K., Vaillancourt, J. (2008) Colibacillosis. In: Diseases of poultry. Saif, Y.M., Fadley, A.M., Clisson, J.R., McDougald, L.R., Nolan, L.K., Swayne, D.E. (eds.). (12th ed.) Iowa State University Press, Ames, IA, USA. p. 691-737.

3. Chuba, P.J., Palchaudhuri, S., Leon, M.A. (1986) Contribution of *traT* and *iss* genes to the serum resistance phenotype of plasmid ColV-K94. Fed Eur Microbiol Soc Microbiol Lett. 37: 135-140.

4. Chuba, P.J., Leon, M.A., Banerjee, A., Palchaudhuri, S. (1989) Cloning and DNA sequence of plasmid determinant *iss*, coding for increased serum survival and surface exclusion, which has homology with lambda DNA. Mol Gen Genet. 216: 287-292.

5. Datsenko, K.A., Wanner B.L. (2000) One-step inactivation of chromosomal genes in *Escherichia coli* K-12 using PCR product. Proc Natl Acad Sci. 97: 6640-6645.

6. Derakhshandeh, A., Zahraei Salehi, T., Tadjbakhsh, H., Karimi, V. (2009) Identification, cloning and sequencing of *Escherichia coli* strain chi1378 (O78: K80) *iss* gene isolated from poultry colibacillosis in Iran. Lett Appl Microbiol. 49: 403-407.

7. Gomis, S., Babiuk, L., Godson, D.L., Allan, B., Thrush, T., Townsend, H., Willson, P., Waters, E., Hecker, R., Potter, A. (2003) Protection of chickens against *Escherichia coli* infections by DNA containing CpG motifs. Infect Immun. 71: 857-863.

8. Gross, W.B. (1994) Diseases due to *Escherichia coli* in poultry. In: *Escherichia coli* in domestic animals and man. Gyles, C.L. (ed.). (1st ed.) CAB International, Wallingford, UK. p. 237-259.

9. Heiat, M., Saadati, M., Hosseini, S.M., Zahraei Salehi, T., Nayeri Fasaei, B., Ahsani Arani, Y., Salehi, A.R., Doroudian, M., Hosseini, E. (2012) Construction and immunogenicity of a genetically mutant of a native Shigella dysenteriae type 1 isolated from an Iranian patient with diarrhea by recombineering. Afr J Microbiol Res. 6: 734-744.

10. Herring, C.D., Glasner, J.D., Blattner, F.R. (2003) Gene replacement without selection: regulated suppression of amber mutations in *Escherichia coli*. Gene. 311: 153-163.

11. Horne, S.M., Pfaff-McDonough, S.J., Giddings, C.W., Nolan, L.K. (2000) Cloning and sequencing of the *iss* gene from a virulent avian *Escherichia coli*. Avian Dis. 46: 179-84.

12. Kariyawasam, S., Johnson, T.J., Nolan L.K. (2006) The pap operon of Avian Pathogenic *Escherichia coli* strain O1:K1 is located on a novel pathogenicity island. Infect Immun. 74: 744-749.

13. Kariyawasam, S., Nolan, L.K. (2009) Pap mutant of avian pathogenic *Escherichia coli* O1, an O1:K1:H7 strain is attenuated in vivo. Avian Dis. 53: 255-260.

14. Kwaga, J.K., Allan, B.J., van der Hurk, J.V., Seida, H., Potter, A.A. (1994) A carAB mutant of avian pathogenic *Escherichia coli* serogroups O2 is attenuated and effective as live oral vaccine against colibacillosis in turkey. Infect Immune. 62: 3766-3772.

15. La Ragione, R.M., Casula, G., Cutting, S.M., Woodward, M.J. (2001) *Bacillus subtilis* spores competitively exclude *Escherichia coli* O78: K80 in poultry. Vet Microbiol. 79: 133- 142.

16. La Ragione, R.M., Narbad, A., Gasson, M.J., Woodward, M.J. (2004) In vivo characterization of *Lactobacillus johnsonii* F19785 for use as a defined competitive exclusion agent against bacterial pathogen in poultry. Lett Appl Microbiol. 38: 197-205.

17. La Ragoine, R.M., Sayers, A.R., Woodward, M.J. (2000) The role of fimbriae and flagella in the colonization, invasion and persistence of *Escherichia coli* O78: K80 in the day-old-chick model. Epidemiol Infect. 124: 351-363.

18. Lee, M.D., Wooley, R.E., Brown, J., Spears, K.R., Nolan, L.K., Shotts, E.B.Jr. (1991) Comparison of a quantitative microtiter method, a quantitative automated method, and the plate-count method for determining microbial complement resistance. Avian Dis. 35: 892-896.

19. Lynne, A.M., Skyberg, J.A., Logue, C.M., Doetkott, C., Foley, S.L., Nolan, L.K. (2007a) Characterization of a series of transconjugant mutants of an avian pathogenic *Escherichia coli* isolate for resistance to serum complement. Avian Dis. 51: 771-776.

20. Lynne, A.M., Skyberg, J.A., Logue, C.M., Nolan, L.K. (2007b) Detection of *Iss* and *Bor* on the surface of *Escherichia coli*. J Appl Microbiol. 102: 660-666.

21. Mellata, M., Dho-Moulin, M., Dozois, C.M., Curtiss, R., Brown, P.K., Arne, P., Bree, A., Desautels, C.,

Fairbrother, J.M. (2003) Role of Virulence Factors in Resistance of Avian Pathogenic *Escherichia coli* to Serum and in Pathogenicity. Infect Immun. 71: 536-540.

22. Nayeri Fasaei, B., Zahraei Salehi, T., Tadjbakhsh, H., Firuzi, R., Casadesus, J. (2009) Construction of genetically defined aroA mutant of a native *E. coli* O78:K80 isolated from avian colibacillosis, in Iran. Comp Clin Pathol.18: 69- 75.
23. Nolan, L.K., Horne, S.M., Giddings, C.W., Foley, S.L., Johnson, T.J., Lynne, A.M., Skyberg, J. (2003) Resistance to serum complement, *iss*, and virulence of avian *Escherichia coli*. Vet Res Commun. 27: 101-110.
24. Nolan, L.K., Wooley, R.E., Cooper, R.K. (1992) Transposon mutagenesis used to study the role of complement resistance in the virulence of an avian *Escherichia coli*. Avian Dis. 36: 398-402.
25. Sharan, S.K., Thomason, L.C., Kuznetsov, S.G., Court, D.L. (2009) Recombineering: a homologous recombination-based method of genetic engineering. Nat Protoc. 4: 206-223.
26. Skyberg, J.A., Johnson, T.J., Nolan, L.K. (2008) Mutational and transcriptional analyses of an avian pathogenic _*Escherichia coli*_ ColV plasmid. BMC Microbiol. 29: 24.
27. Stordeur, P., Bree, A., Mainil, J., Moulin-Schouleur, M. (2004) Pathogenicity of pap negative avian *Escherichia coli* isolated from septicemia lesions. Microbes Infect. 6: 637-645.
28. Tischer, B.K., von Einem, J., Kaufer, B., Osterrieded, N. (2001) Two-step red-mediated recombination for versatile high-efficiency markerless DNA manipulation in *Escherichia coli*. BioTechniques. 40: 191-197.
29. Vandekerchove, D., De Herdt, P., Laevens, H., Pasmans, F. (2004) Colibacillosis in caged layer hens: characteristics of the disease and the aetiological agent. Avian Pathol. 33: 117-125.
30. Vidotto, C.M., Muller, E.E., Freitas, C.J., Alfrieri, A.A., Guimaraes, G.I., Santos, S.D. (1990) Virulence factors of avian *Escherichia coli*. Avian Dis. 34: 531-538.
31. Wooley, R.E., Brown, J., Spears, K.R., Nolan, L.K. (1991) Comparison of chicken plasma and guinea pig serum in a quantitative microtiter method of determining microbial complement resistance. Avian Dis. 35: 897-900.
32. Zahraei Salehi, T., Rajabi, Z., Modirsanei, M. (2004) Evaluation of the immunogenicity of endemic *Escherichia coli* serotypes isolated from poultry in Iran. J Vet Res. University of Tehran. 59: 189-195.
33. Zare, P., Tabatabaei, M., Yousefbeygi, Gh., Jabbari, A.R. (2008) Using red recombinase and PCR product for one-step in-frame inactivation of aroA gene in *Pasteurella multocida* A:1 and evaluation of pathogenicity and immunogenicity. J Anim Vet Adv. 7: 1155-1159.

The prevalence of coronavirus in fecal samples of neonatal calf diarrhea using electron microscopic examination

Davoudi, Y.[1], Nourmohammadzadeh, F.[2*], Abdollahpour, G.[2], Nouri, A.[3], Nowrouzian, I.[4]

[1]*Islamic Azad University, Sarab Branch, Sarab, Iran*

[2]*Department of Internal Medicine, Faculty of Veterinary Medicine, University of Tehran, Tehran, Iran*

[3]*Razi Vaccine and Serum Research Institute, Karaj, Iran*

[4]*Department of Surgery, Faculty of Veterinary Medicine, University of Tehran, Tehran, Iran*

Key words:
calf diarrhea, coronavirus, electron microscopy

Correspondence
Nourmohammadzadeh, F.
Department of Internal Medicine, Faculty of Veterinary Medicine, University of Tehran, Tehran, Iran

Email: fenour@ut.ac.ir

Abstract:

BACKGROUND: Neonatal calf diarrhea (NCD), also known as calf scours, is caused by viruses, bacteria, and parasites. Coronavirus is one of the important causes of NCD syndrome. Electron microcopy has been used for demonstration of viruses in fecal samples of diarrheic calves since 1969. **OBJECTIVES:** The aim of this study was to determine the prevalence of coronavirus in fecal samples of neonatal calf diarrhea using electron microcopy examination of fecal samples. **METHODS:** For the purpose of this study, a total of 100 cases (under 2 months of age) of diarrheic calves from 25 commercial farms in four districts of East Azerbaijan province of Iran were used. Fresh Fecal samples using sterile swab were collected from every calf with clinical diarrhea. All samples were transferred into a sterile container and then were sent to the laboratory to be kept in -20°C freezer until examination. Electron microscopic examination was applied to all fecal samples. Chi-square test was used to analyze the data. **RESULTS:** According to the results of this study, coronavirus was present in 15% of cases and a significant difference was found between the prevalence rate and the seasons ($p<0.05$). The highest prevalence was recorded in winter (28%) and the least prevalence was seen in summer (4%). There was not any significant difference in both age groups and different districts according to the prevalence rate of infection. **CONCLUSIONS:** Neonatal calf diarrhea is a multi-etiological syndrome. Among the viral diarrhea, bovine coronavirus is one of the major causes of this syndrome. For detection of coronavirus in feces, electron microscope examination is a gold standard diagnostic technique. It seems that coronavirus can be considered as one of the important etiologies of neonatal calf diarrhea in east Azerbaijan of Iran.

Introduction

Diarrhea in newborn calves under 30 days of age is one of the most common disease complexes. It is a significant cause of economic loss in both dairy and beef herds. The bovine coronavirus is an important cause of diarrhea in calves from birth to 3 months of age, but mostly between 1 and 2 weeks of age. Coronavirus was first isolated from calves with diarrhea in 1971 during an experimental field trial to evaluate a rotavirus vaccine. All known corona-viruses are single stranded RNA viruses of the

Coronaviridae family (Anderson 1992). Experimental studies showed that the incubation period is 20 to 30 hours. Generally, coronavirus diarrhea is more watery and greater in severity than rotavirus diarrhea, leading more rapidly to dehydration and acidosis (Andrews et al., 2004). The virus can be shed by up to 70% of adult cows despite the presence of specific antibodies in their serum and feces. The peaks of shedding are during the winter and at parturition in North America (Radostits et al., 2007). Calves born from carrier cows are at a higher risk of diarrhea. The pathogenesis of coronaviral enteritis in calves is similar to the rotavirus infection. The villous epithelial cells of the small and large intestines are commonly affected. In 1969, for the first time, electron microcopy was used to show the responsibility of a virus in calf diarrhea (Brugere-Picoux, Tessieer, 2010). Electron microscopy examination is a gold standard diagnostic technique for demonstration of the virus in feces. Subclinical persistence and recurrent infections are also common in both neonatal and older calves. Demonstration of the virus in feces using electron microscopy (EM) has been introduced as a standard diagnostic technique. The EM technique is currently used in Texas Veterinary Medical Diagnostic Laboratory in USA for calf diarrhea pathogen identification (Schroeder et al., 2012). It is easier to see the virus if it has been concentrated by ultracentrifugation or clumped by immune electron microscopy using specific antiserum. With electron microscopy, the virus can be detected for up to 6 to 10 days after the onset of the diarrhea. Immunofluorescent staining is used as another technique for detection of the virus in fecal samples and can be conducted in a few hours. The fluorescent antibody technique can only detect the virus within epithelial cells which are present in the feces for 4 to 6 h after the onset of the diarrhea. However, in some studies the fluorescent antibody technique detects the virus in only 20% of the samples, while electron microscopy detected the virus in about 60% of the samples (Radostits et al., 2007). ELISA technique has also been used for demonstration of coronavirus antibodies in serum samples (Rabbani et al., 2007). More recently, RT-PCR has been introduced as a modern test for detecting RNA of the virus in fecal samples (Zhu et al., 2011). The aim of this study was to determine the prevalence of coronavirus in neonatal calf diarrhea fecal samples in the East Azerbaijan province of Iran, during a 12-month period.

Materials and Methods

For this study, the following solution and materials were prepared, as described previously (Nourmohammadzadeh et al., 2012).

Antibiotic solution: To prevent the growth of the bacteria which can interfere with the existence of the virus in the samples, an antibiotic mixture was prepared and added into each sample. For this purpose, 10ml sterilized purified distilled water was added into a vial containing 1 million units of Penicillin G procaine and 1 gr of streptomycin. The mixture was shaken in order for the antibiotic to be completely dissolved. All sampled calves were located in the Province of Azerbaijan of Iran. The region was divided into four districts: northwest, northeast, southwest, and southeast. The number of the dairy farms in each district was determined, and the sampling of the diarrheic calves was done in a period of twelve months.

Totally, one hundred fecal samples were collected from diarrheic calves of industrial dairy farms within the first week of the onset. Fecal samples were collected after cleaning the anus of the calf. Each fecal sample was taken directly from the rectum of the calf via a sterile swap, transferred into a sterilized glass vessel with lids, on which the number of each calf and the specimen were written. One ml of the antibiotic solution was added into each vessel. After fixing the lid, it was shaken to provide a mixture of the feces with antibiotic solution.

All samples were placed into an ice container at the farm and then within 12 hours transferred into a -20°C freezer until the time of examination. For conducting the electron microcopy examinations, all freezed samples were carried to the Virology section at Razi Vaccine and Serum Research Institute, in Karaj. In general, this process was set up so that each sample group was tested in less than one week.

To prepare the samples for the electron microscope examination, they were taken out of the freezer to be melted at room temperature. When the samples turned from the frozen state into the liquid, 5 mL of each sample was transferred into a centrifuge tube and then spun at 10000 rpm for 15 minutes using a centrifuge. As the viruses are lighter than the other particles in the feces, they floated up to the upper part. One drop of the upper part was spread on the cooper grid. When it became dried, it was dyed by the negative PTA method, as described by Bozzola and Russell, and then observed by the electron microscope (Philips 400) (Bozzola and Russell, 1999). If a sample contained coronavirus virus, it would be photographed.

Results

Among the 100 collected fecal samples, 15 cases were found to have coronavirus using electron microscopic examination. This result indicated that the prevalence of coronavirus contamination in the whole area of East Azerbaijan province of Iran was equal to 15%. The rate of contamination in the dairy farms of northwest, northeast, southwest, and southeast was equal to 10.71%, 20%, 15.38%, and 12.5%, respectively (Table 1) which shows the highest prevalence rate in the northeast and the lowest rate in the northwest area.

Comparing the prevalence of coronavirus infections during the four seasons, as shown in table 2, indicates that the highest prevalence was recorded in winter (28%) and the lowest was found in the summer (4%). There is a significant difference between different seasons ($p<0.05$). Table 3 shows the rate of infection in five age groups, which indicates that the highest prevalence rate was seen at 2 to 4 weeks of age (19.23%) and the least during the first week of age (10%). Figure 1 shows a photograph of a complete and also an empty coronavirus particle from a positive fecal sample.

Discussion

Coronavirus is an important cause of diarrhea in calves with prevalence estimates ranging from 11 to 81%. (Radostits et al., 2007). Coronaviruses are particularly common in 5 to 30 days old calves, and they have been detected in feces of more than 70% of clinically normal cows. Calves born to carrier animals are at a higher risk for developing diarrhea. Calves may be infected with coronavirus by the oral or respiratory route (Smith, 2009). In Australia, it has

Table 1. Prevalence rate of coronavirus in fecal samples in four districts of Eastern Azerbaijan.

District	Number of Samples	Number of positive samples	Prevalence rate %
North - West	28	3	10.71
North - East	30	6	20
South - West	26	4	15.38
South - East	16	2	12.5
Total	100	15	15

Table 2. Prevalence rate of coronavirus in fecal samples in different seasons.

Season	Number of samples	Number of positive samples	Prevalence rate %
Spring	25	3	12
Summer	25	1	4
Autumn	25	4	16
Winter	25	7	28
Total	100	15	15

Table 3. Prevalence rate of coronavirus in fecal samples in different age groups.

Age groups (Week)	Number of samples	Number of positive samples	Prevalence rate %
1	20	2	10
1-2	26	5	19-23
2-4	21	3	14.23
4-6	18	3	16.66
6-8	15	2	13.33
Total	100	15	15

been reported that 21.6% diarrheic calves were infected with coronavirus, using RT-PCR method (Izzo et al., 2011). In another study conducted by Zhu et al., 7.14% of diarrheic calves were found infected with coronavirus, using RT-PCR (Zhu et al., 2011). However, the study of the coronavirus infection using ELISA in India showed that 11.76% of the clinically diarrheic calves were positive (Rai et al., 2011).

In Iran, a study in 2007 showed that coronavirus antibodies are presented in 82% of the diarrheic calves and in 72% of the healthy calves (Rabbani et al., 2007). In an earlier serological study conducted in Markazi Province of Iran, it was shown that 34% of the diarrheic calves younger than 30 days old were positive against coronavirus, using ELISA test (Ghaemmaghami et al., 1999). The Study of coronavirus infection using cELISA in diarrhoic calves in Mashhad district showed that 3.7% of the calves were infected (Mayameei et al., 2010).

In the present study, using fecal electron microscopy examinations, 15% of the diarrheic

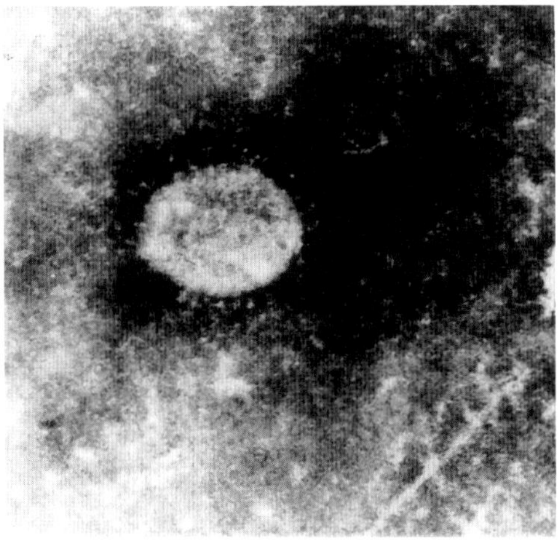

Figure 1. Photograph of coronavirus in fecal sample of a diarrheic calf using negative stain transmission electron microscopy.

calves showed coronavirus infection. Comparing the results of the present study with other studies revealed that the rate of coronavirus infection is different in different geographical and climate conditions. However, the high prevalence rate of coronavirus in serological studies in comparison to the virus detection methods showed that the serological methods could not demonstrate the accurate clinical pattern of the infection.

The results of our study show that the highest prevalence rate of infection was found in the northeast (20%) and the lowest rate was found in the northwest area (10.7%). However, statistical analysis using chi-square test shows that there is no significant difference between districts according to the prevalence rate of coronavirus infection. Nonetheless, results of chi-square test, shown in table 2, reveal that there is a significant difference between the prevalence rate and the season ($p<0.05$). The highest prevalence rate was recorded in winter (28%) and the lowest was found in the summer (4%). The high prevalence of coronavirus infections in winter in the present study is in agreement with other studies (Radostits et al., 2007). It seems that in cold conditions, as in winter, the absorption of the IgG1 by calves is decreased which can cause reduction of the serum IgG level. As a result, this can reduce the immunity of the calves and increase the rate of coronavirus infection in calves born during winter (Badiei et al., 2013).

The results of the present study also indicate that the highest prevalence rate was seen at 2 to 6 weeks of age and the least during the first week of age and 6 to 8 weeks of age. However, statistical analysis of the data shows that there is no significant difference between age groups.

Acknowledgments

The authors would like to acknowledge the Research Vice Chancellors of Tehran University for financial support of this project (218/1/374). The authors would also like to thank Dr. I Nowrouzian for his help on this project.

References

1. Anderson Neil, V. (1992) Veterinary Gastroenterology. (2th ed.) Lea & Febiger, London, UK.
2. Andrews, A.H., Blowey, R.W., Boyd, H., Eddy, R.G. (2004) Bovine Medicine. (2nd ed.) Blackwell publishing. London, UK.
3. Badiei, Kh., ourjfar, M., Ghane, M. (2013) Detection of fecal coronavirus antigen in diarrheic calves of high- and average-producing Holstein dairy cows. Turk J Vet Anim Sci. 37: 296-301.
4. Bozzola, J.J., Russell, L.D. (1999) Specimen staining and contrast methods for transmission elctron microscopy. On: Electron Microscopy, Principles and Techniques for Biologists, Jones and Bartlett Publisher. (2nd ed.) London, UK. p. 130-133.
5. Brugere-Picoux, J., Tessier, P. (2010) Viral gastro-enteritis in domestic animals and zoonoses. Bull Acad Natl Med. 194: 1439-49.
6. Ghaemmaghami, SH., Karegar Moakhar, R., Niroumand, H., Sadri, R. (1999) Study on prevalence of rotavirus, coronavirus, *E. coli* K99 and cryptosporidium in calf diarrhea using ELISA test. Pejouhesh & Sazandegi. 43: 60-66.
7. Izzo, M.M., Kirkland, P.D., Mohler, V.L., Perkins, N.R., Gunn, A.A., House, J.K. (2011) Prevalence of major enteric pathogens in Australian dairy calves with diarrhoea. Aust Vet J. 89: 167-173.
8. Mayameei, A., Mohammadi, Gh., Yavari, S., Afshari, E., Omidi, A. (2010) Evaluation of relationship between Rotavirus and Coronavirus infections with calf diarrhea by capture ELISA, Comp Clin Pathol. 19: 553-557.
9. Nourmohammadzadeh, F., Davoudi, Y., Abdol-

lahpour, G., Nouri, A. (2012) The prevalence of rotavirus in neonatal calf diarrhoea, using electron microscopic examination. Comp Clin Pathol. 21: 1231-1234.

10. Rabbani, M., Mokhber Dezfuli, M.R., Zahraie Salehi, T., Yoosefi Ramandi, A., Bahonar, A.R., Rezazadeh, F. (2007) Detection on anti ELISA, Rotavirus and coronavirus antibodies in sera samples of diarrheic and normal calves under 1 months of age. J Vet Res. 62: 145-149.
11. Radostits, O.M., Gay, C.C., Hinchcliff, K.W., Constable, P.D. (2007) Veterinary Medicine. (10th ed.) Elsevier. Philadelphia, USA.
12. Rai, R.B., Hansha, A., Rai, S., Singh, B., Kumar, H., Singh, A.K., Damodaran, T., Dhama, K. (2011) Prevalence of rota and coronavirus infections in calves of Barabanki and Raebareli districts of Uttar Pradesh. Indian J Vet Pathol. 35: 73-74.
13. Schroeder, M.E., Bounpheng, M.A., Rodgers, S., Baker, R.J., Black, W., Naikare, H., Velayudhan, B., Sneed, L., Szonyi, B., Clavijo, A. (2012) Development and performance evaluation of calf diarrhea pathogen nucleic acid purification and detection workflow. J Vet Diagn Invest. 24: 945-953.
14. Smith, B.P. (2009) Large Animal Internal Medicine. (4th ed.) Elsevier, St. Louis, Missouri, USA.
15. Zhu, W., Dong, J., Haga, T., Goto, Y., Sueyoshi, M. (2011) Rapid and sensitive detection of bovine coronavirus and group a bovine rotavirus from fecal samples by using one-step duplex RT-PCR assay. J Vet Med Sci. 73: 531-534.

Molecular detection of *Babesia* spp in sheep and vector ticks in North Khorasan province, Iran

Seidabadi, M.[1], Razmi, Gh.R.[2*], Naghibi, A.[2]

[1] *Graduated from the Faculty of Veterinary Medicine, Ferdowsi University of Mashhad, Mashhad, Iran*

[2] *Department of Pathobiology, Faculty of Veterinary Medicine, Ferdowsi University of Mashhad, Mashhad, Iran*

Key words:
Babesia spp., Ixodid ticks, semi-nested PCR, sheep

Correspondence
Razmi, Gh.R.
Department of Pathobiology, Faculty of Veterinary Medicine, Ferdowsi University of Mashhad, Mashhad, Iran

Email: razmi@um.ac.ir

Abstract:

BACKGROUND: Babesiosis is an important tickborne disease in the sheep of Iran. **OBJECTIVES:** A molecular study was carried out in North Khorasan province, Iran in 2010-2011, designed to identify *Babesia* spp. infection of both sheep and ticks. **METHODS:** Ninety sheep from different flocks were clinically examined and blood samples were collected with ixodid ticks . The collected ticks were separated into 82 tick pools and the salivary glands were dissected out in 0.85% (w/v) saline under a stereomicroscope. The blood and the salivary glands were examined using semi-nested PCR. **RESULTS:** Piroplasm infection was detected in 37 blood smears using microcopic examination while 80 blood samples were piroplasm positive in the first round of semi-nested PCR and *Babesia ovis* was only detected in 6 (6.6%) of positive samples in the second round of semi-nested PCR. Of the 434 ticks that were collected, the most prevalent species was *Rhipicephalus turanicus* (69.3%) followed by *Hyalomma marginatum turanicum* (18.4%), *Dermacentor marginatus* (6.4%) and *Rhipicephalus bursa* (5.7%). One pool of *H. m. turanicum* salivary glands and one pool of *R.turanicus* were infected with *B. ovis*. **CONCLUSIONS:** Based on these results, it is concluded that *B.ovis* has a low prevalence among the sheep of North Khorasan province and *H. m. turanicum* and *R. turanicus* may be the vectors of *B.ovis* in this area.

Introduction

Babesiosis is a haemoparasitic disease of domestic and wild animals in tropical and subtropical countries. The *Babesia* spp. is transmitted by hard ticks and causes fever,anemia,haemoglobinuria and icterus in small ruminants (Soulsby,1986). Babesia species of small ruminants are commonly grouped together, but this may be an oversimplification, as the susceptibility of sheep and goats is highly variable (Uilenberg, 2006). *Babesia ovis* and *B.motasi* are generally regarded as valid taxa. Two other parasites have also been described; i.e., *B. taylori* and *B. foliata*, but their validity is doubtful" (Uilenberg, 2001, 2006). *B. crassa* is isolated from Iran for the first time, it is a large *Babesia* spp and mostly crosses piriforms in erythrocytes (Hashemi-Fesharki and Uilenberg, 1981).

B. ovis, *B. motasi*, and *B. crassa* have been reported in sheep and goats in Iran (Hashemi-Fesharaki, 1997). The seroprevalence of *Babesia ovis* infection is also variable, from 12 to 58% in different geographic areas of Iran (Tavassoli and Rahbari, 1998; Hashemzadeh et al., 2006). *B.ovis* was also identified using PCR (Shayan and Rahbari, 2005; Sadeghi Dehkordi et al., 2010) and RLB (Ranjbar-Bahdori et al., 2012) in infected sheep in Iran. In addition, molecular studies have demonstrated that *R. bursa*, *R. turanicus*, and *R.sanguineus* can serve as vectors for *B.ovis* in Iran (Shayan et al., 2007).

The large Khorasan region includes three

provinces in the north, center and south. The climate of the north of the Khorasan Province is mountainous and is different from the center and south areas with desert and semidesert climates. The epidemiological aspect of ovine babesiosis is poorly understood in the North Khorasan Province. The aim of the study was to identify *Babesia* species and vector ticks in sheep by using microscopic examination and semi-nested PCR in North Khorasan province.

Materials and Methods

Field study area: North Khorasan Province is located in northeastern Iran between 36°37´-38°17´ N latitudes and 55°53´-58°20´ E longitudes with an area of more than 28,400 km2. It is situated next to the north eastern border of Iran, level with the southern Caspian sea and south of Turkmenistan (Figure 1). The province has mountainous areas and receives about 250 mm of rainfall annually.

Boold samples collecting: Sheep flocks were randomly selected by the local veterinary service of Bojonord, Shirvan and Faroj areas. Each flock was visited during the seasons of tick activity from 2010 to 2011. First, a number of sheep were clinically examined; five sheep with clinical signs such as anemia and icterus were selected and blood smears were prepared from capillary veins of the ear. In addition, the blood of sheep was drawn by syringe from jugular veins and collected in EDTA tubes. Simultaneously, the body of animals were inspected and attached ticks were collected into labelled specimen tubes. The blood and ticks specimens were kept cool and transferred to the parasitology laboratory in the Faculty of Veterinary Medicine.

Examination of blood smears: The smears were fixed in methanol and stained in 10% Giemsa solution in phosphate buffered saline (PBS) pH 7.2. The slides were examined with oil immersion lens at a total magnification of ×1000.

Tick examination: The ticks were counted and speciation was done by using the identification keys (Hoogstraal, 1956; Walker et al., 2003; Estrada- Peña et al., 2004). The collected ticks were grouped into 82 pools with five ticks according to their species. Then, the salivary glands of each pool tick were dissected out in 0.85% saline solution under stereo microscope. Then, the salivary gland samples were kept at -20°C until they were used for PCR.

Semi- nested PCR: Total DNA was extracted from EDTA blood and tick samples using a DNA isolation kit (Cinna gene, Iran) Then, a semi nested PCR was performed according to the method of Shayan and Rahbari (2005). Briefly, in the first round of the amplification of semi nested PCR, two oligonucleotide PCR primers Forward primer (P1): 5'-CACAGGGAGGTAGTGACAAG-3', and the reverse (p2): 5'-AAGAATTTCACCTATGACAG-3' were used to differentiate *Theileria* spp and *Babesia* spp. In the second round of the amplification of the internal primers used to detect *B.ovis* were: forward primer (P3) 5'-TGCGCGCGGCCTTTGCGT-3' and reverse primer (P2) 5'-AAGAATTTCACCTATGACAG-3' and to detect *B.motasi* were forward primer (P4) 5'-CGCGATTCCGTTATTGGAG-3' and reverse primer (P2) 5'-AAGAATTTCACCTATGACAG-3'. Amplification was conducted in 20 µL reaction volumes (Accupower PCR premix kit, Bioneer®, South Korea) with a final concentration of each dNTP of 250 µM in 10mM Tris-HCl pH 9.0, 30mM KCl and 1·5mM MgCl2, 1U Taq DNA polymerase and 10 pmol of each PCR primer (Takapouzist Co. Iran). Then 1 µL of DNA template (was added to each reaction and the remaining 20 µL reaction volume was filled with sterile distilled water. The reactions were subjected to the following cycling conditions using a BioRad thermocycler: 95°C for five min, 36 cycles with denaturing at 94°C for 45 s, primer annealing at 54-58°C for 45 s and extension step at 72°C for 45s, followed by final extension at 72°C for 10 min. The products were then chilled to 4°C. The PCR products were electrophoresed in a 1.5% agarose gel with TBE buffer and visualized using ethidium bromide and UV-elimintor. A visible band at 389-402 for *Babesia* spp was produced in the first round of PCR. The second round was done on the positive PCR products with the same reaction in the first round. The PCR products were also electrophoresed through a 1.5% agarose gel to assess the presence of a special band of *B.ovis* (186bp) and *B.motasi* (205bp).

Results

Piroplasm infections were microscopically detected in 37 (41.1%) of blood smears with low

Table1. Results of Molecular and microscopic examination of piroplasm infection in sheep of different areas in North Khorasan Province.

Areas	Seminested PCR (First round) No (%)	Seminested PCR No (%)			Microscopic examination No (%)	Total
	Piroplasm	*B. ovis*	*B.motasi*	Total	Piroplasm infections	
Bojnord	30	1	0	1	14	30
Shirvan	26	2	0	2	11	30
Farooj	24	3	0	3	12	30
Total	80 (88)	6 (6.6)	0 (0)	6 (6.6)	37 (41.1)	90

Table2. Frequency of tick infestation and results of semi-nested PCR for detection *Babesia* spp in salivary glands of Ixodid ticks.

Tick Species	Ticks No (%)	Tick pool S. glands No	Semi-nested PCR No(%)			Total
			B.ovis	*B.motasi*	Mixed	
R. turanicus	301 (69.3)	30	1	0	0	1
H. m.turanicum	80 (18.4)	10	1	0	0	1
D. marginatus	28 (6.4)	2	0	0	0	0
R. bursa	25 (5.7)	2	0	0	0	0
Total	434	44	2 (4.5%)	0 (0%)	0(0%)	2

parasitemia (0.2 -0.01%). In the first round of seminested PCR, 80 (88.8%) of blood samples were positive for *Theileria* spp and *Babesia* spp. In the second round, B .ovis was detected in 6 (6.6%) of positive samples (Table 1) (Figure 2).

In this study, 434 ixodid ticks were collected from different areas of the North Khorasan Province. The most common tick species was *R. turanicus* 301 (69%), followed by *H. m. turanicum* 80 (18.4%), *D. marginatus* 28 (6.4%) and *R. bursa* 25 (5.7%). Two pools belong to the salivary glands of *H. m. turanicum* and *R. turanicus* salivary gland were positive with *B.ovis* (Table 2).

Discussion

In this study, piroplasm infection was microscopically observed in 41% of blood smears. The parasitemia of blood smears was low and it is virtually impossible to distinguish between *Theileria* spp. and *Babesia* spp upon morphology and size criteria in sheep. The frequency of piroplam infection was also deteced in 88% of blood samples in the first round of seminested-PCR. The results confirmed the high sensitivity and specificity of molecular method in comparison with the microscopical examination. In the second round of the seminested-PCR , *B. ovis* was detected in 6.6% of positive samples. The frequency of *B.ovis* was lower than the frequency of *B.ovis* infection as reported in the sheep of the Khorasn Province using microscopic examination (Razmi et al., 2002; Razmi et al., 2003). Microscopic examination has a little value for the specific differentiation between *Theileria* spp. and *Babesia* spp. in small ruminants, especially when parasitemia was low (Schnittger et al., 2004). Therefore, *Babesia* spp may be wrongly detected in many blood smear samples, while actually having been *Theileria* spp. A low prevalence of *B.ovis* has been reported in 5.8% of sheep in Iran (Sadeghi Dehkordi et al., 2010) and other countries such as Turkey (Atlay et al., 2007) and Greece (Theodoropoulos et al., 2006) using molecular methods.

In the present study, *B.motasi* was neither detected by microscopy nor by semi-nested PCR. *B. motasi* was reported upon morphological parameters in the sheep of Iran (Razmi et al., 2002, Razmi et al., 2003). However, some molecular studies have revealed that the genes of the reported *B. motasi* in Iran are the same as *B. ovis* (Shayan et al., 2008; Sadeghi Dehkordi et al., 2010; Ranjbar-Bahdori et al., 2012). They concluded that a morphological polymorphism of *B. ovis* may be the main problem in differentiation between *B. ovis* and *B. motasi* by Geimsa staining.

In the present study, *R. turanicus*, *H. m. turanicum*, *D. marginatus* and *R. bursa* were found in the sheep and *R.turanicus* had the highest frequency in comparison with other ixodid ticks.

So far, *R. turanicus* has been reported abundant in the ticks of the sheep of the large Khorasan (Rahbari et al., 2007; Razmi et al., 2011). *B. ovis* infection was

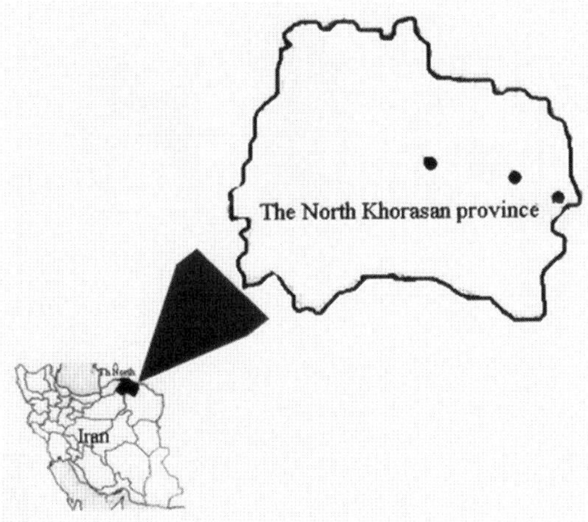

Figure 1. Locality where the fields work was carried out in North khorasan Province, Iran.

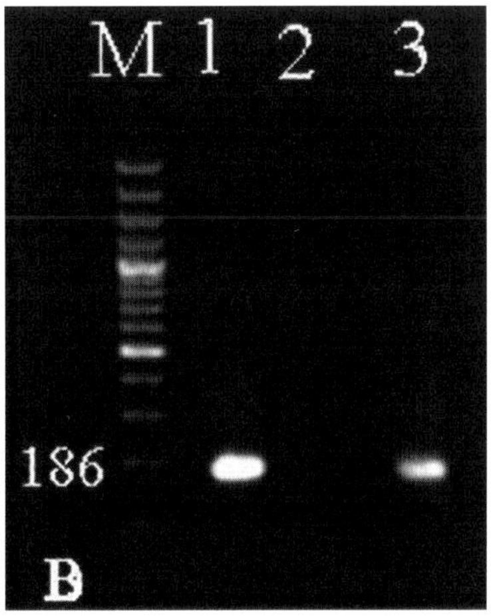

Figure 2. PCR product of *B.ovis*, ladder marker (lane M), Positive control (lane 1, 186bp), Negative control (lane 2), Positoive (lane4 ,186).

detected in the salivary glands of *R. turanicus* and *H. m. turanicum* by semi-nested PCR. *R.turanicus* is seen in different climates and many animals may be infested with *R. turanicus*, but high infestation is found in sheep (Estrada- Peña et al., 2004). A similar study shows that *R. turanicus* could be the vector of *B.ovis* in Iran (Shayan et al. 2007). *H. m. turanicum* is known as pale legged Hyalomma and originates from the Middle East. Adult ticks feed on cattle, sheep, goats, horses and large wild herbivores. *H. m. turanicum* is not known to be a main vector pathogen disease to domestic animals, but is considered a vector of the virus causing Crimean-Congo hemorrhagic fever in humans (Estrada- Peña et al., 2004). The kinetes of *Babesia* spp were detected in the haemolymph of *H. marginatum* collected from an infected sheep with *B. ovis* (Razmi et al., 2002). However, *H. marginatum* could not transovarially transmit *B.ovis* to sheep (Razmi and Nouroozi, 2010).

Based on the results, it is concluded that *B.ovis* has a low ferquency in the sheep of the North Khorasn Province and *R. tuanicus* and *H. m. turanicum* could act as vectors of *B.ovis* in the sheep.

Acknowledgements

We are really grateful to H. Eshrati for his technical assiatance. The author would like to thank North Khorasan Veterinary office for providing information about sheep flocks and the logistic support.

References

1. Altay, K., Aktas, M., Dumanli, N.(2007) Molecular identification, genetic diversity and distribution of *Theileria* and *Babesia* species infecting small. Vet Parasitol. 147: 161-165.
2. Estrada- Peña, A., Bouattour, A., Camicas, J.L., Walker, A.R. (2004) Ticks of domestic animals in Mediterranean region, a guide to identification of species. (1st ed.) Univerity of Zaragoza, Spain.
3. Hashemi-Fesharki, R., Uilenberg, G. (1981) *Babesia crassa* n. sp. (Sporozoa, Babesiidae) of domestic sheep in Iran. Vet Quarterly . 3: 1-8.
4. Hashemi-Fesharki, R. (1997) Tick-borne disease of sheep and goats and their related vectors in Iran. Parassitology. 39: 115-117.
5. Hashemzadeh, F., Nabavi, L., Seyfabad Shapouri, M.F., Rahbari, S., Azizi, F. (2006) Development of an ELISA technique for the detection of *B. ovis* and serological survey of the parasite in Khuzestan province, southern Iran. Iran J Vet Res. 7: 53-58.
6. Hoogstraal, H. (1956) African ixodidae. In: Ticks of the Sudan, Research report, Vol. 1. (1st ed.) Novel Medical, Washington, USA.
7. Rahbari, S., Nabian, S., Shayan, P. (2007) Primary report on distribution of tick fauna in Iran. Parasitol Res. 101: (Suppl 2)S175-S177.
8. Ranjbar-Bahadori, S., Eckert, B., Omidian, Z., Sadr Shirazi, N., Shayan, P. (2012) *Babesia ovis* as the main causative agent of sheep babesiosis in Iran. Parasitol Res. 110: 1531-1536.
9. Razmi, G.R., Naghibi, A., Aslani, M.R., Dastjerdi,

K., Hosseini, H. (2003) An epidemiological study on Babesia infection in small ruminants in Mashhad suburb, Province of Khorasan, Iran. Small Rum Res. 50: 39-44.

10. Razmi,G.R., Naghibi, A., Aslani, M.R., Fathivand, M., Dastjerdi, K. (2002) An epidemiological study on ovine babesiosis in the Mashhad suburb area, province of Khorasan, Iran. Vet Parasitol. 108: 109-115.

11. Razmi, G.R., Najarnejad, V., Rashtibaf, M. (2011) Determination the frequency of Ixodid ticks on the sheep in Khorasan Razavi province, Iran. Arch Razi Inst. 66: 129-132.

12. Razmi, G.R., Nouroozi, E. (2010) Transovarial Transmission of *Babesia ovis* by *Rhipicephalus sanguineus* and *Hyalomma marginatum*. Iran J Parasitol. 5: 35-39.

13. Sadeghi- Dehkordi, Z., Zakeri, S., Nabian, S., Bahonar, A., Ghasemi, F., Noorollahi, F., Rahbari, S. (2010) Molecular and biomorphometrical identification of ovine babesiosis in Iran. Iran J Parasitol. 5: 21-30.

14. Schnittger, L., Yin, H., Qi, B., Gubbels, M.J., Beyer, D., Niemann, S., Jongejan, F., Ahmed, J.S. (2004) Simultaneous detection and differentiation of *Theileria* and *Babesia parasites* infecting small ruminants by reverse line blotting. Parasitol Res. 92: 189-196.

15. Shayan, P., Hooshmand, E., Nabian, S., Rahbari, S. (2008) Biometrical and genetical characterization of large *Babesia ovis* in Iran. Parsitolol Res. 103: 217-221.

16. Shayan, P., Hooshmand, E., Nabian, S., Rahbari, S. (2007) Determination of *Rhipicephalus* spp. as vectors for *Babesia ovis* in Iran. Parasitol Res. 101: 1029-33.

17. Shayan, P., Rahbari, S. (2005) Simultaneous differentiation between *Theileria* spp. and *Babesia* spp. on stained blood smear using PCR. Parasitol Res. 97: 281-286.

18. Soulsby, E.J.L. (1986) The Helminths, Arthoropods and Protozoa of Domestic Animal. (7th ed.) Bailliere & Tindall. London, UK.

19. Tavassoli, M., Rahbari, S. (1998) A seroepidemiological survey on *Babesia ovis* in different geographical region of Iran. J Vet Res. (in Persian, with English abstract). 53: 55-59.

20. Theodoropoulos, G., Gazouli, M., Ikonomopoulos, J.A., Kantzoura, V., Kominakis, A. (2006) Determination of prevalence and risk factors of infection with Babesia in small ruminants from Greece by polymerase chain reaction amplification. Vet Parasitol. 135: 99-104.

21. Uilenberg, G. (2006) Babesia-A historical overview. Vet Parasitol. 138: 3-10.

22. Uilenberg, G. (2001) Babesiosis. In: Encyclopedia of Arthropod-Transmitted Infections of Man and Domesticated Animals. Service, M.W. (es.). (1st ed.) Wallingford: CABI Publishing, UK. p. 53-60.

23. Walker, A.R., Bouattour, A., Camicas, J.L., Estrada-Pena, A., Horak, I.G., Latif, A., Pegram, R.G., Preston, P.M. (2003) Ticks of Domestic Animals in Africa, A guide to Identification of Species. (1st ed.) Biosience Reports, UK.

Synovial fluid inflammatory cytokines and proteins in clinically healthy and arthritic joint of dromedary camels (*Camelus dromedarius*)

Najizadeh, M.H., Pourjafar, M.*, Chalmeh, A., Badiei, Kh., Nazifi, S., Naghib, M.

Department of Clinical Sciences, School of Veterinary Medicine, Shiraz University, Shiraz, Iran

Key words:
acute phase proteins, arthritis, dromedary camel, inflammatory cytokines, synovial fluid

Correspondence
Pourjafar, M.
Department of Clinical Sciences,
School of Veterinary Medicine,
Shiraz University, Shiraz, Iran

Email: dmp4m@yahoo.com

Abstract:

BACKGROUND: Background: Analyzing the synovial fluid is one of the common methods to diagnose the articular problems to detect the stage and express the prognosis. Such gross, cytological, and biochemical analysis of synovial fluids can aid in the diagnosis of various joint diseases. **OBJECTIVES:** Normal values for synovial fluid in the camels have been described previously; however, there are no reports regarding concentr-ation of acute phase proteins and inflammatory cytokines in camelids synovial fluid. Hence, the present study tried to compare the synovial fluid inflammatory cytokines and acute phase proteins in clinically healthy and arthritic tarsal joints of dromedary camels. **METHODS:** 46 male dromedary camels, 5 to 10 years old, were used in this study. 33 camels did not have any clinical articular abnormalities while 13 camels had gross articular problems such as lameness and swollen tarsal joints. Collecting the synovial fluids was extracted from the healthy and arthritic tarsal joints immediately after slaughter. Then, the concentration of haptoglobin, serum amyloid A, tumor necrosis factor-alpha, and interferon-gamma were measured in samples. **RESULTS:** Concentration of all measured parameters in arthritic joints were significantly higher than clinically healthy joints ($p<0.05$). The synovial fluid concentration of serum amyloid A, haptoglobin, tumor necrosis factor-alpha, and interferon-gamma were 5.379, 4.285, 25.503, and 1.904 times higher in arthritic joints than normal joints, respectively. **CONCLUSIONS:** The articular inflammatory processes can increase the synovial fluid concentration of acute phase proteins and inflammatory cytokines. Information about the normal values of these parameters and their changing patterns may help camel rearing systems during arthritis by assessing the health status of joints in the camels; in addition, the information about normal values can be diagnostically valuable when considering diseased animals.

Introduction

The joints of camels, as in other animals, are susceptible to a variety of infectious and noninfecti-ous disorders that may affect their racing perform-ance. In addition, camels serve as an important food source in many parts of the world. Early diagnosis of articular problems is a principal part of treatment. Synovial fluid analysis remains one of the most important diagnostic tools in abnormalities that affect the joint space. It also provides valuable information about the stage and prognosis of the articular abnormalities (Al-Rukibat et al., 2006). Synovial fluid is a plasma dialysate modified by constituents secreted by the joint tissues; hence, alterations in synovial fluid are indications of articular problems. Such gross and cytological analysis of synovial fluids can aid in the diagnosis of various joint diseases, including ligament damage, trauma, neoplasia, infectious and non-infectious synovitis and arthritis, osteoarthritis, and immune-mediated polyarthritis (Madison et al., 1991). The normal values for synovial fluid analysis in the adult dromedarian camel (Nazifi et al., 1998) and llama and alpaca (Waguespack et al., 2002) have been described. Nonetheless, to the best of the authors' knowledge, there are no reports in the literature regarding concentration of acute phase proteins and inflammatory cytokines in camelids synovial fluid.

The purpose of the present study was to determine and compare the concentrations of acute phase proteins (serum amyloid A and haptoglubin) and inflammatory cytokines (tumor necrosis factor-alpha and interferon-gamma) in synovial fluid from the clinically healthy and arthritic tarsal joint of adult male dromedary camels. Furthermore, the data reported here could be used as reference values for assessing articular abnormalities in this species.

Materials and Methods

The study was carried out in November 2010. 46 male dromedary camels (Camelus dromedarius), 5 to 10 years of age, were used in this study. The camels were presented for slaughter to the Meibod abattoir, Yazd province, Iran. The slaughterhouse authorities gave permission to use the animals in this study. Before slaughtering, the animals were visually examined for abnormalities in musculoskeletal system. From all animals, 33 camels did not have any clinical articular abnormalities whereas 13 camels had gross problems such as lameness and swollen tarsal joints. Based on clinical signs and disease history, these animals were suspected to arthritis. An 18 gauge, 1.5 inch needle attached to a 5 milliliters syringe, was used to collect synovial fluid from the healthy and arthritic tarsal joints immediately after the camels were slaughtered. To collect the sample aseptically, the skin covering each joint was clipped and scrubbed using povidone-iodine solution. The needle was inserted into the medial pouch of the tarsal joint. Only blood-free samples were included in the analysis. In cases that blood contamination was suspected based on visual examination, the sample was discarded and a second sampling was attempted at a remote site in the joint. Five milliliters of synovial fluid were collected from each joint and placed in the plain and anticoagulant-coated tubes. Samples of synovial fluids were stored at -20°C until assay.

Haptoglobin (Hp) was measured according to prevention of peroxidase activity of hemoglobin, which is directly proportional to the amount of Hp (Tridelta Development Plc, Wicklow, Ireland). Serum amyloid A (SAA) was measured by a solid phase sandwich ELISA (Tridelta Development Plc, Wicklow, Ireland). Tumor necrosis factor-alpha (TNF-α) and interferon-gamma (IFN-γ) were measured by a solid phase sandwich ELISA (AbC 606 and AbC 607, respectively; Votre fournisseur AbCys S.A. Paris, France).

Data were expressed as mean ± standard deviation (SD). Two independent samples t-test was used to compare the synovial fluid parameters between clinically healthy and arthritic tarsal joints. Statistical analyses were performed by SPSS software (SPSS for Windows, version 11.5, SPSS Inc, Chicago, Illinois). The level of significance was set at $p<0.05$.

Results

The values (mean±SD) of synovial fluid concentration of SAA, Hp, TNF-α and IFN-γ in clinically healthy and arthritic tarsal joints of male dromedary camels are presented in Table 1. Concentration of these parameters in arthritic joints was significantly higher than clinically healthy joints ($p<0.05$). Based on our findings, the synovial fluid concentration of SAA, Hp, TNF-α and IFN-γ in arthritic joints were 5.379, 4.285, 25.503, and 1.904 times higher than normal joints, respectively.

Discussion

Currently, reference values for synovial fluid concentration of inflammatory cytokines and acute phase proteins from camels are interpreted based on values from ruminants (Bani Ismail and Al-Rukibat,

Table 1. Synovial fluid concentrations (mean±SD) of acute phase proteins and inflammatory cytokines in clinically healthy and arthritic tarsal joints of male dromedary camels.

	Clinically healthy tarsal joints (n=33)	Arthritic tarsal joints (n=13)
Serum amyloid A (μg/mL)	0.124±0.015	0.667±0.016
Haptoglubin (g/L)	0.007±0.001	0.030±0.008
Tumor necrosis factor-alpha (pg/dL)	7.474±0.737	19.061±4.318
Interferon-gamma (pg/dL)	1.351±0.191	2.573±0.375

2006). There are literatures on physical, biochemical, and cytologic properties of blood and synovial fluid in clinically normal adult camels (Nazifi et al., 1998; Bani Ismail and Al-Rukibat, 2006; Al-Rukibat et al., 2006); however, there are few or no information about synovial fluid inflammatory cytokines, acute phase proteins, and their changes in arthritic joints in dromedary camels. Bani Ismail et al. (2007) studied the synovial fluid analysis and bacterial population in clinically arthritic joints of juvenile male camel calves; however, synovial fluid concentration of inflammatory cytokines and acute phase proteins were not determined in their study. In the present study, we described, for the first time, the reference values of synovial fluid concentration of inflammatory cytokines and acute phase proteins from the tarsal joints of clinically healthy adult male dromedary camels and their comparison with the arthritic joints.

Acute phase proteins and their changes have been intensively studied in response to various inflammatory and non-inflammatory conditions, in many animal species (Eckersall, 2000; Petersen et al., 2004; Murata, 2007). Acute phase proteins assessment is more sensitive than hematological and clinical tests for diagnosis of diseases. Furthermore, acute phase proteins increase during the progressive stage of disease and decrease in the recovery stage; therefore, it helps to diagnose the disease in the early stages (Nazifi et al., 2008). SAA and Hp as well as other acute phase proteins have been proposed as stress markers in animals (Pineiro et al., 2007). SAA is an apolipoprotein of high-density lipoprotein and is considered as one of the major acute phase proteins in vertebrates. Determination and evaluation of SAA showed that this protein could be a valuable factor in the diagnosis of infection (Gruys et al., 1994). Hp is an alpha2-globulin synthesized in the liver and is used as another major acute phase protein in numerous species of productive and companion animals. In ruminants, the level of circulating Hp is negligible in normal animals but increases over 100-fold with immune stimulation (Feldman et al., 2000). Furthermore, Hp is a clinically useful parameter for the evaluation of the occurrence and severity of inflammatory diseases in large animals (Skinner and Roberts, 1994). To the best of the authors' knowledge, there are no reports on synovial fluid concentration of SAA and Hp in clinically healthy and arthritic joints of dromedary camels. Based on the findings of the present study, synovial fluid concentration of acute phase proteins in arthritic tarsal joints were significantly ($p<0.05$), and several times, higher than clinically healthy similar joints.

TNF-α is a cytokine involved in systemic inflammation and a member of a group of cytokines that stimulate the acute phase response. In the liver, TNF-α stimulates the acute phase response, leading to an increase in acute phase proteins. TNF-α, in particular, has been amply implicated in deleterious host responses (Heinzel 1990). IFN-γ is a dimerized soluble cytokine that is the only member of the type II class of interferons. IFN-γ is a cytokine that is critical for innate and adaptive immunity against viral and intracellular bacterial infections. Endotoxin activates macrophage microbicidal effector functions and production of proinflammatory cytokines, such as IFN-γ (Schroder et al., 2004). The ability of IFN-γ has been described to increase macrophage TNF-α production by both transcriptional and translational mechanisms (Burchett et al., 1988). In the present study, for the first time, we compared the synovial fluid concentration of TNF-α and IFN-γ in clinically healthy dromedary camels with these cytokines in arthritic synovial fluid. The results of the present study showed that the synovial fluid concentration of inflammatory cytokines in clinically healthy tarsal joints was significantly ($p<0.05$), and several times, lower than similar arthritic joints.

Several studies on measuring acute phase response proteins and cytokines have mentioned that increasing the amount of these factors takes place immediately after commencement of inflammatory processes (Nazifi et al., 2008; Chalmeh et al., 2013a-c). Hence, it could be stated that evaluating acute phase response biomarkers can be used for early diagnosis of camel inflammatory joint diseases.

In conclusion, the data provided here are the first reference values of synovial fluid concentration of acute phase proteins and inflammatory cytokines in clinically healthy tarsal joints of dromedary camels. These data showed that the articular inflammatory processes could increase the synovial fluid acute phase response biomarkers such as acute phase proteins and inflammatory cytokines. Information about the normal values of these parameters and their changing patterns may help camel rearing systems during arthritis by assessing the health status of joints in the camels; in addition, the information about normal values can be diagnostically valuable when considering diseased animals.

Acknowledgments

The authors would like to appreciate all the staff of the Veterinary Organization of Yazd Province for their valuable collaborations.Conflict of interest statement: The authors have declared no conflicts of interest.

References

1. Al-Rukibat, R.K., Bani Ismail, Z.A., Al-Zghoul, M.B. (2006) Cytologic analysis of synovial fluid in clinically normal tarsal joints of young camels (*Camelus dromedarius*). Vet Clin Pathol. 35: 326-328.
2. Baghshani, H., Nazifi, S., Saeb, M., Saeb, S. (2010) Influence of road transportation on plasma concentrations of acute phase proteins, including fibrinogen, haptoglobin, serum amyloid A, and ceruloplasmin, in dromedary camels (*Camelus dromedarius*). Comp Clin Pathol. 19: 193-198.
3. Bani Ismail, Z., Al-Rukibat, R. (2006) Synovial fluid cell counts and total protein concentration in clinically normal fetlock joints of young dromedarian camels. J Vet Med A Physiol Pathol Clin Med. 53: 263-265.
4. Bani Ismail, Z., Al-Rukibat, R., Al-Tarazi, Y., Al-Zghoul, M.B. (2007) Synovial fluid analysis and bacterial findings in arthritic joints of juvenile male camel (*Camelus dromedarius*) calves. J Vet Med A Physiol Pathol Clin Med. 54: 66-69.
5. Burchett, S.K., Weaver, W.M., Westall, J.A., Larsen, A., Kronheim, S., Wilson, C.B. (1988) Regulation of tumor necrosis factor/cachectin and IL-1 secretion in human mononuclear phagocytes. J Immunol. 140: 3473-3481.
6. Chalmeh, A., Badiei, K., Pourjafar, M., Nazifi, S. (2013a) Anti-inflammatory effects of insulin regular and flunixin meglumine on endotoxemia experimentally induced by *Escherichia coli* serotype O55: B5 in an ovine model. Inflamm Res. 62: 61-67.
7. Chalmeh, A., Badiei, K., Pourjafar, M., Nazifi, S. (2013b) Acute phase response in experimentally *Escherichia coli* serotype O55: B5 induced endotoxemia and its comparative treatment with dexamethasone and flunixin meglumine in Iranian fat-tailed sheep. Vet Arhiv. 83: 301-312.
8. Chalmeh, A., Badiei, K., Pourjafar, M., Nazifi, S. (2013c) Modulation of inflammatory responses following insulin therapy in experimentally bolus intravenous *Escherichia coli* lipopolysaccharide serotype O55:B5 induced endotoxemia in Iranian fat-tailed sheep. Small Rumin Res. 113: 283-289.
9. Eckersall, P.D. (2000) Recent advances and future prospects for the use of acute phase proteins as markers of disease in animals. Rev Med Vet. 151: 577-584.
10. El-Boshy, M., Abbas, H., El-Khodery, S., Osman, S. (2009) Cytokine response and clinicopathological findings in Brucella infected camels (*Camelus dromedarius*). Vet Med-Czech. 54: 25-32.
11. Feldman, B.F., Zinkl, J.G., Jain, N.C. (2000) Schalm's Veterinary Hematology. (1st ed.) Philadelphia, Lippincott Williams and Wilkins. Philadelphia, USA.
12. Gruys, E., Obwolo, M.J., Toussaint, M.J.M. (1994) Diagnostic significance of the major acute phase proteins in veterinary clinical chemistry: a review. Vet Bull. 64: 1009-1018.
13. Heinzel, F.P. (1990) The role of IFN-γ in the pathology of experimental endotoxemia. J Immunol. 145: 2920-2924.
14. Madison, J.R., Sommer, M., Spencer, P.A. (1991) Relations among synovial membrane histopathologic findings, synovial fluid cytologic findings, and bacterial culture results in horses with suspected infectious arthritis: 64 cases (1979-1987). J Am Vet Med Assoc. 198: 1655-1661.
15. Murata, H. (2007) Stress and acute phase protein response: an inconspicuous but essential linkage. Vet

J. 173: 473-474.
16. Nazifi, S., Rezakhani, A., Gheisari, H.R. (1998) Physical, biochemical and cytologic properties of blood and synovial fluid in clinically normal adult camel (*Camelus dromedarius*). J Vet Med A. 45: 155-160.
17. Nazifi, S., Khoshvaghti, A., Gheisari, H.R. (2008) Evaluation of serum and milk amyloid A in some inflammatory diseases of cattle. Iran J Vet Res. 9: 222-226.
18. Petersen, H.H., Nielsen, J.P., Heegaard, P.M.H. (2004) Application of acute phase protein measurements in veterinary clinical chemistry. Vet Res. 35: 163-187.
19. Pineiro, M., Pineiro, C., Carpintero, R., Morales, J., Campbell, F.M., Eckersall, P.D., Toussaint, M.J., Lampreave, F. (2007) Characterization of the pig acute phase protein response to road transport. Vet J. 173: 669-674.
20. Schroder, K., Hertzog, P.J., Ravasi, T., Hume, D.A. (2004) Interferon-γ: an overview of signals, mechanisms and functions. J Leukocyte Biol. 75: 163-189.
21. Skinner, J.G., Roberts, L. (1994) Haptoglobin as an indicator of infection in sheep. Vet Rec. 134: 33-36.
22. Waguespack, R.W., Belknap, E.B., Spano, J.S., Wenzel, J.G., Pugh, D. (2002) Analysis of synovial fluid from clinically normal alpaca and llamas. Am J Vet Res. 63: 576-578.

Phylogenetic study based on the phosphoprotein gene of Iranian Newcastle disease viruses (NDV) isolates, 2010 -2012

Ghalyanchi Langroudi, A.[1*], Hosseini, H.[2], Karimi, V.[3], Madadgar, O.[1], Hashemzadeh, M.[4], Ghafouri, S.A.[5], Bagheri Ghadikolaei, S.S.[6], Vahedi, S.M.[6]

[1]*Department of Microbiology and Immunology, Faculty of Veterinary Medicine, University of Tehran, Tehran, Iran*

[2]*Department of Clinical Sciences, Faculty of Veterinary Medicine, Islamic Azad University, Karaj Branch, Karaj, Iran*

[3]*Department of Poultry Diseases, Faculty of Veterinary Medicine, University of Tehran, Tehran, Iran*

[4]*Department of Research & Production of Veterinary and Poultry Vaccines, Razi Vaccine and Serum Research Institute, Karaj, Iran*

[5]*Department of Poultry Health and Diseases, Iranian Veterinary Organization, Tehran, Iran*

[6]*Students' Scientific Association of Microbiology, Faculty of Veterinary Medicine, University of Tehran, Tehran, Iran*

Key words:
Newcastle disease, phosphoprotein, phylogenetic study

Correspondence
Ghalyanchi Langeroudi, A.
Department of Microbiology and Immunology, Faculty of Veterinary Medicine, University of Tehran, Tehran, Iran

Email: ghalyana@ut.ac.ir

Abstract:

BACKGROUND: Newcastle disease virus (NDV) is the causative agent of the Newcastle disease (ND), a highly contagious disease in birds that causes significant economic losses to the poultry industry worldwide. ND is endemic in Iran and outbreaks are reported regularly in commercial poultry flocks and different species of birds. **OBJECTIVES:** The current study was carried out to characterize NDV based on phosphorprotein (P) gene from recent outbreaks in Iran, 2010-2012. **METHODS:** The P gene fragment of NDV isolates of five chickens, 1 ostrich, and 1 Pigeon paramyxovirus-1 was obtained by RT-PCR and sequenced. **RESULTS:** Phylogenetic analysis of sequences revealed that chicken and ostrich NDV isolates were closely related and placed in the genotype VII and Pigeon Paramyxovirus-1 was located in the genotype V. **CONCLUSIONS:** This is the first report of Phosphoprotein gene sequences of NDV strains isolated in Iran. This study will help us to understand the epidemiology and molecular characteristics of Newcastle disease virus in Iran.

Introduction

Newcastle disease (ND), caused by Newcastle disease virus (NDV), is a highly contagious respiratory, enteric or neurological viral disease and an OIE notifiable devastating disease that is found in most avian species, especially in chickens (Miller et al., 2009).

The NDV is a member of avian paramyxovirus serotype-1 (APMV-1), which belongs to the genus Avulavirus and Paramyxoviridae family. The NDV has RNA genome (a negative-sense single stranded, 15 Kb), which codes for an RNA-directed RNA polymerase (L), hemagglutinin-neuraminidaseprotein (HN), fusion protein (F), matrixprotein (M), phosphoprotein (P), and nucleoprotein (*NP*) (Alexander et al., 1997).

All NDV isolates are classified as three pathotypes based on the disease severity: mesogenic, velogenic, and lentogenic. Genetic and antigenic analyses of NDV isolates have determined the existence of two main classes I and II, which could be divided into ten genotypes (1-10 in class I and I-X in class II): The genotypes VI and VII being further divided into seven (VIa-VIg) and five (VIIa-VIIe) sub-genotypes respectively (Miller et al., 2010).

The phosphoprotein, or P protein, of NDV, has the critical role in replication and transcription and has multiple functions. For example, the P protein also acts as a chaperone to prevent uncontrolled encapsidation of non-viral RNA by the NP protein (Jahanshiri et al., 2005; Locke et al., 2000; Smith and Hightower, 1981). ND is endemic in Iran and we have some reports for incidence of ND in every year. In the past few decades, implementations of extensive vaccination programs in commercial poultry farms, and to some extent in small rural poultry flocks have reduced the number of epizootics outbreaks of ND in Iran(Bozorgmehri-Fard and Keyvanfar, 1979; Rezaeianzadeh et al., 2011). No data is available about the P gene of Iranian NDV isolates till now. The study is the first report on P gene characterization of Iranian NDV isolates and provides a suggestion on NDV data collection to increase future virus evolutionary analysis.

Materials and Methods

Samples: We worked on six velogenic NDV isolates and one Pigeon Paramyxovirus -1 (approved by analyses of sequences of Fusion gene) that were isolated form different outbreaks in broiler and breeder farms, ostrich and pigeon case. Ten-day-old SPF embryonated chicken eggs (Allantoic cavity) were inoculated. These eggs were incubated at 37 C for up to 2 days, embryonic death was monitored, and then allantoic fluid was collected under routine conditions. All data of mentioned isolates are available in Table 1.

RNA extraction and RT-PCR: RNA is extracted from allantoic fluid through QIAamp virus spin kit (QIAGEN, USA) and stored at -70°C. Reverse transcription was done by using random hexamer with revert aid first strand cDNA synthesis Kit (Fermentas Co, Canada) (OIE, 2012). Amplification of the P gene was carried out by PCR as described by using one pair of specific primers of phosphopotein gene (NDF: ACCAGYGGRACTGTCATHGAC, NDR: CGGACAGTGTCCYTCTCYAC).The PCR amplification was carried out in a 50 μL reaction mixture containing 0.2 lM dNTP, 0.5 mM MgCl2, 0.2 lM each primer, 19 PCR buffer and 1 U of Taq polymerase. Reactions were performed according to the following protocol: 95 °C for 5 min, followed by 35 cycles (95°C for 45 s, 58°C for 45 s, 72 °C for 1 min) and a final extension step of 10 min at 72 °C.

Sequencing and bioinformatics study: The PCR products were purified with the AccuPrep® PCRPCR Purification kit (Bioneer Co, South Korea) and sent to Source BioScience Company (UK) for DNA sequencing. The primary sequence analyses and edition were carried out in the CLC sequence viewer (Ver. 6.0.2). Multiple amino acid alignments were performed on P genes representative viruses using Clustal W (MEGA5) (Tamura et al., 2011) on current study isolates and other NDV isolates from Gene bank (Table 2). Phylogenetic trees were drawn from nucleotide sequences based on the sequence of phosphprotein gene using Neibor-Joining method with MEGA5.Model with 1000 bootstrapping replications in molecular evolutionary genetics analysis (MEGA5). The structure of the NDV that were sequenced and analyzed in this study has been submitted to GeneBank under the accession numbersKF824513-KF824519 (Table 1).

Results

The partial sequences of phosphoprotein gene of six Iranian NDV isolates were amplified and sequenced. MEGA5 program were used to determine the sequence similarity and homology of the p gene among them. Results indicate that nucleotide homology among six NDVs isolates with P genes is between 99.6% and 99.9%. The percent identify based on amino acid is between 99.3%- 99.8 %. In BLAST result NDVs isolates have high nucleotide identities (97%) with JSG0210 (JF340367), chicken/TC/9/2011 (KC461214), JSD0812 (GQ849007). Pigeon Paramyxovirus-1 has 94% nucleotide identities with Pigeon paramyxovirus-1 strain AV324/96(GQ429292). A phylogenetic tree (Figure 1) was constructed based on the aminoacidemia sequences of the P genein allisolates and one and the corresponding region of the other NDV strains retrieved from Gene Bank (Table 2). All six NDV fleld isolates, isolated in 2010-2012 outbreaks, were classifled into genotype VII and one Pigeon Paramyxovirus-1 was located in the genotype V.

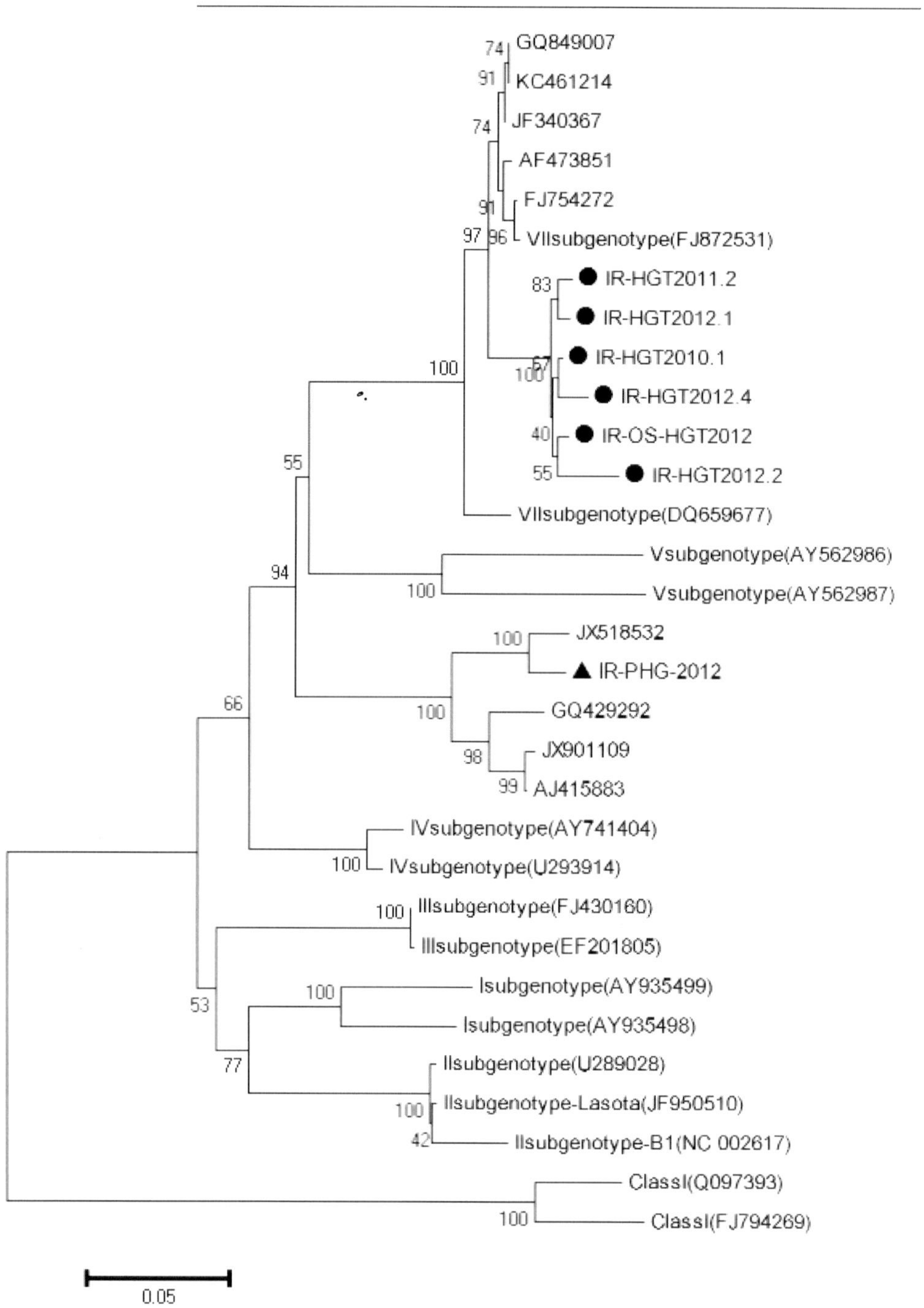

Figure 1. Nucleic acid Phylogenetic relationships of phosphoprotein gene of Newcastle disease genome isolated from broilers and pigeon, Iran. The Phylogenetic tree was generated using Neibor Joining model with MEGA (version 5.1 beta). Numbers below branches indicate bootstrap value from 1000 replicates, bootstrap values. Horizontal distances are proportional to the minimum number of nucleic acid differences required to join nodes. The vertical lines are for spacing branches and labels. Analysis was based on complete open reading frames of all gene segments. The scale bar represents the distance unit between sequence pairs. The virus genome of broiler characterized in this report is indicated as Black Circle. Black triangle is indicated for pigeon isolate. The sequences obtained from Gene Bank.

Discussion

Newcastle disease (ND) has a destructive economic effect on commercial farms in Iran; thus, it is necessary to identify the ecology and transmission dynamics in order to improve disease control measures. This study was conducted to characterize

Table 1. The characteristic of Iranian Newcastle disease virus isolates (2010-2012).

No	Strain Name	Accession Number (Fusion Protein)	Accession Number (Phospho protein)	Isolation from Species	Clinical sign	Year	Province/Iran	Sample
1	IR-HGT2010.1	JX131352	KF824516	Broiler	Neurological	2010	Gilan	Brain
2	IR-HGT2011.1	JX131355	KF824517	Broiler	Neurological	2011	Mazandaran	Brain
3	IR-HGT2012.1	JX131357	KF824513	Broiler	Digestive	2012	Alborz	Cecal tonsil
4	IR-HGT2012.2	JX131358	KF824514	Broiler	Neurological	2012	Isfahan	Brain
5	IR-HGT2012.4	JX131360	KF824515	Breeder	Neurological	2012	Mazandaran	Brain
6	IR-OS-HGT2012	JX131350.1	KF824518	ostrich	Neurological	2012	Tehran	Brain
7	IR-PHG-2012	No submission	KF824519	Pigeon	Neurological	2012	Tehran	Brain

Table2. List of Newcastle disease viruses' characteristics that included in the phylogenetic.

Accession Number	Strain Name	Class	Sub-Genotype
AY935499	I-2	II	I
AY935498	99-1435	II	I
EU289028	VG/GA	II	II
NC_002617	B1	II	II
JF950510	Lasota	II	II
FJ430160	JS/9/05/Go	II	III
EF201805	Mukteswar	II	III
AY741404	Herts/33	II	IV
EU293914	Italien	II	IV
AY562986	Anhinga/U.S.(Fl)/44083/93	II	V
AY562987	Gamefowl/U.S.(CA)/211472/02	II	V
JX518532	Pigeon paramyxovirus	II	V
GQ429292	AV324/96	II	V
JX901109	PMV-1/Belgium/98-238/1998	II	V
AJ415883	Pigeon paramyxovirus-1	II	V
AY562985	Cockatoo/Indonesia/14698/90	II	VI
AJ880277	Pigeon paramyxovirus 1	II	VI
FJ872531	Muscovy duck/China(Fujian)/FP1/02	II	VII
DQ659677	NA-1(Goose)	II	VII
AF473851	SF02/Goose	II	VII
FJ754272	WF00D	II	VII
JF340367	JSG0210	II	VII
KC461214	chicken/TC/9/2011	II	VII
JSD0812	GQ849007	II	VII
DQ097393	DE-R49/99	I	--
FJ794269	NDV08-004	I	--

NDVs isolated from five chicken, one ostrich and one Pigeon paramyxovirus-1. Phylogenetic analysis of sequences revealed that chicken and ostrich origin NDV isolates were closely related and placed in the genotype VII and Pigeon Paramyxovirus-1 was located in the genotype V. It is similar to pervious results of researches of Iranians on F (Kianizadeh et al., 2002) and M gene (Langeroudi et al., 2012). Ebrahimi et al. (2012), based on F gene of Iranian NDV isolates, reported that they were representing sub-genotype VIIb (Ebrahimi et al., 2012). According to the results of our study, it is the first report that mentioned Iranian NDV strains were located in genotype VIId. Aboshah (2012), working on NDV isolates from Iranian commercial farms, been revealed that these isolates were located in VIIb subgenotype (Abdoshah, 2012). Esmaealzadeh and co-investigators showed that the 6 Iranian isolates examined share significant similarity with 2 Russian isolates, Sterna- Astr/ 2755/ 2001 and VOL95 (Esmaelizad et al., 2012).The results also indicate that genotype VII was the most prevalent isolate in Iran during the recent years. Genotype VII of NDV in Asia has been traced back to 1984 in Taiwan and to 1985 in Japan (Yang et al., 1999). According to Munir et al. (2012) the P gene was the most variable gene among the six NDV genes when compared with representatives of each genotype. Therefore, it is believed that the P gene is an evolutionary strategy of the virus that increases the coding capacity of the genome (Munir et al., 2012). It is the first report for characterization and phylogenic analysis of Pigeon Paramyxovirus-1In Iran. The data revealed that Iranian pigeon paramyxovirus-1 belongs to Genotype V beside other related pigeon Paramyxovirus-1. The presence of multiple NDV strains in Iran, the Far East and highly transmissible nature of the virus can complicate and increase the cost of attempts to prevent the spread of infection to the other parts of the world. In accordance with high occurrence of ND in pigeon population in Iran, more detailed studies should be carried out on their isolates. Finally, we suggest that researchers perform full length characterization on Iranian NDV isolates in recent years to reach more details of molecular epidemiology. In conclusion, our results reveal that NDV surveillance would be helpful to expand the understanding of NDV epidemiology in endemic regions.

Acknowledgments

The authors would like to acknowledge Mr. Ahmad Vahedi for his technical assistance.

References

1. Abdoshah, M., Pourbakhsh, S., Peighambari, S., Shojadoost, B., Momayez, R., Mojahedi, Z. (2012) Pathogenicity indices of Newcastle disease viruses isolated from Iranian poultry flocks in Iran. J Vet Res. 67: 159-164.
2. Alexander, D.J., Manvell, R.J., Lowings, J.P., Frost, K.M., Collins, M.S., Russell, P.H., Smith, J.E. (1997) Antigenic diversity and similarities detected in avian paramyxovirus type 1 (Newcastle disease virus) isolates using monoclonal antibodies. Avian pathol. 26: 399-418.
3. Bozorgmehri-Fard, M.H., Keyvanfar, H. (1979) Isolation of Newcastle disease virus from teals (Anas crecca) in Iran. J Wildlife Dis.15: 335-337.
4. Ebrahimi, M.M., Shahsavandi, S., Moazenijula, G., Shamsara, M. (2012) Phylogeny and evolution of Newcastle disease virus genotypes isolated in Asia during 2008-2011. Virus genes. 45: 63-68.
5. Esmaelizad, M., Ashtiani, M.P., Jelokhani-Niaraki, S., Hashemnejad, K. (2012) Identification of 23 specific nucleotide patterns in the HN gene of Newcastle disease viruses isolated from Iran. Turk J Biol. 36: 135-142.
6. Jahanshiri, F., Eshaghi, M., Yusoff, K. (2005) Identification of phosphoprotein: phosphoprotein and phosphoprotein:nucleocapsid protein interaction domains of the Newcastle disease virus. Arch Virol. 150: 611-618.
7. Kianizadeh, M., Aini, I., Omar, A.R., Yusoff, K., Sahrabadi, M., Kargar, R. (2002) Sequence and phylogenetic analysis of the fusion protein cleavage site of Newcastle disease virus field isolates from Iran. Acta Virologica. 46: 247-251.
8. Kianizadeh, M., Ideris, A., Shahrabadi, M.S., Kargar, R., Pourbakhsh, S.A., Omar, S., Yusoffi, A. (1999) Biological and Molecular characterization of Newcastle disease virus Isolated from Iran. Arch Razi Ins. 50: 1-10.
9. Langeroudi, A.G., Hosseini, H., Karimi, V., Hashemzadeh, M., Estabragh, A.S., Madadgar, O., (2012) Phylogenetic study base on matrix gene of Iranian Newcastle disease virus isolates, 2011-2012. Comp Clin Pathol. p.1-5.
10. Locke, D.P., Sellers, H.S., Crawford, J.M., Schultz-Cherry, S., King, D.J., Meinersmann, R.J., Seal, B.S., (2000) Newcastle disease virus phosphoprotein gene analysis and transcriptional editing in avian cells. Virus Res. 69: 55-68.
11. Miller, P.J., Decanini, E.L., Afonso, C.L. (2010) Newcastle disease: evolution of genotypes and the related diagnostic challenges. Infection, genetics and evolution. J Mol Epidemiol Evol Genet Infect Dis. 10: 26-35.
12. Miller, P.J., Kim, L.M., Ip, H.S., Afonso, C.L. (2009) Evolutionary dynamics of Newcastle disease virus. Virology. 391: 64-72.
13. Munir, M., Zohari, S., Abbas, M., Berg, M. (2012) Sequencing and analysis of the complete genome of Newcastle disease virus isolated from a commercial poultry farm in 2010. Arch Virol. 157: 765-768.
14. OIE, A. (2012) Manual of Diagnostic Tests and Vaccines for Terrestrial Animals. Office international des epizooties, Paris, France.
15. Rezaeianzadeh, G., Dadras, H., Ali, A.S.M., Nazemshirazi, M. (2011) Serological and molecular study of Newcastle disease virus circulating in village chickens of Fars province, Iran. J Vet Med Anim Health. 3: 105-111.
16. Smith, G.W., Hightower, L.E. (1981) Identification of the P proteins and other disulfide-linked and phosphorylated proteins of Newcastle disease virus. J Virol. 37: 256-267.
17. Tamura, K., Peterson, D., Peterson, N., Stecher, G., Nei, M., Kumar, S. (2011) MEGA5: molecular evolutionary genetics analysis using maximum likelihood, evolutionary distance, and maximum parsimony methods. Mol Biol Evol. 28: 2731-2739.
18. Yang, C.Y., Shieh, H.K., Lin, Y.L., Chang, P.C. (1999) Newcastle disease virus isolated from recent outbreaks in Taiwan phylogenetically related to viruses (genotype VII) from recent outbreaks in western Europe. Avian Dis. 43: 125-130.

Identification of *Coxiella burnetii* by touch-down PCR assay in unpasteurized milk and dairy products in North - East of Iran

Khanzadi, S.[1*], Jamshidi, A.[1], Razmyar, J.[2], Borji, Sh.[3]

[1] *Department of Food Hygiene and Aquaculture, Faculty of Veterinary Medicine, Ferdowsi University of Mashhad, Mashhad, Iran*

[2] *Department of Clinical Sciences, Faculty of Veterinary Medicine, Ferdowsi University of Mashhad, Mashhad, Iran*

[3] *Graduated from the Faculty of Veterinary Medicine, Ferdowsi University of Mashhad, Mashhad, Iran*

Key words:
Coxiella burnetii, milk, touch-down PCR, unpasteurized dairy products

Correspondence
Khanzadi, S.
Department of Food Hygiene and Aquaculture, Faculty of Veterinary Medicine, Ferdowsi University of Mashhad, Mashhad, Iran

Email: khanzadi@um.ac.ir

Abstract:

BACKGROUND: *Coxiella burnetii* is the causative agent of the zoonotic disease Q fever, and ruminants being considered as the main source for human infection. Although the main route of infection in human is inhalation of contaminated aerosols, oral transmission by contaminated raw milk or unpasteurized dairy products is also a possible route of infection. Raw milk or dairy products produced from unpasteurized milk may contain virulent *C. burnetii*. **OBJECTIVES:** This study aimed to determine the contamination rate of milk and unpasteurized dairy products with *C. burnetii*. **METHODS:** Touch-down PCR was used to examine the presence of *C. burnetii* on 147 dairy product samples collected from local traditional and commercial markets in Mashhad-Khorasan Razavi province- Iran. **RESULTS:** 2 of 28 (7.14%) cheese samples, 2 of 26 (7.69%) yoghurt samples, 8 of 23 (34.78%) sheep milk samples, and 2 of 60 (3.33%) cow milk samples were found to be positive for *C. burnetii* DNA. However, 10 goat milk samples were found to be negative. **CONCLUSIONS:** The results of this study indicate that the clinically healthy dairy livestock and their dairy products are important sources of *C. burnetii* infection.

Introduction

Coxiella burnetii is strictly intracellular Gram-negative bacteria, a short (0.3 to 1.0 μm) and pleomorphic rod organism. It is the causative agent of a zoonotic disease that occurs in human (Q fever) and animals (coxiellosis). *C. burnetii* is extremely resistant to heat, pressure, and chemical stress and can survive for months in stressful environments (Rahimi et al., 2010). This organism is also highly infectious. In experimental conditions, only one organism is required to produce infection (Ormsbee et al., 1978).

Q fever is a worldwide zoonotic disease and has been reported from most countries except New Zealand (Fournier et al., 1998). Recent studies show that Q fever is a considerable public health problem in many countries, especially people who are in direct contact with domestic animals. People who are in contact with animals, including veterinarians, farm workers, slaughterhouse workers, and laboratory personnel working with infected animals are at higher risk (Maurin and Raoult, 1999; Kirkan et al., 2008).

Cattle, sheep, and goats are the major reservoirs of *C. burnetii*. Also a wide variety of other animals can be infected with *C. burnetii*, including dogs, cats, non-human primates, wild rodents, small mammals, big game wildlife, non-mammalian animals, including reptiles, amphibians, domesticated and wild birds, fish, and ticks (Parker et al., 2006). Ticks are normally the primary reservoir of these bacteria and also the distributer of bacteria in wild and domestic animals (Abbasi et al., 2011).

The organism is shed via urine, feces, and milk of infected animals and has a particularly high concentration during parturition. Shedding into the environment occurs mainly by birth products, particularly the placenta. In the chronic phase, the uterus and mammary glands are primary sites of infection for *C. burnetii* (Maurin and Raoult, 1999; Kim et al., 2005). The main transmission route of *C. burnetii* for human is respiratory aerosols or dust contaminated with birth fluid, placenta, urine, and feces of infected animals.

Although animals are often the main source of infection for human, they do not show the coxiellosis symptoms clearly, except in cases of abortion in the last weeks of pregnancy, infertility (which has been reported in cattle and its occurrence has not been reported in sheep), metritis, mastitis, and stillbirth. Abortion occurs in sheep and goat, but less frequently in cattle (Barlow et al., 2008; Kirkan et al., 2008). In human, Q fever is most often asymptomatic, but acute disease (mainly a limited flu-like illness, pneumonia or hepatitis) or chronic disease (chronic fatigue syndrome or endocarditis) can occur (Fournier et al., 1998).

The gastrointestinal route (consumption of row milk and unpasteurized dairy products) is of minor importance (Rahimi et al., 2010). It has been reported that up to 105 cfu ml-1 coxiellae can be shed in bovine milk during several lactation periods (Biberstein et al., 1974). Therefore, a specific and sensitive diagnostic system is necessary to detect even small numbers of this microorganism.

In previous studies, serological tests were the main way to determine the prevalence of *C. burnetii* infection (Berri et al., 2000), however, it may indicate a history of previous exposure to *C. burnetii*. Cell culture is a sensitive method for detection of *C. burnetii*, but this method is time-consuming. Capture enzyme-linked immunosorbent assay (ELISA) method is faster than cell culture; however, considering the low level of shedding and the minimum infectious dose of *C. burnetii*, the detection limit is not completely satisfactory (Lorenz et al., 1998). Polymerase chain reaction (PCR) is a highly sensitive and specific detection method that has been used for screening (Kim et al., 2005; Ongor et al., 2004) and determining the presence of the bacteria in milk, feces, or vaginal swabs (Berri et al., 2000).

The objective of the present study was to determine the presence of *C. burnetii* in raw milk and dairy products that are made from unpasteurized milk, in Mashhad using a touchdown PCR assay.

Materials and Methods

Sampling: From January to May 2012, a total of 147 samples of raw milk or dairy product which were prepared from unpasteurized milk were collected from dairy farms and retail stores in different areas in Mashhad city, Khorasan-Razavi province of Iran. The samples included 10 goat' raw milk, 23 sheep's raw milk, 60 cow's raw milk, 28 cheese samples (100 gram each) which were made from sheep milk and 26 yoghurt samples with the same origin. Samples were collected aseptically and placed in a cooler box with ice packs and immediately transferred to the laboratory. The samples were processed within an hour of collection or stored at -20°C until use.

DNA extraction from raw milk: Bacterial DNA from milk samples were extracted by centrifuging and removing the cream and milk layers as described previously by Berri et al., (2003) with some modifications. Briefly, 50ml of each milk sample was transferred to the 50 ml falcon tube and centrifuged 3 times at 3000 g for 10 minutes. Each time the supernatant was discarded and replaced by phosphate buffered saline (PBS). Purification of DNA was achieved using a genomic DNA extraction kit (Bioneer, South Korea) according to the manufacturer's instruction, and the total DNA was measured at 260 nm optical density according to the method described by Sambrook and Russell (2001).

DNA extraction from cheese and yoghurt: Briefly, 5g of cheese or 5ml of yoghurt were transferred to the stomacher bag, then 45 ml of the diluent (0.5% w/v sodium chloride, 1% w/v casitone, 2% w/v sodium citrate) were added and the bags were squeezed manually to dispense the diluent. The bags were placed into stomacher and stomached for 5 min, then heated at 50°C for 2 h; this step was repeated 4 times (Hirai et al., 2012). The rest of the process was the same as raw milk processing.

DNA amplification (trans-PCR): In this study, a polymerase chain reaction (PCR) assay targeting a transposon-like repetitive region of the bacterial genome (IS1111 gene) was used to detect *C. burnetii*. Trans-1 and trans-2 primers with the following sequence were used from the published data. Trans-1 (5'-TAT GTA TCC ACC GTA GCCAGT C-3') and trans-2 (5'-CCC AAC AACACC TCC TTA TTC-3') (Hoover et al., 1992). Primers were synthesized by Bioneer Co. (South Korea). These primers amplify a 687-bp fragment of the target sequence. PCR assay was performed as described previously (Vaidya et al., 2008). The PCR mixture (25µL) included 2.5µL of 10×PCR buffer (100 mM Tris-HCl buffer, pH 8.3, 500 mM KCl, 15 mM MgCl2, and 0.01% gelatin), 200 µM deoxynucleoside triphosphate mix, 2µM of each primers, 0.3 U of Taq DNA polymerase, 3µL of template DNA, and high pure double sterilized water to make up the reaction mixture volume. The amplification was performed in a personal thermo-cycler (TECHNE TC- 5 UK). The cycling denaturation of DNA at 95°C for 2 min, followed by five cycles at 94°C for 30s, 66 to 61°C (the temperature was decreased by 1°C between consecutive steps) for 1 min, and 72°C for 1 min. These cycles were followed by 35 cycles consisting of 94°C for 30 s, 61°C for 30 s, and 72°C for 1 min and then a final extension step of 10 min at 72°C (Hoover et al., 1992).

After electrophoresis of amplicons in agarose gel and staining with ethidium bromide at concentration of 0.5 mg mL-1, they visualized under UV illumination.

After confirmation of the first positive PCR product as *C. burnetii* by sequence analysis, it was used as positive control, and for negative control deionized distilled water was used.

Sequence analysis: The first positive PCR product was purified using the Roche purification kit (Roche Molecular Biochemicals, Mannheim, Germany) and submitted for automated sequencing in both directions at the Eurofins MWG Operon (Martinsried, Germany) using PCR primers as sequencing primers. Nucleotide and predicted amino acid sequence data were aligned with the clustal alignment algorithm. Phylogenetic analysis based on nucleotide sequences was conducted using a distance method, unweighted pair group with arithmetic mean, by calculating boots trap values for 1000 replicates in CLC main Workbench Package Version 5 (CLC Bio, Aarhus, Denmark).

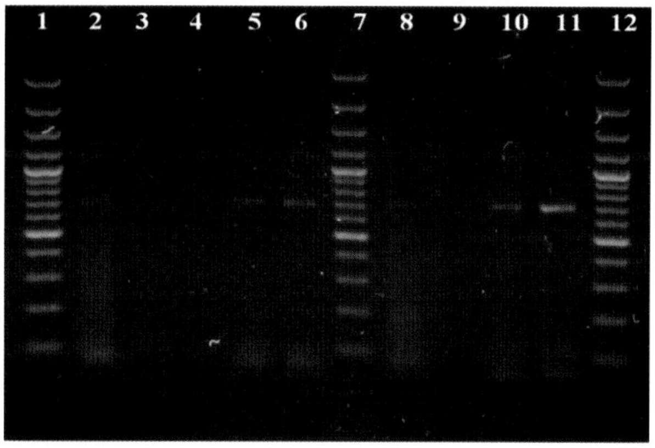

Figure 1. Detection of *Coxiella burnetii* in milk and dairy products using touch-down PCR assay, amplifying a 687 bp segment of the IS1111 gene: Lanes 1, 7, 12 100bp markers. Lane 2 positive control. Lane 3 negative control (DW). Lanes 5, 6 positive samples for *C. burnetii* in bovine milk samples. Lanes 8, 10, 11 positive samples for *C. burnetii* in yoghurt samples.

Results

The presence of *C. burnetii* was evaluated in sheep, goat and cow raw milk and also cheese and yoghurt samples which were made from sheep milk. After the DNA extraction, touch-down PCR assay targeting the IS1111 gene of the organism by Trans-1 and trans-2 primers resulted in 2 of 28 cheese samples (7.14%), 2 of 26 yoghurt samples (7.69%), 8 of 23 sheep milk samples (34.78%), and 2 of 60 (3.33%) bovine milk samples as positive for *C. burnetii*, whereas all 10 goat milk samples were detected as negative. A sample photograph of gel electrophoresis is shown in Figure 1.

For positive control, the 687 base pairs of the amplified gene fragment were successfully sequenced from the first PCR-positive sample and by comparing to the published sequences of *C. burnetti* in Gene bank. No differences in nucleotide and deduced amino acid were found.

Discussion

The most commonly identified sources of human infections with *C. burnetti* are farm animals such as cattle, goats, and sheep. Mammals can shed *C. burnetii* in milk, and thus consumption of raw milk and dairy products which are made from unpasteurized milk could be a source of infection

(Fournier et al., 1998).

In order to identify *C. burnetii* in milk and dairy products, the PCR method is a safe and useful method, whereas conventional isolation of *C. burnetii* is hazardous, difficult, and time-consuming; besides, the isolation of this microorganism must be performed in biosafety-level 3 laboratories (Barlow et al., 2008; Khalili et al., 2011; Arricau-Bouvery and Rodolakis, 2005). Although this method could not determine the viability of the organisms in raw milk and dairy products, some studies have compared results of PCR detection of *C. burnetii* in milk with bacterial viability assay by mouse inoculation (Rahimi et al., 2010; Hoover et al., 1992). While these studies demonstrated PCR positive milk samples contained viable organisms, additional studies are needed to determine how PCR based detection relates to the potential infectiousness of *C. burnetii* in milk samples, and the sensitivity and specificity of PCR relative to inoculation or antigen detection assays (Barlow et al., 2008). Only a few studies have described the presence of *C. burnetii* in dairy products such as cheese (Hirai et al., 2012). Furthermore, there have been no reports on detection of *C. burnetii* in yoghurt by PCR assay and this study is the first report in detection of DNA *C. burnetii* in yoghurt.

In this study, for detection of *C. burnetii* in raw milk and dairy produts, PCR assay was used for targeting the repetitive transposon-like region of *C. burnetii* (Trans-PCR). The efficiency of the method for detection of Coxiella in milk samples was further improved and one *C. burnetii*-cell could be detected in 1 ml of milk (Berri et al., 2000) and it has been proved that trans-PCR has a high sensitivity and specificity (Kim et al., 2005; Barlow et al., 2008; Kirkan et al., 2008; Berri et al., 2009).

In order to prepare the PCR mixture and excluding the PCR inhibitors which might be present in raw milk and dairy products, samples were centrifuged three times and each time the pellet were resuspended in PBS. It has been reported that, the detection limit for *C. burnetii* in PBS was 10-fold higher than that in milk (Muramatsu et al., 1997).

According to these findings, DNA sequence of *C. burnetii* has been detected in 3.33% of cow milk, 34.78% of ovine milk, 7.14% of cheese and 7.69% of yoghurt samples. The size of this survey does not allow any statistical statement, and possibly because of our sample size, goat's milk samples were detected as negative. These data only show the shedding of *C. burnetii* through bovine and ovine milk and consequently the presence of their DNA sequence in milk products.

Other studies have reported a different range of the presence of this microorganism in milk. 1.8% in goat milk and 0% in Iranian sheep milk (Rahimi et al., 2010), 3.5% of ovine milk samples from Turkey (Maurin and Raoult, 1999) and 0% of goat and sheep milk from Switzerland (Kim et al., 2005; Fretz et al., 2007), whereas 83.8% of cow milk from France (Berri et al., 2000), 53.7% from Japan (Maurin and Raoult 1999) and 14.3% from Italy (Ongor et al., 2004) were positive for *C. burnetii*. However, for the presence of this microorganism in cheese the only report is 17.1% from Japan (Hirai et al., 2012).

It should be considered that *C. burnetii* might shed by other routes such as vaginal mucus, feces, urine, placenta, or birth fluids. Testing an animal based on only milk sample can lead to misclassify the status of the animal. Sheep shed *C. burnetii* mainly in feces and vaginal mucus; whereas, cow shed *C. burnetii* mainly in milk and goat excrete *C. burnetii* in their vaginal discharges, feces, and milk. Furthermore, the infected animals may not persistently shed this microorganism (Guatteo et al., 2007).

The results of this study indicate a potential risk to the public health associated with the presence of *C. burnetii* in raw milk and unpasteurized dairy products in this area of Iran, which may be viable and infectious.

Acknowledgments

The authors wish to thank Mr. Ali Kargar for his technical help. This research was supported by a grant no. 22659/2 from the Research Council of the Ferdowsi University of Mashhad.

References

1. Abbasi, S., Farzan, R., Momtaz, H. (2011) Molecular detection of *Coxiella burnetii* in goat bulk milk samples in some provinces of Iran. Afr J Biotechnol. 10: 18513-18515.
2. Arricau-Bouvery, N., Rodolakis, A. (2005) Is Q fever

an emerging or re-emerging zoonosis?. Vet Res. 36: 327-349.

3. Barlow, J., Rauch, B., Welcome, F., Kim, S.G., Dubovi, E., Schukken, Y. (2008) Association between *Coxiella burnetii* shedding in milk and subclinical mastitis in dairy cattle. Vet Res. 39: 23-32.
4. Biberstein, E.L., Behymer, D.E., Bushnell, R., Crenshaw, G., Riemann, H.P., Franti, C.E. (1974) A survey of Q fever (*Coxiella burnetii*) in California dairy cows. Am J Vet Res. 35: 1577-1582.
5. Berri, M., Arricau-Bouvery, N., Rodolakis, A. (2003) PCR-based detection of *Coxiella burnetii* from clinical samples. Methods Mol Biol. 216: 153-161.
6. Berri, M., Laroucau, K., Rodolakis, A. (2000) The detection of *Coxiella burnetii* from ovine genital swabs, milk and fecal samples by the use of a single touchdown polymerase chain reaction. Vet Microbiol. 15: 285-293.
7. Berri, M., Rekiki, A., Sidi Boumedine, K., Rodolakis, A. (2009) Simultaneous differential detection of Chlamydophila abortus, Chlamydophila pecorum and *Coxiella burnetii* from aborted ruminant's clinical samples using multiplex PCR. BMC Microbiol. 9: 130-138.
8. Fournier, P.E., Marrie, T.J., Raoult, D. (1998) Diagnosis of Q fever. J Clin Microbiol. 36: 1823-1834.
9. Fretz, R., Schaeren, W., Tanner, M., Baumgartner, A. (2007) Screening of various foodstuffs for occurrence of *Coxiella burnetii* in Switzerland. Int J Food Microbiol. 116: 414-418.
10. Guatteo, R., Beaudeau, F., Joly, A., Seegers, H. (2007) *Coxiella burnetii* shedding by dairy cows. Vet Res. 38: 849-860.
11. Hirai, A., Nakama, A., Chiba, T., Kai, A. (2012) Development of a method for detecting *Coxiella burnetii* in cheese samples. J Vet Med Sci. 74: 175-180.
12. Hoover, T.A., Vodkin, M.H., Williams, J.C. (1992) A *Coxiella burnetii* repeated DNA element resembling a bacterial insertion sequence. J Bacteriol. 174: 5540-5548.
13. Khalili, M., Sakhaee, E., Aflatoonian, M.R, Shahabi-Nejad, N. (2011) Herd-prevalence of *Coxiella burnetii* (Q fever) antibodies in dairy cattle farms based on bulk tank milk analysis. Asian Pac J Trop Med. 4: 58-60.
14. Kim, S.G., Kim, E.H., Lafferty, C.J. Dubovi, E. (2005) *Coxiella burnetii* in bulk tank milk samples, United States. Emerg Infect Dis. 11: 619-621.
15. Kirkan, S., Kaya, O., Tekbiyik, S., Parin, U. (2008) Detection of *Coxiella burnetii* in cattle by PCR. Turk J Vet Anim Sci. 32: 215-220.
16. Lorenz, H., Jager, C., Willems, H., Baljer, G. (1998) PCR detection of *Coxiella burnetii* from different clinical specimens, especially bovine milk, on the basis of DNA preparation with a silica matrix. Appl Environ Microbiol. 64: 4234-4237.
17. Maurin, M., Raoult, D. (1999) Q fever. Clin Microbiol Rev. 12: 518-553.
18. Muramatsu, Y., Yanase, T., Okabayashi, T., Ueno, H., Morita, C. (1997) Detection of *Coxiella burnetii* in cow's milk by PCR-Enzyme-Linked Immunosorbent Assay combined with a novel sample preparation method. Appl Environ Microbiol. 63: 2142-2146.
19. Ormsbee, R., Peacock, M., Gerloff, R., Tallent, G., Wike, D. (1978) Limits of rickettsial infectivity. Infect Immun. 19: 239-245.
20. Ongor, H., Cetinkaya, B., Karahan, M., Açik, M.N., Bulut, H., Muz, A. (2004) Detection of *Coxiella burnetii* by immunomagnetic separation-PCR in the milk of sheep in Turkey. Vet Rec.154: 570-572.
21. Parker, N.R., Barralet, J.H., Bell, A.M. (2006) Q-fever. Lancet. 367: 679-688.
22. Rahimi, E., Doosti, A., Ameri, M., Kabiri, E., Sharifian, B. (2010) Detection of *Coxiella burnetii* by Nested PCR in bulk milk samples from dairy bovine, ovine, and caprine herds in Iran. Zoonoses Public Health. 57: 38-41.
23. Sambrook, J., Russell, D.W. (2001) Molecular Cloning: A laboratory Manual. (3rd ed.) Cold Spring Harbor Laboratory Press, Cold Spring Harbor, New York, USA.
24. Vaidya, V.M., Malik, S.V., Kaur, S., Kumar, S., Barbuddhe, S.B. (2008) Comparison of PCR, immunofluorescence assay and pathogen isolation for diagnosis of Q fever in humans with spontaneous abortions. J Clin Microbiol. 46: 2038-2044.

Betaine as a methyl donor and an antioxidant agent in levodopa-induced hyperhomocysteinemia and oxidative stress in rat's kidney

Alirezaei, M.[*]

Division of Biochemistry, School of Veterinary Medicine, Lorestan University, Khorram Abad, Iran

Key words:
benserazide, betaine, homocysteine, kidney, levodopa

Correspondence
Alirezaei, M.
Division of Biochemistry, School of Veterinary Medicine, Lorestan University, Khorram Abad, Iran

Email: alirezaei_m54@yahoo.com

Abstract:

BACKGROUND: Betaine has been shown to be antioxidant and methyl donor effects in our recent studies. **OBJECTIVES:** In the present study, the antioxidant and methyl donor properties of betaine in levodopa/benserazide-mediated hyperhomocysteinemia and levodopa-induced oxidative stress in rat's kidney were examined. **METHODS:** Sprague-Dawley male rats were divided into levodopa (LD), Betaine (Bet.), levodopa plus betaine (LD/Bet.), levodopa plus benserazide (LD/Ben.), levodopa plus betaine-benserazide (LD/Bet.-Ben.), and control groups. The experimental groups received LD (3×100 mg/kg), Bet. (1.5% w/w of the total diet), Ben. (3×25 mg/kg), and distilled water was given to controls for 10 consecutive days, orally by gavage. **RESULTS:** Plasma total homocysteine (tHcy) concentration decreased significantly in Bet.-, LD/Bet.-, and LD/Bet.-Ben.-treated rats compared to LD/Ben. group. Thiobarbituric acid reactive substances concentration (as a lipid peroxidation marker) in renal tissue reduced statistically in betaine group in comparison with LD and LD/Ben. groups. Renal catalase activity increased significantly in LD-treated rats when compared to controls. Renal superoxide dismutase activity significantly decreased in LD-treated group when compared to LD/Ben. group. However, there was not any significant difference in renal glutathione peroxidase (GPx) activity among the groups. **CONCLUSIONS:** These findings indicate that LD and LD/Ben. have side effects in kidney due to induction of hyperhomocysteinemia and oxidative stress. In contrast, betaine acts as a promising antioxidant and methyl donor agent versus LD-induced complications.

Introduction

Oxidative stress is a hypothesis for the association of reactive oxygen species (ROS) with neurodegenerative and inflammatory diseases such as Parkinson's disease (PD), chronic renal failure, and end-stage renal disease (ESRD) (Alirezaei et al., 2011; Neamati et al., 2011). ROS such as superoxide anion, hydrogen peroxide and hydroxyl radical are generated during oxidative metabolism and can inflict damage on all classes of macromolecules, eventually leading to cell death (Bergamini et al., 2004; Smith et al., 2005; Alirezaei et al., 2011). Regarding oxidative stress, betaine has recently been shown antioxidant and methyl donor effects in our previous reports (Alirezaei et al., 2011, 2012b,c,d, 2014a,b; Kheradmand et al., 2013). Betaine (trimethylglycine) transfers a methyl group via the enzyme betaine homocysteine methyl transferase (BHMT) to become dimethylglycine (Alirezaei et al.,

2011, 2012b,c). BHMT is the only known enzyme that uses betaine as a substrate, mediates the transfer of a methyl group from betaine to homocysteine (Hcy), forming methionine and dimethylglycine (Alirezaei et al., 2011; Fridman et al., 2012). BHMT activity in rat kidney in several orders of magnitude lower than that in rat's liver and only restricted to the renal cortex (Fridman et al., 2012). Betaine also acts as osmolyte in kidney medulla, protecting cell from high extracellular osmolarity (Fridman et al., 2012).

It is interesting to note that chronic and acute repeated intake of levodopa (LD) elevates total homocysteine (tHcy) concentration, and hyperhomocysteinemia is known as a side effect of LD consumption (Muller et al., 2011). LD is the most effective dopaminergic agent for PD, it is available in immediate and controlled release forms and is routinely combined with a dopa-decarboxylase inhibitor (DDI) such as benserazide to reduce its peripheral metabolism so as to avoid peripheral toxicity and to enhance its brain penetration (Muller et al., 2011; Schapira et al., 2008). Although chronic intake of LD/DDI improves motor complications in PD patients according to the concept of continuous dopaminergic stimulation, PD patients receive several grams of LD/DDI daily (Schapira et al., 2008). This regimen elevates tHcy as a risk factor for cardiovascular and neurodegenerative diseases, as well as renal diseases (McGregor et al., 2002; Alirezaei et al., 2011). Plasma tHcy increases as renal function declines and more than 80% of people with ESRD are hyperhomocysteinemic. Another concern regarding LD is the potential to induce ROS-mediate damage and thereby induce and or accelerate renal cell dysfunction and death (McGregor et al., 2002).

Taking the above-mentioned issues into consideration, we decided to determine whether oral administration of betaine concomitant with LD and LD/DDI could act as an antioxidant agent to prevent oxidative stress in kidney of rats. We also examined possible protective effects of betaine in a LD-induced hyperhomocysteinemia model by measuring tHcy in plasma of rats.

Materials and Methods

Materials: MADOPAR® (Levodopa 100 mg+ Benserazide [as a dopa-decarboxylase inhibitor] 25 mg) was obtained from Roche Company, New Zealand. Betaine (Betafin® 96%) was prepared from Biochem Company (Brinkstrasse 55, D-49393 Lohne, Germany). GPx and SOD kit were obtained via Randox® Company (Randox, UK). The homocysteine enzymatic kit was prepared by Axis® Homocysteine (Axis-Shield AS, UK). Levodopa kindly provided by JALINOOS Pharmacy (Karaj, Alborz province, Iran). The other chemicals used were of analytical grade.

Animals: Sprague-Dawley rats (weighing 150-170 g, obtained from Shiraz University of Medical Sciences, Animal House Center, Iran) were housed in temperature-controlled conditions under a 12:12-h light/dark with food and tap water supplied ad libitum. All rats were treated in compliance with the recommendations of Animal Care Committee for Lorestan University of Medical Sciences (Khorramabad, Iran). All experimental procedures were carried out between 08.00 am and 17.00 pm for prevention of circadian rhythm changes among days.

Experimental design: The rats were divided into six equal groups (n=7 rats per group), weight gain and food consumption were determined at 5-day intervals and treated for 10 consecutive days orally by gavage in the following order: control group received 1 mL distilled water, the levodopa (LD) group were treated with LD (3 × 100 mg/kg p.o. at 8.5 am, 12.5 am, and 16.5 pm.), the betaine (Bet.) group received betaine (1.5% w/w of the total diet dissolved in distilled water was given orally by gavage at 8.00 am), the levodopa plus betaine (LD/Bet.) group were treated by LD (3 × 100 mg/kg p.o. at 4 hour intervals) plus betaine (1.5% w/w of the total diet at 8.00 am), the levodopa plus benserazide (LD/Ben.) group received MADOPAR® (3 × (LD 100 mg + Ben. 25 mg) at 4 hour intervals), and the final group, levodopa plus betaine-benserazide (LD/Bet.-Ben.), was treated via MADOPAR® (3×(LD 100 mg + Ben. 25 mg) at 4 hour intervals) and betaine (1.5% w/w of the total diet as betaine group at 8.00 am). Betaine, LD, and LD/Ben. were dissolved in distilled water before administration, daily. Doses of levodopa and benserazide were determined according to a previous report (Nissinen et al., 2005), and betaine was found in our previous works (Alirezaei et al., 2011, 2012b,c). 2 hours after the last gavage, the rats were sacrificed upon light diethyl ether anesthesia (Dagenham, UK). Blood samples were collected via cardiac puncture, whole blood containing EDTA was centrifuged at 3,000 RPM for 10 min and plasma was removed in aliquot microtubes. The right kidneys were removed and carefully cleaned of fat and adhering, and then plasma and kidney samples were stored at -70°C until biochemical analysis.

Tissue preparation for protein measurement, TBARS detection and enzyme assay: Rat kidneys were thawed and manually homogenized in cold phosphate buffer (0.1 M, pH 7.4), containing 5 mM EDTA, and debris was removed by centrifugation at 2000× g for 10 min (Centrifuge 5415 R; Rotofix 32A, Germany). Supernatants were recovered and used for antioxidant enzyme activities, TBARS concentrations and protein measurement. Protein content of tissue homogenates was determined using a colorimetric method of Lowry with bovine serum albumin as a standard (Lowry et al., 1951).

Measurement of tHcy concentration: Total homocysteine of plasma which refers to the sum of protein-bound, free-oxidized, and reduced species of homocysteine was determined by the Axis® Homocysteine enzymatic kit (Golbahar et al., 2005; Karthikeyan et al., 2007; Alirezaei et al., 2011). tHcy concentration was expressed as micromoles per liter (μmol/L) of plasma.

Measurement of lipid peroxidation: The amount of lipid peroxidation was indicated by the content of thiobarbituric acid reactive substances (TBARS) in the kidney. Tissue TBARS was determined by following the production of thiobarbituric acid reactive substances as described previously (Subarao et al., 1990); it was reported previously in our laboratory (Alirezaei et al., 2011, 2012a, b). In short, 40 μL of homogenate was added to 40 μL of 0.9% NaCl and 40 μL of deionized H2O, resulting in a total reaction volume of 120 μL. The reaction was incubated at 37° C for 20 min and stopped by the addition of 600 μL of cold 0.8 M hydrochloride acid, containing 12.5% trichloroacetic acid. Following the addition of 780 μL of 1% TBA, the reaction was boiled for 20 min and then cooled at 4° C for 1 h. In order to measure the amount of TBARS produced by the homogenate, the cooled reaction was spun at 1500× g in a microcentrifuge for 20 min and the absorbance of the supernatant was read spectrophotometrically (S2000 UV model; WPA, Cambridge, UK) at 532 nm, using an extinction coefficient of 1.56×10^5/M Cm. The blanks for all of the TBARS assays contained an additional 40 μL of 0.9% NaCl instead of homogenate as just described. TBARS results were expressed as nanomoles per milligram of tissue protein (nmol/mg protein).

Measurement of CAT activity: Tissue catalase activity was assayed using the method described previously (Claiborne, 1986). The reaction mixture (1 mL) consisted of 50 mM potassium phosphate (pH 7.0), 19 mM H2O2, and a 20-50 μL sample. The reaction was initiated by the addition of H2O2, and absorbance changes were measured at 240 nm (25 °C) for 30 s. The molar extinction coefficient for H2O2 is 43.6/M Cm. The CAT activity was expressed as the unit that is defined as μ mol of H2O2 consumed per min per milligram of tissue protein (U/mg protein).

Measurement of SOD activity: The activity of superoxide dismutase (SOD) was evaluated with Randox® SOD detection kit according to the manufacturer's instructions, was reported previously in our laboratory (Alirezaei et al., 2011, 2012a,b). The role of SOD is to accelerate the dismutation of the toxic superoxide (O2-) produced during oxidative phosphorylation in electron transport chain to hydrogen peroxide and molecular oxygen. This method employs xanthine and xanthine oxidase to generate superoxide radicals which react with 2-(4-iodophenyl)-3-(4-nitrophenol)-5- henyltetrazolium chloride (I.N.T.) to form a red formazan dye. The SOD activity is then measured by degree of inhibition of this reaction. One unit of SOD is that which causes 50% inhibition of the rate of reduction of INT under the conditions of the assay. SOD levels were recorded at 505 nm and through a standard curve and expressed as unit per milligram of tissue protein (U/mg protein).

Measurement of GPx activity: The activity of glutathione peroxidase (GPx) was evaluated with Randox® GPx detection kit according to the manufacturer's instructions, was reported previously in our laboratory (Alirezaei et al., 2011, 2012a,b). GPx catalyze the oxidation of glutathione (GSH) by cumene hydroperoxide. In the presence of glutathione reductase (GR) and NADPH, the oxidised glutathione (GSSG) is immediately converted to the reduced form with a concomitant oxidation of NADPH to NADP+. The decrease in absorbance was measured spectrophotometrically against blank at 340 nm. One unit (U) of GPx was defined as 1 μmol of oxidized NADPH per min per milligram of tissue protein. The GPx activity was expressed as unit per milligram of tissue protein (U/mg protein).

Statistical analysis: Statistical analysis was performed using the statistical package GraphPad PRISM version 5 (GraphPad Software Inc., San Diego, CA, USA). All variables were tested for normal and homogeneous variances by Leven's statistic test. All results are presented as mean± (S.E.M.). The statistical differences were applied among the all groups by one-way analysis of variance (ANOVA) with Tukey's post hoc analysis. A calculated P value of less than 0.05 was considered statistically significant.

Results

Treatment of rats with MADOPAR® (levodopa plus dopa-decarboxylase inhibitor) significantly increased tHcy in plasma of the LD/Ben. group compared to the other groups, while administration of betaine to the Bet. and LD/Bet. groups could suppress tHcy increasing ($p<0.05$; Figure 1).

Regarding lipid peroxidation, treatment of rats with levodopa, and levodopa plus benserazide significantly increased TBARS concentration in the LD- and LD/Ben.-treated rats when compared to the control and betaine groups ($p<0.05$). However, the concentration of TBARS in the LD/Bet.-Ben. group was slightly lower compared with the LD/Ben.-treated rats ($p>0.05$; Figure 2).

The mean values (±SEM) of the catalase (CAT), superoxide dismutase (SOD), and glutathione peroxidase (GPx) activities of the kidney tissue from experimental groups are presented in figures 3, 4, and 5. CAT activity was significantly higher in the LD group compared to the control, and there was not any significant difference among the other groups for CAT activity ($p>0.05$). SOD activity was significantly higher in the LD/Ben. group compared to the LD-treated rats ($p<0.05$). However, SOD activity was insignificantly higher in the betaine group compared to the LD and LD/ Bet. groups ($p>0.05$). Although the activity of the GPx in the LD group was slightly lower compared to the other groups, these reductions were not statistically significant ($p>0.05$). Indeed, when betaine was administered with LD and LD/Ben., it could increase the level of GPx activity near to the control group (Figure 5).

Discussion

This report is, to the best of our knowledge, the first to have evaluated the effects of betaine on levodopa/ benserazide (LD/Ben.)-mediated hyperhomocysteinemia and levodopa (LD)- induced oxidative stress in kidney tissue. Our data show that LD/Ben. treatment, as a new drug for Parkinson's disease (PD), induces hyperhomocysteinemia and this effect is more noticeable than is the LD treatment. Based on the present results, betaine is not only a methyl donor, but also it is as an antioxidant agent versus oxidative stress mediated by LD and LD/Ben. Treatment in the rat kidney. Although the primary role of betaine in the kidney is likely to be as an osmoprotectant, the methyl donor and antioxidant properties of betaine are promising, particularly in management of hyperhomocysteinemia and oxidative stress in kidney tissue. Indeed, it seems that combination of betaine with LD or LD/Ben. is promising to reduce the drug side effects.

In recent years, there has been increasingly more evidence to show LD-induced hyperhomocysteinemia (Nissinen et al., 2005; Muller et al., 2011; Schapira et al., 2008). LD, the most effective drug known in the treatment of PD, has been observed to induce elevations in plasma tHcy concentrations (Nissinen et al., 2005). LD is metabolized by four major metabolic pathways including: decarboxylation, O-methylation, transamination, and oxidation. The principal path is decarboxylation, whereby dopamine is formed by aromatic amino acid decarboxylase (Muzzi et al., 2008; Schapira et al., 2008). Methoxylation of LD to 3-O-methyldopa (3-O-MD) by catechol-O-methyltransferase (COMT) is a second less prominent metabolic pathway. Transamination and oxidation are additional metabolic pathways (Muzzi et al., 2008). In the present study, LD is administered with a peripheral-acting dopa decarboxylase inhibitor (DDI), benserazide, in order to prevent its metabolism to dopamine so as to enhance brain penetration. The administration of benserazide with LD results in increased metabolism of LD to 3-O-MD via the enzyme COMT in peripheral tissues

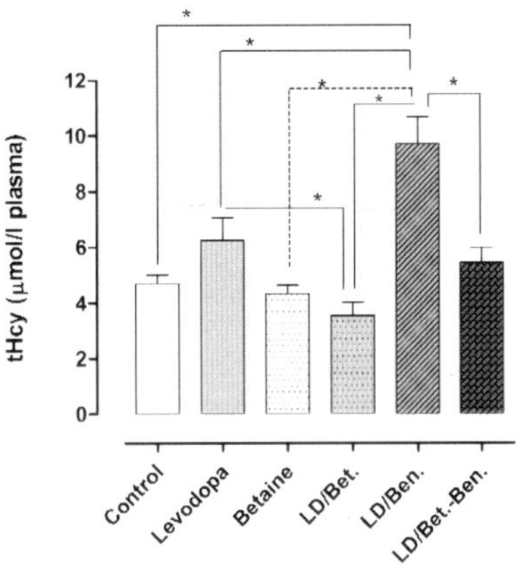

Figure 1. Comparison of plasma total homocysteine (tHcy) concentration among the control and treated groups. Values represent mean± SEM of tHcy (μmol/L of plasma). Asterisk indicates statistically difference among the groups ($p<0.05$). LD; levodopa, Bet.; betaine, Ben.; benserazide.

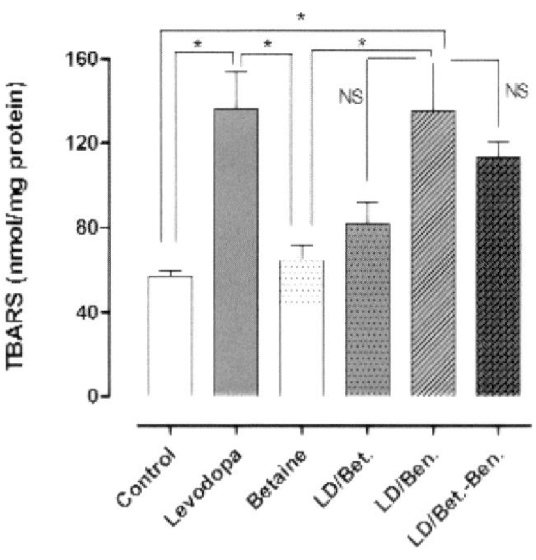

Figure 2. Comparison of thiobarbituric acid reactive substances (TBARS) concentration among the control and treated groups. Values represent mean±SEM of TBARS (nanomoles per milligram protein of kidney tissue). Asterisk indicates statistically difference among the groups ($p<0.05$). There is no significant difference between levodopa and LD/Bet. groups ($p>0.05$). NS; not significant. LD; levodopa, Bet.; betaine, Ben.; benserazide.

(Nissinen et al., 2005; Muller et al., 2011). It is known that COMT activity requires S-adenosyl-L-methionine (SAM) as the methyl donor and this leads to the formation of Hcy (Nissinen et al., 2005). Thus, in the present study tHcy increased in LD/Ben.-treated rats according to the above-mentioned processes. However, tHcy increased slightly in LD-treated rats in comparison with controls and betaine could suppress tHcy increasing in LD/Bet.-Ben. group when compared to the LD/Ben.-treated rats (Figure 1).

As LD is used chronically in the treatment of PD, we studied the effect of LD concomitant with betaine. It has been shown that the elevated plasma Hcy levels found in PD patients treated with LD are associated with a nearly two-fold increased prevalence of coronary artery diseases (Rogers et al., 2003; Nissinen et al., 2005). Previous reports also suggest that elevated plasma Hcy levels may be a risk factor for neuropsychiatric disorders such as dementia, depression and PD (Nissinen et al., 2005; Alirezaei et al., 2011). The high prevalence of hyperhomocysteinemia in the population and its easy treatment make Hcy an interesting amino acid for studies in the prevention of degenerative brain disorders such as PD (Sachdev et al., 2005; Alirezaei et al., 2011). In the present study, betaine, a methyl donor that continuously generates SAM, is shown to lead to long-term lowering of tHcy during supplementation in the dietary intake range of 1.5% (w/w) of total diet (Alirezaei et al., 2011). BHMT has been shown to be expressed at high levels in the livers of all vertebrate species tested. In mammalian liver, BHMT represents 1% or more of the total soluble protein (Barak et al., 2002; Fridman et al., 2012). BHMT activity also exists in the renal cortex and BHMT activity was found about 1-2% of the BHMT specific activity as that found in liver (Fridman et al., 2012). Betaine can also be endogenously produced in the liver and kidney cortex from its metabolic precursor choline via choline oxidase (Fridman et al., 2012). Betaine regulates cell volume by counteracting changes in extracellular tonicity and stabilizing macromolecules against a variety of physiological perturbations (Alirezaei et al., 2011; Fridman et al., 2012). Based on our results, tHcy concentration decreased moderately in betaine group in comparison with LD-treated rats, while tHcy concentration in the plasma of LD/Ben.-treated rats due to lack of SAM elevated significantly. LD is predominantly metabolized to 3-OMD in the presence of a DDI, like benserazide, by COMT. COMT is the essential enzyme for this O-methylation of LD, which demands for a methyl group transfer from the donor SAM (Muzzi et al., 2008; Muller et al., 2011). As one consequence, SAM is transformed into the short living S-adenosyl-homocysteine and then to Hcy. Thus, we assume that a certain balance between LD and betaine is developed during this treatment protocol. Because Hcy synthesis represents a

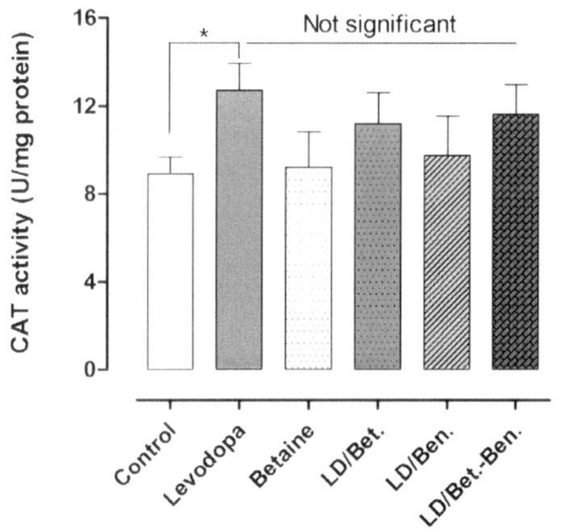

Figure 3. Comparison of CAT activity among the control and treated groups. Values represent mean±SEM of enzyme activity (unit/mg protein of kidney tissue). Asterisk indicates statistically difference between control and levodopa groups ($p<0.05$) while, there is not any significant difference among the other groups ($p>0.05$). LD; levodopa, Bet.; betaine, Ben.; benserazide.

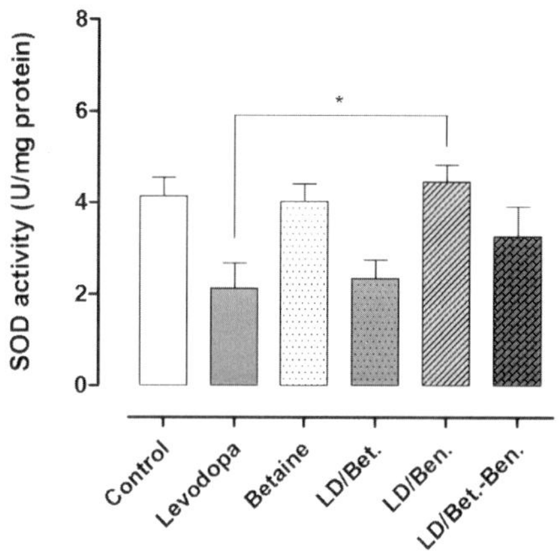

Figure 4. Comparison of SOD activity among the control and treated groups. Values represent mean±SEM of enzyme activity (unit/mg protein of kidney tissue). Asterisk indicates statistically difference between levodopa and LD/Ben. groups ($p<0.05$) while, there is not any significant difference among the other groups ($p>0.05$). LD; levodopa, Bet.; betaine, Ben.; benserazide.

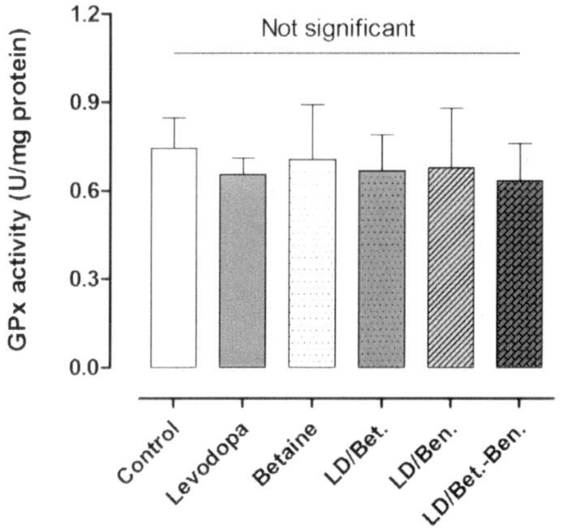

Figure 5. Comparison of GPx activity among the control and treated groups. Values represent mean±SEM of enzyme activity (unit/mg protein of kidney tissue). There is not any significant difference among the groups ($p>0.05$). LD; levodopa, Bet.; betaine, Ben.; benserazide.

secondary reaction product of O-methylation of LD to 3-OMD, one may hypothesize that betaine/or methyl donors supplementation may exert a certain preventive effect on the onset of hyperhomocysteinemia during LD/Ben. administration.

There is abundant evidence for oxidative stress in substantia nigra area of brain in PD patients (Nissinen et al., 2005; Muller et al., 2011; Schapira et al., 2008). Nevertheless, it remains unknown whether an increased oxidative load produced by LD would induce oxidative stress in kidney tissue of PD patients. It is known that LD administration produces dopamine in peripheral tissues and in the dopaminergic cells of the substantia nigra pars compact it converts to dopamine (Schapira et al., 2008). Dopamine may undergo autooxidation, semiquinone formation, and polymerization with the production of ROS (Tse et al., 1976; Fahan et al., 2005; Schapira et al., 2008). Dopamine can also be metabolized by monoamine oxidase-B to produce hydrogen peroxide (H2O2) which can then, in the presence of iron, be converted by the Fenton reaction to produce the highly reactive hydroxyl radical (Schapira et al., 2008). The potential pro-oxidant actions of LD have added to the debate over the role of oxidative stress in PD and its role in disease progression (Fahan et al., 2005; Shulman et al., 2000, Weiner et al., 2000). Hyperhomocysteinemia also inhibits the expression of antioxidant enzymes which might potentiate the toxic effects of ROS (Bleich et al., 2004; Alirezaei et al., 2011). In addition, auto-oxidation of homocysteine is known to generate ROS, whereby the prevention of LD-induced toxicity by catalase suggests that hydrogen peroxide acted as a mediator of oxidative injury, leading to oxidative stress in the rat kidney (Austin et al., 1998; D'Emilia and Lipton, 1999). In this regard, only catalase activity was significantly higher in the LD group compared to the controls (Figure 3). It seems that the elevation of CAT activity is a compensatory mechanism. It is known that LD can act both as a pro-oxidant and anti-oxidant molecule depending on circumstances. "For example, low concentrations of LD can induce an up-regulation in glutathione (GSH) molecule possibly because the drug acts as a minimal stressor that enhances the production of protective molecules" (Schapira et al., 2008). Indeed, catalase prevented H_2O_2 accumulation and elevated its activity (in order compensatory) to suppress oxidative stress in the LD group; however, this elevation was not able to prevent lipid peroxidation in the rat kidney.

LD has the potential to increase free radical generation through oxidative pathways and thereby could theoretically contribute to the lipid peroxidation and potentially accelerate oxidative stress in kidney. Betaine is believed to play a significant role in maintaining the structural and functional integrity of cell membranes. Previous studies have demonstrated that betaine, through its participation in sequential methylation within the cellular membranes, maintains a proper balance between phosphotidyl ethanolamine and phosphotidyl choline, thus sustaining proper membranes (Kharbanda et al., 2007; Ganesan et al., 2010; Alirezaei et al., 2011). In our study, LD and LD/Ben. consumption caused significantly increased TBARS concentration (as a lipid peroxidation marker) in the LD- and LD/Ben.-treated rats and betaine treatment restored this elevated TBARS concentration in the LD/Bet. group near the control group (Figure 2). On the other hand, there were significant differences among the control and betaine with LD and LD/Ben. groups, indicating the occurrence of oxidative stress in LD- and LD/Ben.-treated rats.

All cells are able to defend themselves from damaging effects of oxygen radicals by their own antioxidant mechanisms, including enzymatic and non-enzymatic antioxidant systems (Alirezaei et al., 2011; Neamati et al., 2011). GPx and CAT are two key antioxidant enzymes that can decompose hydrogen peroxide to water (Alirezaei et al., 2011; Kheradmand et al., 2013). SOD, another antioxidant enzyme in cells, rapidly converts superoxide anion (O_2^-) to less dangerous H_2O_2 then GPx, and CAT can decompose H_2O_2 to water. Although H_2O_2 is not a reactive product, it can be reduced to the highly reactive metabolites hydroxyl radicals (Alirezaei et al., 2012c; Neamati et al., 2011). The increase in SOD activity in our investigation for LD/Ben.-treated rats (Figure 4) correlates well with the increase of lipid peroxidation in renal tissue. SOD shifts highly reactive O_2^- to H_2O_2 and thus prevents the renal cell membrane damage caused by this highly toxic anion. It seems that elevation of SOD activity in LD/Ben. group is a compensatory mechanism that was not able to prevent lipid peroxidation in the kidney. In this context, Masella et al. (2004) have expressed that "antioxidant responsive elements (AREs) are present in the promoter regions of many of the genes inducible by oxidative and chemical stresses". Thus, it appears that in the present study the consumption of LD and LD/Ben. (both oxidative agents) can increase the activity of the antioxidant enzymes such as CAT and SOD by a compensatory mechanism via AREs.

Although the mean activity of GPx in our study was slightly lower in the LD and LD/Ben. groups than betaine group, these differences were not statistically significant (Figure 5). Possibly, prolonged treatments by LD or higher doses are needed to induce greater activity of GPx for suppression of oxidative stress in the kidney. On the other hand, as indicated in Figure 5, GPx seems to be less affected by LD and LD/Ben., and these drugs could not influence renal GPx activity markedly.

As mentioned above, this is the first in vivo study to show that betaine treatment results in an overall decrease in the lipid peroxidation in rat's kidney. Betaine is a methyl donor agent like SAM, and it also stabilizes SAM levels via BHMT pathway (Alirezaei et al., 2011; 2012b,c,d, 2014a,b). In addition, it reduces Hcy concentration (as an oxidative agent) via BHMT. With regard to BHMT, which is abundant in primates, The beneficial properties of betaine are promising and reduce the elevated plasma Hcy concentrations via the BHMT pathway (Alirezaei et al., 2011; 2012b,c). Although betaine demonstrated as a potential methyl donor and antioxidant agent for prevention of hyperhomocysteinemia and oxidative stress, further studies including evaluation of kidney function and histochemical techniques are needed to clarify protective effects of betaine in the kidney tissue.

Acknowledgments

This study was financially supported by Lorestan

University, Khorram Abad, Iran. We are most grateful to the members and manager of JALINOOS Pharmacy (Tehran, Iran) for providing levodopa.

Conflict of interest: The author declares that there is no conflict of interest in the present study.

References

1. Alirezaei, M., Dezfoulian, O., Kheradmand, A., Neamati, S., Khonsari, A., Pirzadeh, A. (2012a) Hepatoprotective effects of purified oleuropein from olive leaf extract against ethanol-induced damages in the rat. Iran J Vet Res. 13: 218-226.
2. Alirezaei, M., Jelodar, G., Ghayemi, Z. (2012b) Antioxidant defense of betaine against oxidative stress induced by ethanol in the rat testes. Int J Pept Res Ther. 18: 239-247.
3. Alirezaei, M., Jelodar, G., Ghayemi, Z., Khordad Mehr, M. (2014a) Antioxidant and methyl donor effects of betaine versus ethanol-induced oxidative stress in the rat liver. Comp Clin Pathol. 23: 161-168.
4. Alirezaei, M., Jelodar, G., Niknam P., Ghayemi Z., Nazifi, S. (2011) Betaine prevents ethanol-induced oxidative stress and reduces total homocysteine in the rat cerebellum. J Physiol Biochem. 67: 605-612.
5. Alirezaei, M., Jelodar G., Niknam, P., Khoshdel, Z., Yavari, M. (2014b) Nutritional effects of betaine on weight and length of rat offspring. Comp Clin Pathol 1-6. DOI 10.1007/s00580-012-1650-z
6. Alirezaei, M., Niknam, P., Jelodar, G. (2012c) Betaine elevates ovarian antioxidant enzyme activities and demonstrates methyl donor effect in non-pregnant rats. Int J Pept Res Ther. 18: 281-290.
7. Alirezaei, M., Saeb, M., Javidnia, K., Nazifi, S., Saeb, S. (2012d) Hyperhomocysteinemia reduction in ethanol-fed rabbits by oral betaine. Comp Clin Pathol. 21: 421-427.
8. Austin, R.C., Sood, S.K., Dorward, A.M., Singh, G., Shaughnessy, S.G., Pamidi, S., Outinen, P.A., Weitz, J.I. (1998) Homocysteine-dependent Alterations in Mitochondrial Gene Expression, Function and Structure. Homocysteine and H2O2 act synergistically to enhance mitochondrial damage. J Biol Chem. 273: 30808-30817.
9. Barak, A.J., Beckenhauer, H.C., Tuma, D.J. (2002) Methionine synthase a possible prime site of the ethanolic lesion in liver. Alcohol. 26: 65-67.
10. Bergamini, C.M., Gambetti, S., Dondi, A., Cervellati, C. (2004) Oxygen, reactive oxygen species and tissue damage. Curr Pharm Des. 10: 1611-1626.
11. Bleich, S., Degner, D., Sperling, W., Bönsch, D., Thürauf, N., Kornhuber, J. (2004) Homocysteine as a neurotoxin in chronic alcoholism. Prog Neuropsychopharmacol Biol Psychiat. 28: 453-464.
12. Claiborne A (1986) Catalase activity. In: CRC Handbook of Methods for Oxygen Radical Research. Greenwald, R.A. (ed.).Vol 1.CRCPress, Boca Raton, Florida, USA. p. 283-284.23.
13. D'Emilia, D.M., Lipton, S.A. (1999) Ratio of S-nitrosohomocyst (e) ine to homocyst (e) ine or other thiols determines neurotoxicity in rat cerebrocortical cultures. Neurosci Lett. 265: 103-106.
14. Fahn, S. (2005) Does levodopa slow or hasten the rate of progression of Parkinson´s disease? J Neurol. 252: iv37-iv42.
15. Fridman, O., Morales, A.V., Bortoni, L.E., Turk-Noceto, P.C., Prieto, E.A. (2012) Corticoadrenal activity regulates in rat betaine-homocysteine S-methyltransferase expression with opposites effects in liver and kidney. J Biosci. 37: 115-123.
16. Ganesan, B., Buddhan, S., Anandan, R., Sivakumar, R., Anbinezhilan, R. (2010) Antioxidant defense of betaine against isoprenaline-induced myocardial infarction in rats. Mol Biol Rep. 37: 1319-1327.
17. Golbahar, J., Aminzadeh, M.A., Hamidi, S.A., Omrani, G.R. (2005) Association of red blood cell 5-methyltetrahydrfoate folate with bone mineral density in postmenopausal Iranian women. Osteop Int. 16: 1894-1898.
18. Karthikeyan, G., Thachil, A., Sharma, S., Kalaivani, M., Ramakrishnan, L. (2007) Elevated high sensitivity CRP levels in patients with mitral stenosis and left atrial thrombus. Int J Cardiol. 122: 252-254.
19. Kharbanda, K.K., Mailliard, M.E., Baldwin, C.R., Beckenhauer, H.C., Sorrell, M.F., Tuma, D.J. (2007) Betaine attenuates alcoholic steatosis by restoring phosphatidylcholine generation via the phosphatidylethanolamine methyltransferase pathway. J Hepatol. 46: 314-321.
20. Kheradmand, A., Alirezaei, M., Dezfoulian, O. (2013) Cadmium-Induced Oxidative Stress in the Rat Testes: Protective Effects of Betaine. Int J Pept Res Ther. 19: 337-344.
21. Lowry, O.H., Rosebrough, N.J., Farr, A.L., Randal, R.J. (1951) Protein measurement with the Folin phenol reagent. J Biol Chem. 193: 265-275.

22. Masella, R., Vari, R., D'Archivio, M., Di Benedetto, R., Matarrese, P., Malorni, W., Scazzocchio, B., Giovannini, C. (2004) Extra virgin olive oil biophenols inhibit cell-mediated oxidation of LDL by increasing the mRNA transcription of glutathione-related enzymes. J Nutr. 134: 785-791.
23. McGregor, D.O., Dellow, W.J., Robson, R.A., Lever, M., George, P.M., Chambers, S.T. (2002) Betaine supplementation decreases post-methionine hyperhomocysteinemia in chronic renal failure. Kidney Int. 61: 1040-1046.
24. Muller, T., Jugel, C., Ehret, R., Ebersbach, G., Bengel, G., Muhlack, S., Klostermann, F. (2011) Elevation of total homocysteine levels in patients with Parkinson´s disease treated with duodenal levodopa/carbidopa gel. J Neural Transm. 118: 1329-1333.
25. Muzzi, C., Bertocci, E., Terzuoli, L., Porcelli, B., Ciari, I., Pagani, R., Guerranti, R. (2008) Simultaneous determination of serum concentrations of levodopa., dopamine., 3-O-methyldopa and O-methyldopa by HPLC. Biomed Pharmacotherap. 62: 253-258.
26. Neamati, S., Alirezaei, M., Kheradmand, A. (2011) Ghrelin acts as an antioxidant agent in the rat kidney. Int J Pept Res Ther. 17: 239-245.
27. Nissinen, E., Nissinen, H., Larjonmaa, H., Vaananen, A., Helkamaa, T., Reenila, I., Rauhala, P. (2005) The COMT inhibitor, entacapone, reduces levodopa-induced elevations in plasma homocysteine in healthy adult rats. J Neural Transm. 112: 1213-1221.
28. Rogers, J.D., Sanchez-Saffon, A., Frol, A.B., Diaz-Arrastia, R. (2003) Elevated plasma homocysteine levels in patients treated with levodopa: association with vascular disease. Arch Neurol. 60: 59-64.
29. Sachdev, P.S. (2009) Homocysteine and brain atrophy. Prog Neuropsychopharmacol Biol Psychiat. 29: 1152-1161.
30. Schapira, A.H.V. (2008) The clinical relevance of levodopa toxicity in the treatment of Parkinson's disease. Mov Disord. 23: S515-S520.
31. Shulman, L.M. (2000) Levodopa Toxicity in Parkinson Disease: Reality or Myth?: Reality--Practice Patterns Should Change. Arch Neurol. 57: 406-407.
32. Smith, A.M., Zeve, D.R., Grisel, J.J., Chen, W.J.A. (2005) Neonatal alcohol exposure increases malondialdehyde (MDA) and glutathione (GSH) levels in the developing cerebellum. Dev Brain Res. 160: 231-238.
33. Subbarao, K.V., Richardson, J.S., Ang, L.C. (1990) Autopsy samples of Alzheimer's cortex show increased peroxidation in vitro. J Neurochem. 55: 342-345.
34. Tse, D.C.S., McCreery, R.L., Adams, R.N. (1976) Potential oxidative pathways of brain catecholamines. J Med Chem. 19: 37-40.
35. Weiner, W.J. (2000) Is levodopa toxic? Arch Neurol. 57: 408.

Visceral coccisdiosis in a common mynah (*Acridotheres tristis*) due to *Isospora* sp. infection

Arabkhazaeli, F.[1*]**, Madani, S.A.**[2]

[1] *Department of Parasitology, Faculty of Veterinary Medicine, University of Tehran, Tehran, Iran*

[2] *Department of Avian Diseases, Faculty of Veterinary Medicine, University of Tehran, Tehran, Iran*

Key words:
Atoxoplasma, *Isospora*, pet bird, visceral coccidiosis

Correspondence
Arabkhazaeli, F.
Department of Parasitology, Faculty of Veterinary Medicine, University of Tehran, Tehran, Iran

Email: farab@ut.ac.ir

Abstract:

A captive adult common mynah (*Acridotheres tristis*) died shortly after a course of seizure and opisthotonous with an illness characterized by severe lethargy, depression, loss of appetite, polyurate, and urate discoloration. Abdominal distention and hepatomegly, visible over the abdominal skin, were noticed clinically. At necropsy, severe enlargement of liver with general discoloration was obvious. Histopathological findings included schizonts and gametes in the intestine, especially in the duodenum. Cytology from impression smears revealed intracytoplasmic Atoxoplasma-like zoites in the inflammatory cells especially macrophages within the liver and in the contact smears prepared from the liver, lung, and spleen. Based on postmortem findings of the organisms in blood mononuclear cells and in impression smears of liver and Giemsa stained impression smears of liver, the spleen and lung atoxoplasmosis caused by *Isoapora* sp. was specified as the cause of death. According to the literature, visceral coccidiosis (atoxoplasmosis), described here, could be considered as one of the severe causes of mortality among captive birds.

Case History

A captive adult common mynah (*Acridotheres tristis*) was referred with a history of severe lethargy, depression, and loss of appetite. Clinical signs and histopathological findings associated with *Isospora* (*Atoxoplasma*) infection in a common mynah in Iran are described.

Clinical Presentations

Abdominal distention and hepatomegaly were clinically visible over the abdominal skin. Polyurate and urate discoloration were noticed. The bird died shortly after a course of seizure and opisthotonous.

Diagnostic Tests

At necropsy, severe enlargement of liver with general discoloration of both lobes, as distribution of pale and congested areas, was observed (Figure 1). Intestinal distension especially in duodenum along with moderate thickening of the intestinal mucosa was obvious.

Liver cytology revealed typical vacuolization of the hepatocytes and large number of inflammatory cells especially macrophages containing circular light blue objects with purple-red center resembling *Atoxoplasma* zoites caused indention of the cells' nuclei (Figure 2A). The same intracytoplasmic parasites were seen in the lung and the spleen impression smears; however, the number of infected cells were typically lower in these two organs (Figures 2 B & C). Some degrees of erythrocyte polychromasia were seen in the lung cytology. In histological section of the liver, hepatocyte vacuolization, severe disseminated necrosis without particular lobular pattern, and parasitic interacytoplasmic inclusion bodies were numerously noted.

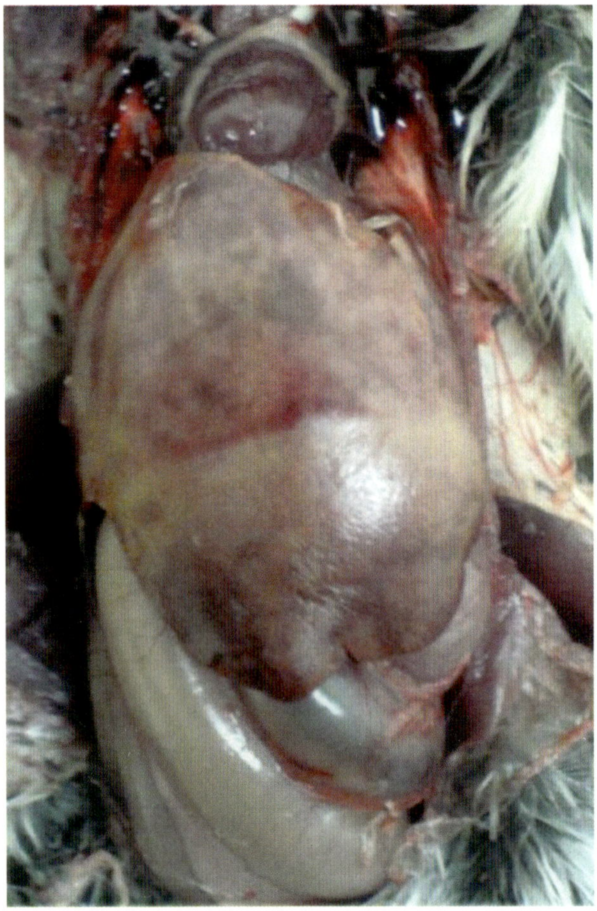

Figure 1. Severe enlargement of the liver with general discoloration of both lobes.

The parasites were also observed in the section derived from spleen. The presence of schizonts and gametocytes in the intestine, especially in the duodenum was recorded (Figure 2D).

Assessments

Atoxoplasma-like infections have been reported in several species of passerine birds, including greenfinches (*Carduelis chloris*), house sparrows (*Passer domesticus*), Bali mynahs (*Leucopsar rothschildi*), bullfinches (*Pyrrhula pyrrhula*), canaries (*Serinus canaria*) (Martinez and Munoz, 1998; Sa´nchez-Cordo´n et al., 2007; Maslin and Latimer, 2009), and rarely in raptors (Remple, 2004). To the best knowledge of the authors, there were no reports of atoxoplasmosis (with extra-intestinal merogony) from Iran, and up until now in the world in common mynah. There are reports of *Isopora* species from birds of the Sturnidae family, solely identified on the basis of the morphology of the oocysts in the feces and no *Atoxoplasma*-like organisms were found in the blood smears (Berto et al., 2011); as was the case for Tavasoli and Dastjerd (2000) who detected Isosporan oocysts in %47.6 of examined canary feces; however, they could not find mononuclear merozoites at necropsy.

Atoxoplasmosis, the cause of frequent mortalities among captive pet birds, is sometimes called "going light" as infected birds may stop eating and lose weight (Greiner, 2008). Affected birds have heavy extraintestinal merogonic infection (Gill and Paperna, 2008), often accompanied by the presence of fecal oocysts (Greiner, 2008). Following the ingestion of isosporoid (disporous tetrazoic) oocysts, coccidiosis due to *Isospora* (formerly known as *Atoxoplasma*) occurs in passerine birds, with a life cycle including invasion to both the reticulo-endothelial system and the intestinal epithelium (Pereira et al., 2011; Schrenzel et al., 2005; Adkesson et al., 2005). Merogony (asexual reproduction) occurs in both intestinal and lymphoid-macrophage cells, resulting in the presence of merozoites in the mononuclear leukocytes of the peripheral blood and dissemination to other viscera. Gametogenesis occurs in the intestinal cells of the same host (Adkesson et al., 2005). Some species of among many described *Isospora* species from birds have endogenous stages only in small intestine epithelium, while other species form extraintestinal stages in mononuclear phagocytes in different organs. The species with extraintestinal stages were suggested to be named *Atoxoplasma* (Dolnik et al., 2009). However until now, it has been sugessted that *Isospora* spp. and *Atoxoplasma* spp. in passerine birds are a unified group of organisms with intestinal and extra-intestinal forms that cause significant morbidity and mortality (Schrenzel et al., 2005). *Atoxoplasma* infections have been diagnosed using histopathologic examination of tissue samples, buffy coat smears, impression smears of organs, transmission electron microscopy and polymerase chain reaction (PCR) analysis (Adkesson et al., 2005; Greiner, 2008; Remple, 2004). Definitive taxonomic classification of *Isospora* remained ambiguous for many years and still there are many elusive aspects of the parasite pathobiology, namely the clonal expansion of the infected lymphocytes (Maslin and

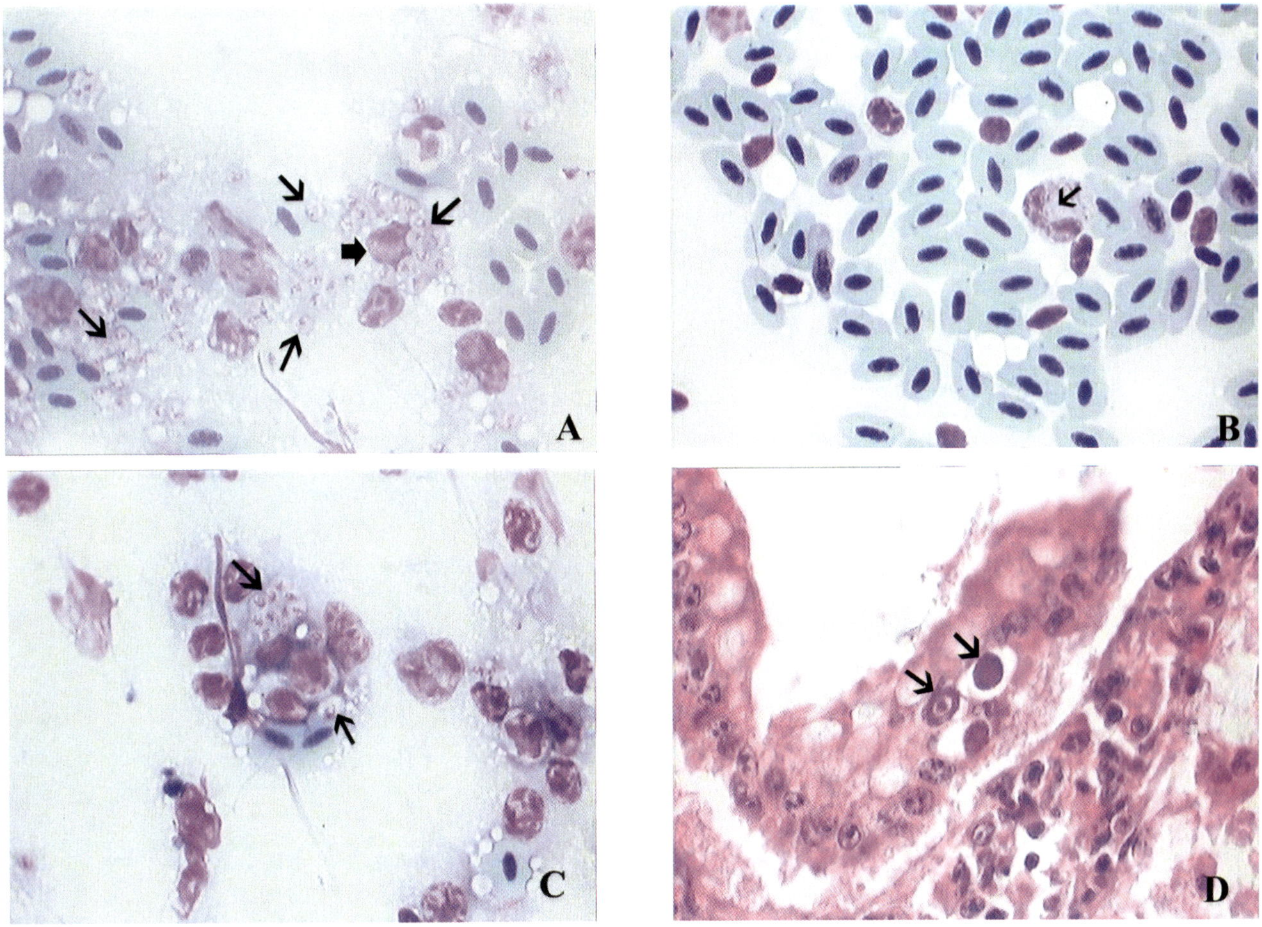

Figure 2. Impression smears of the liver, lung and spleen and histopathologic section of the duodenum from a naturally-infected common mynah: (A) Impression smear of the liver. Note the typical vacuolization of the hepatocytes and *Atoxoplasma* zoites (thin arrows) causing indention of the cells' nuclei (thick arrow) (1000x), (B) Impression smear of the lung. *Atoxoplasma* zoite (arrow) within a macrophage (1000x), (C) Spleen cytology. *Atoxoplasma* zoites (arrows) are clearly visible (1000x), (D) Histologic section of the intestine (H&E). Gametocytes (arrows) are shown in the intestinal mucosa (400x).

Latimer, 2009).

Identification of avian coccidian species is mainly based on oocysts morphology. However, regarding molecular methods, DNA derived from both species having intestinal and extra-intestinal life cycle may be present in pooled fecal samples, which limits the strength of PCR as a single diagnostic tool in species determination (Adkesson et al., 2005; Dolnik et al., 2009).

Considering the non-specific symptoms and small size of the parasite, diagnosis of *Atoxoplasma* infection is challenging. The organism may be easily missed, especially in low-grade subclinical infections (Adkesson et al., 2005), like the case for which we did not have the oocysts, and species determination was impossible.

Antemortem diagnosis of atoxoplasmosis is generally based on the finding of swollen and darkened liver through the skin, the organisms in blood mononuclear cells and less practically in impression smears of liver biopsy. At necropsy, Giemsa stained impression smears of liver, spleen, heart, or pancreas provide an effective means of diagnosis (Maslin and Latimer, 2009). As reported, standard anticoccidial drugs are ineffective against the tissue stages of the parasite, but sulfachlorpyrazine appears to decrease oocysts output in the adults, which will minimize exposure and infection in young birds. Cleanliness is also important in minimizing exposure to the oocysts (Maslin and Latimer, 2009; Adkesson et al., 2005). It is necessary for the veterinarians to consider the symptoms of visceral coccidiosis as a cause of illness in pet and wild passerines.

References

1. Adkesson, M.J., Zdziarski, J.M., Little, S.E. (2005) Atoxoplasmosis in tanagers. J Zoo Wildl Med. 36: 265-272.
2. Berto, P.B., Flausino, W., McIntosh, D., Teixeira-Filho, W.L., Lppes, C.W.G. (2011) Coccidia of new world passerine birds (Aves: Passeriformes): a review of Eimeria and Isospora Schneider,•1881 (Apicomplexa: Eimeriidae). Syst Parasitol. 80: 159-204.
3. Dolnik, O.V., Palinauskas, V., Bensch, S. (2009) Individual oocysts of isospora (Apicomplexa: Coccidia) parasites from avian feces: from photo to sequence. J Parasitol. 95: 169-174.
4. Gill, H., Paperna, I. (2008) Proliferative visceral isoapora (atoxoplasmosis) with morbid impact on the Israeli sparrow *Passser domesticus* biblicus Hartert, 1904. Parasitol Res. 103: 493-499.
5. Greiner, E.C. (2008) *Isospora*, *Atoxoplasma*, and *Sarcocystis*. In: Parasitic Diseases of Wild Birds. Atkinson, C.T., Thomas, N.J., Hunter, D.B. (eds.). Wiley-Blackwell, Ames, Iowa, USA. p. 108-119.
6. Martinez, F., Munoz, E. (1998) *Atoxoplasma* spp. in a hybrid passerine (*Serinus canaries×Carduelis cannabina*). Avian Pathol. 27: 420-422.
7. Maslin, W.R., Latimer, K.S. (2009) Atoxoplasmosis in canary fledglings: severe lymphocytic enteritis with preferential parasitism of B lymphocytes. Avian Dis. 53: 473-476.
8. Pereira, L.Q., Berto, B.P., Flausino, W., Lovato, M., Lopes, C.W.G. (2011) *Isospora bocamontensis* n. sp. (Apicomplexa: Eimeriidae) from the yellow cardinal *Gubernatrix cristata* (Vieillot) (Passeriformes: Emberizidae) in South America. Syst Parasitol. 78: 73-80.
9. Remple, J.D. (2004) Intracellular hematozoa of raptors: A review and update. J Avian Med Surg. 18: 75-88.
10. Sa´nchez-Cordo´n, P.J., Go´mez-Villamandos, J.C., Gutie´rrez1, J., Sierra, M.A., Pedrer, M., Bautista, M.J. (2007) *Atoxoplasma* spp. infection in captive canaries (*Serinus canaria*). J Vet Med A. 54: 23-26.
11. Schrenzel, M.D., Maalouf, G.A., Gaffney, P.M., Tokarz, D., Keener, L.L., McClure, D., Griffey, S., McAloose, D., Rideout, B.A. (2005) Molecular characterization of isosporoid coccidia (*Isospora* and *Atoxoplasma* spp.) in passerine birds. J Parasitol. 91: 635-647.
12. Tavasoli, M., Dastjerd, A. (2000) Gastrointestinal parasite of aviary and pet birds in Urimia, Iran. Pajuhesh Va Sazandegi (In persian). 62: 37-39.

Evaluation of dysrhythmias and myocardial biomarkers in high and low-yielding dairy cows

Jafari Dehkordi, A.[1*], Mohebbi, A.N.[2], Balali Dehkordi, Sh.[3]

[1] *Department of Large Animal Internal Medicine, Veterinary Faculty of Shahrekord University, Shahrekord, Iran*

[2] *Department of Veterinary Clinical Pathology, Veterinary Faculty of Shahrekord University, Shahrekord, Iran*

[3] *Graduated from the Faculty of Veterinary Medicine, Shahrekord University, Shahrekord, Iran*

Key words:
dairy cows, dysrhythmias, myocardial biomarkers

Correspondence
Jafari Dehkordi, A.
Department of Large Animal Internal Medicine, Veterinary Faculty of Shahrekord University, Shahrekord, Iran

Email: jafari-a@vet.sku.ac.ir

Abstract:

BACKGROUND: Cardiovascular system is a very important organ that plays a vital role in tissue function. In farm animals, the growth and high milk production depends on function of cardiovascular system. **OBJECTIVES:** Cardiovascular health in high and low-yielding dairy cows was investigated. **METHODS:** Fifty 4-year-old high- yielding Holstein dairy cows and fifty 4-year-old low- yielding Holstein dairy cows were used in this study. Electrocardiogram was recorded by a base- apex lead, and blood samples were collected from the jugular vein for the measurement of cardiac biomarkers (CK (Creatine Kinase), CK-MB (Creatine Kinase-Myocardial Band), LDH (Lactate Dehydrogenase), and AST (Aspartate Aminotransferase) and troponin I). **RESULTS:** Cardiac dysrhythmias were detected more in low- yielding Holstein dairy cows (62%) compared to high-yielding Holstein dairy cows (46%). The cardiac dysrhythmias that were observed in low- yielding Holstein dairy cows included sinus arrhythmia (34.7%), wandering pacemaker (22.45%), sinus bradycardia (18.37%), sinus tachycardia (10.20%), atrial premature beat (2.04%), sinoatrial block (2.04%), atrial fibrillation (8.16%), and atrial tachycardia (2.04%). The cardiac dysrhythmias were observed in high- yielding Holstein dairy cows, including sinus arrhythmia (86.95%) and wandering pace maker (13.05%). Also, notched P wave was observed in high- and low- yielding Holstein dairy cows, 30% and 14% respectively. The amount of cardiac biomarkers in the low yielding cows was significantly higher than that of the high yielding cows. Further more, there was not any detectable significant difference of serum concentration of total CK between the high and low- yielding Holstein cows. **CONCLUSIONS:** Despite significant differences in cardiac biomarkers and based on the normal range of cardiac biomarkers in both groups, the increase in cardiac dysrhythmias in low- yielding Holstein dairy cows may be metabolic and electrolyte disorders.

Introduction

The primary function of the cardiovascular system is to ensure an adequate circulation of blood so that nutrients are delivered, waste products are removed, and a homeostatic milieu is maintained at the organ and cellular level. An inadequate circulation interferes with nutrient delivery and waste product removal, and ultimately leads to circulatory failure, the primary concept in diseases of the cardiovascular system (Radostits et al., 2007).

ECG is the best way to measure and diagnose abnormal rhythm of the heart, particularly abnormal rhythm caused by damage to the conductive tissue that carries electrical signals, or abnormal rhythm caused by electrolyte imbalances. In a myocardial infarction (MI), the ECG can identify if the heart muscle has been damaged in specific areas, though not all areas of the heart are covered. The ECG device detects and amplifies the tiny electrical changes on the skin that are caused when the heart muscle depolarizes during each heartbeat (Smith, 2009; Rezakhani et al., 2010).

The electrocardiogram (ECG) is used primarily to detect cardiac arrhythmias in large animals. For this purpose, a single channel machine can be used, and the lead system chosen can be any that generates distinctive QRS and T complexes. Two leads commonly used for the diagnosis of cardiac arrhythmias are the base-apex lead I and the Y lead of the orthogonal lead system arrhythmias result from abnormalities of impulse generation or impulse conduction or a combination of both. A variety of mechanisms can cause abnormal impulse generation or conduction. Abnormal impulse generation occurs because of localized changes in ionic currents that flow across the membranes of single cells or groups of cells. Abnormal impulse generation can be seen as automatic (normal and abnormal) or triggered activity (Edwards, 1993; Rezakhani et al., 2004; Radostits et al., 2007; Smith, 2009).

Cardiac markers are biomarkers measured to evaluate heart function. They are often discussed in the context of myocardial infarction; however, there are other conditions that can lead to an elevation in cardiac marker level. Most of the early markers identified were enzymes, and as a result, the term "cardiac enzymes" is sometimes used. However, not all of the markers currently used are enzymes. For example, in formal usage, troponin would not be listed as a cardiac enzyme (Laterza et al., 2008; Leonardi et al., 2008).

Therefore, a number of tissue enzymes are valuable tools as diagnostic agents for heart disease such as: AST, LDH, CK, CK- MB, and troponin (Fredericks et al., 2001).

The serum concentration of cardiac troponin I provides an excellent cardiac biomarker in large animals, providing a sensitive and persistent indicator of cardiac injury. Troponin I, T, and C are components of the tropomyosin - troponin complex in cardiac and skeletal muscle, with cardiac troponin I and T having different amino acid sequences at the N- terminal and compared to skeletal muscle troponin I and T. This means that an immunoassay directed at the N- terminal end will be able to differentiate between cardiac and skeletal muscle isoforms and the site of injury (Roberts, 1998; Radostits et al., 2007; Serra et al., 2010).

Serum activities of cardiac isoenzymes of creatine kinase (creatine kinase isoenzyme) MB (CK-MB) and lactate dehydrogenase (isoenzymes 1 and 2) have been used in the past as indices of cardiac disease in large animals (Reimers et al., 1997; Radostits et al., 2007).

Cardiovascular system is a very important organ that plays a vital role in tissue function. In farm animals, the growth and high milk production depends on the function of cardiovascular system. Therefore, it is important to investigate cardiovascular health in high and low-yielding dairy cows based on determination of dysrhythmias and cardiac biomarkers in high and low-yielding dairy cows.

Materials and Methods

Fifty 4-year-old high- yielding Holstein dairy cows and fifty 4-year-old low- yielding Holstein dairy cows were used in this study (the animals were healthy without clinical signs of any organ abnormalities in the clinical examination). All work was performed in a large dairy farm (Zagros Dairy farm, Shahrekord, Iran).

The average 305- day milk yield of high- yielding and low- yielding Holstein dairy cows were 10600 and 6000 kg, respectively, with 3.5% fat and 3.25% protein (100 days in milk). Cows were fed according to their requirements for maintenance and milk production (NRC, 2001). The ration consisted of high quality roughages (maize silage and sugar beet pulp), soybean meal, concentrates (corn, barley), and mineral and vitamin supplement.

For ECG recording, each cow was kept in a stock and allowed to settle for 10 minutes. The base-apex lead was used to detect the arrhythmias; it was attached using positive, negative, and ground leads as follows:

a) The positive electrode was attached to the skin over the left fifth intercostal space at the point of maximal intensity (PMI) of the apex beat; using lead I, this is the left arm electrode.

b) The negative electrode was attached to the skin of the left jugular furrow two thirds of the distance from the ramus of the mandible to the thoracic inlet; using lead I, this is the right arm.

c) The earth electrode was placed to the skin of the left flank.

After spraying the area with ethanol as a degreasing agent, we attached the electrodes to the specific position.

The ECG was recorded from 3 to 5 minutes (Animal in a relaxed state) while the cows kept in a standing position. The ECGs were obtained on a single channel machine (Kenz-ECG 110 Class I, Japan) with the paper speed 25mm/sec and calibration of 10 mm equal to 1mV. All of the ECGs were inspected by two of the authors independently, and finally both authors explained all dysrhythmias together. Blood samples were collected from the jugular vein and delivered to laboratory. The serum was separated and stored at -20°C until measurement of cardiac biomarkers.

The following step by-step approach can be used:

1. Identify all the QRS complexes. Each QRS complex should be followed by a T wave, and the QT interval should be similar for all QRS configurations, unless there is a marked change in heart rate. Identify the remaining complexes. Are P waves, "F" (flutter) waves, or "f" (fibrillation) waves present? Are there any artifacts?

2. Determine the atrial and ventricular rates. Are they identical? Is one too fast or too slow? This step determines whether there is a tachycardia or bradycardia.

3. Are the P-P and R-R intervals regular? Determine whether an irregular rhythm has underlying regularity that is interrupted by irregular intervals or whether the rhythm is consistently irregular. Second-degree AV block and atrial and ventricular premature beats are arrhythmias with underlying regularity, whereas atrial fibrillation, sinus arrhythmia, and sinus arrest are truly irregular rhythms.

4. Are P waves present? If so, is there a P wave preceding every QRS complex? If not, there are premature depolarizations, escape beats, or atrial fibrillation. Are all P waves followed by QRS complexes? If not, second degree AV block may be present. Is the resultant P-R interval constant? If not, there may be a first-degree AV block.

5. Are all P waves and QRS complexes identical or normal in contour? If not, this signifies more than one pacemaker, premature depolarizations, or escape beats (Radostits et al., 2007; Smith, 2009).

Blood samples were collected from the jugular vein after recording ECG. The blood serum and plasma were obtained by centrifugation at 2500g for 15 minutes. The serum and plasma samples were preserved at -20 °C until analysis. The activity of AST, LDH, CK, CK- MB, and troponin I were determined. Serum aspartate aminotransferase (AST), creatine kinase (CK), and myocard originating creatine kinase (CK - MB) levels were measured spectrophotometrically by IFCC method using commercial test kits (pars azmoon kits Commpany, Iran) as instructed by producers. Serum lactate dehydrogenase (LDH) was measured spectrophotometrically by using commercial test kit (Darman kave kit Commpany, Iran) as instructed by producers. Concentration of troponin I was determined by ultra immunoassay with commercial test kit (Monobind Inc. Lake Forest, CA 92630, USA) [normal range, less than 1.3 ng/mL].

Data were analyzed by one-way ANOVA to determine significant difference. Probability of $p<0.05$ was considered to be statically significant.

Results

ECGs were recorded from fifty 4-year-old high-yielding Holstein dairy cows and fifty 4-year-old low- yielding Holstein dairy cows. The types and number of cardiac dysrhythmias in both groups are given in Table 1. The mean concentration of CK, CK-MB, LDH, AST, and troponin I in both groups are given in Table 2.

Cardiac dysrhythmias were detected more in the low- yielding Holstein dairy cows (62%) as compared to the high- yielding Holstein dairy cows (46%).

The cardiac dysrhythmias that were observed in the low- yielding Holstein dairy cows included sinus arrhythmia (34.7%) Figure 1, wandering pace maker

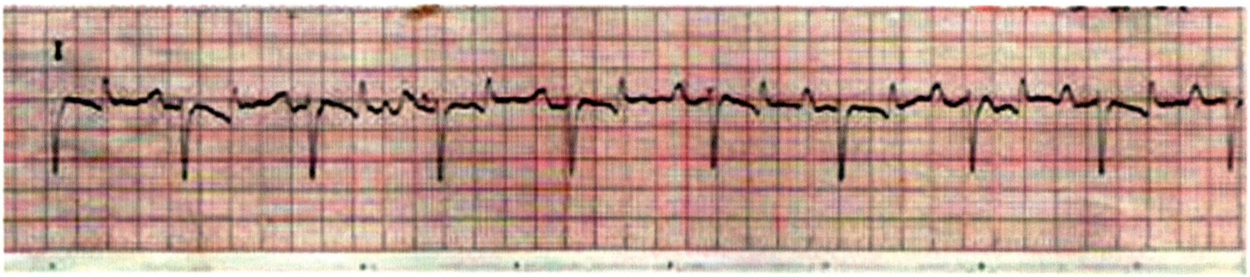

Figure 1. Sinus arrhythmia and wandering pace maker in high yielding Holstein cow.

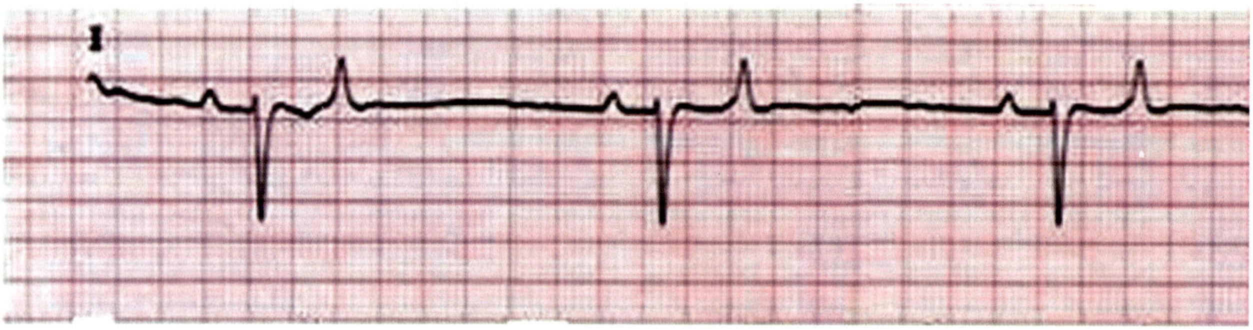

Figure 2. Bradycardia in low yielding Holstein cow.

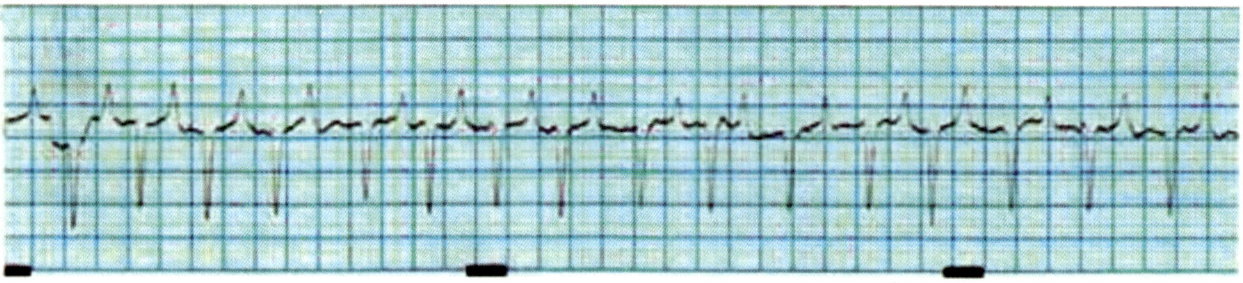

Figure 3. Atrial tachycardia in low yielding Holstein cow.

(22.45%) Figure 1, bradycardia (18.37%) Figure 2, tachycardia (10.20%) Fig. 3, atrial premature beat (2.04%) Figure 4, sinoatrial block (2.04%) Figure 5, atrial fibrillation (8.16%) Figure 6, and atrial tachycardia (2.04%) Figure 7. The cardiac dysrhythmias were observed in the high- yielding Holstein dairy cows included sinus arrhythmia (86.95%) and wandering pace maker (13.05%). Also, notched P wave was observed in both high- and low-yielding Holstein dairy cows, 30% and 14% respectively Figure 8.

The results of this study have shown significant difference ($p<0.05$) between serum concentration of CK- MB, LDH, AST, and troponin I in the high and

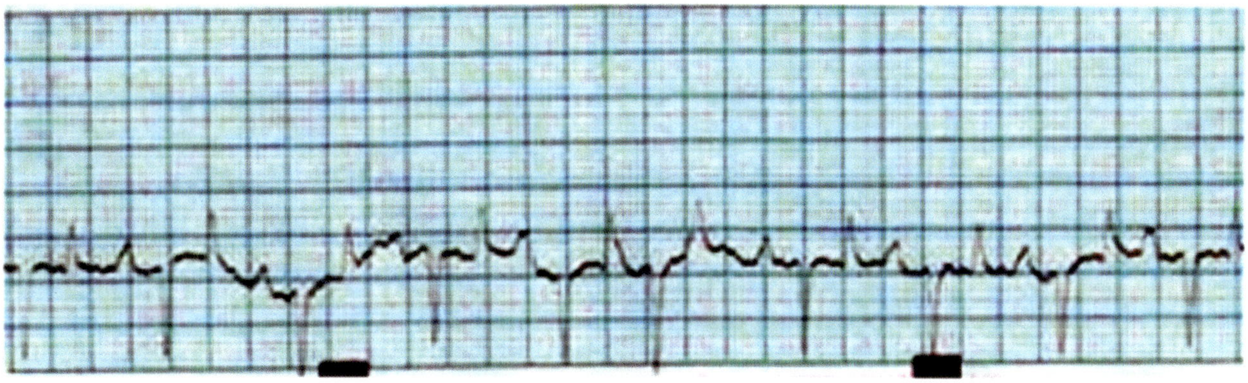

Figure 4. Atrial premature complex in low yielding Holstein cow.

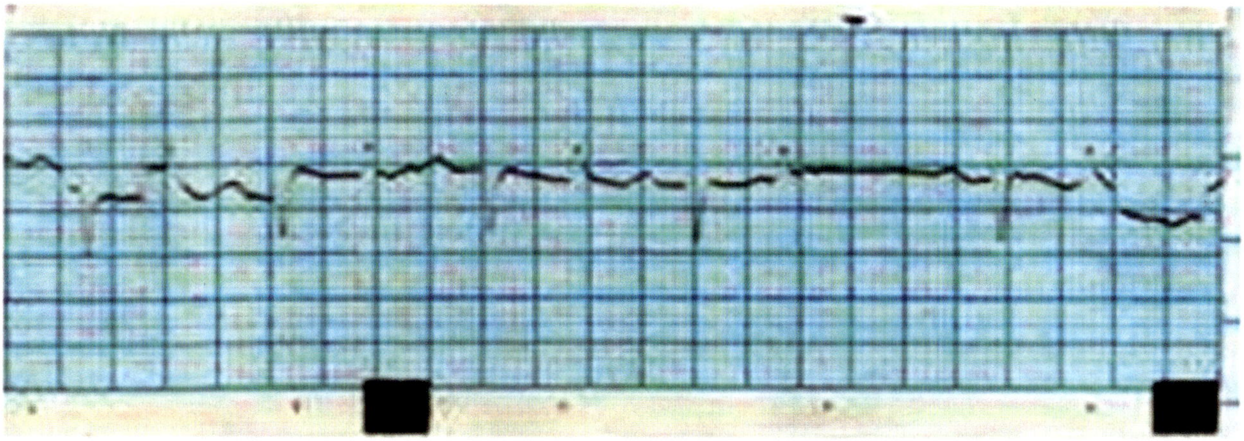

Figure 5. SA block in low yielding Holstein cow.

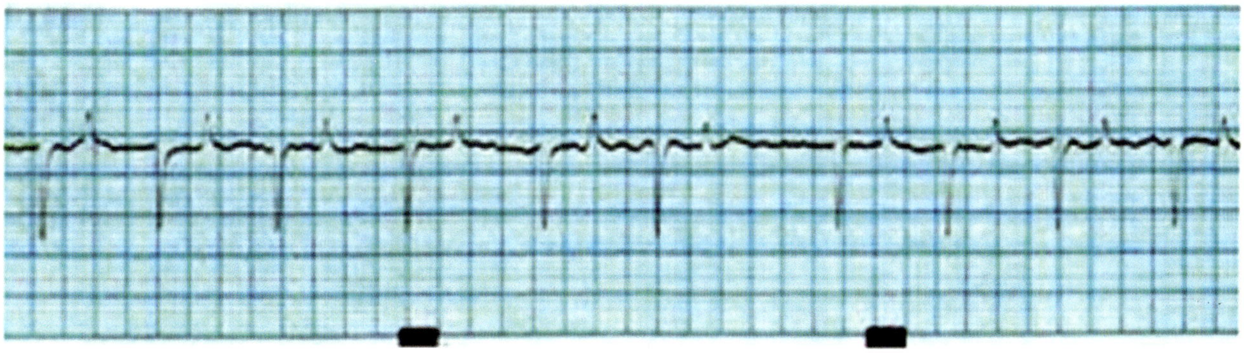

Figure 6. Atrial fibrillation in low yielding Holstein cow.

low yielding cows. According to these results, the amount of cardiac biomarkers in the low yielding cows was higher than that of the high yielding cows. Furthermore, there was not any detectable significant difference of serum concentration of total CK between the high and low- yielding Holstein cows.

Discussion

Cardiac dysrhythmias or arrhythmias are defined as disturbances of impulse formation, disorders of impulse conduction, or both. In the present study, Cardiac dysrhythmias were detected more in the low-yielding Holstein dairy cows (62%) as compared to

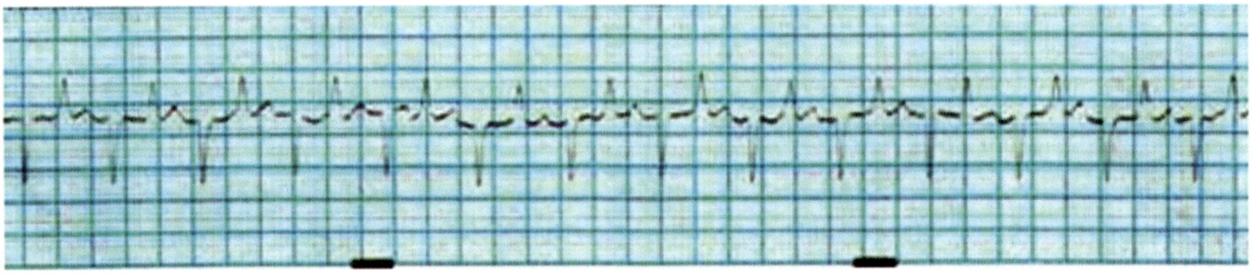

Figure 7. Sinus tachycardia in low yielding Holstein cow.

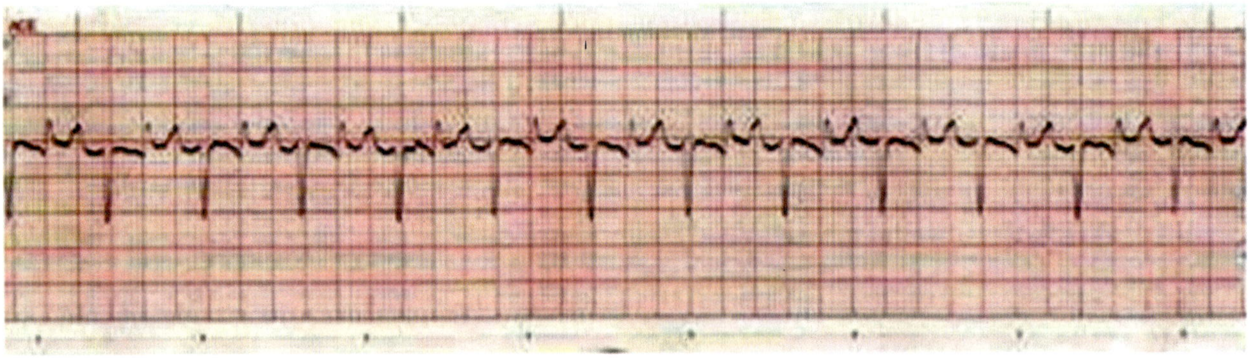

Figure 8. Notch P wave in high and low yielding Holstein cow.

the high- yielding Holstein dairy cows (46%). Eight types of dysrhythmias, either alone or in combination with another type, were observed in the low- yielding Holstein dairy cows, whereas two types of dysrhythmias determined in the high- yielding Holstein dairy cows.

Among biochemical parameters for the diagnosis of cardiac muscular disease, CK- MB, LDH, and AST have been used commonly. However, many disadvantageous of these parameters have been reported, and thus these parameters were replaced with newly developed cardiac markers such as cardiac troponin I (CTnI) and cardiac troponin T (CTnT) (McLaurin et al., 1997; Leonardi et al., 2008; O Brien, 2008; Aldous, 2012).

In this study, troponin I in both high and low yielding Holstein cows was found to be 0.55±0.02 and 0.67±0.04 ng/mL, respectively. Therefore, the serum concentration of troponin I in low yielding Holstein cows was higher than that of high yielding Holstein cows significantly ($p<0.05$). Therefore, according to the normal range of troponin I, less than 1.3 ng/ml, it can be concluded that the increase of cardiac dysrhythmias in low yielding Holstein cows may be resulted from metabolic and electrolyte disorders. Troponin is released from injured myocardiocytes in to the circulation within hours, peaks within 2 days, and remains elevated for as long as the injury continues (Willis et al., 2007; Varga et al., 2009). Cardiac troponin I and T parameters are usually investigated for cardiac muscle injuries. Although CTnT was claimed to be specific for cardiac muscle, CTnI was reported to have high sensitivity in the diagnosis of cardiac disease (Antman et al., 1996; Apple et al., 1998; Willis et al., 2007). This protein is the gold- standard biomarker of myocardial injury in humans and animals because of its high tissue specificity and persistence in the blood. (Wells and Sleeper, 2008; Varga et al., 2009) To date, the protein has been studied in rats, mice, rabbits,

Table 1. Mean±SEM of serum concentration of cardiac biomarkers in high and low yielding Holstein cows. (*)Values are significant at $p<0.05$.

Parameters	High yielding cows	Low yielding cows
AST U/L	67.25±9.21	127.89±13.16(*)
LDH U/L	117.167±1005.9	1402.96±153.14(*)
CK U/L	57.23±11.96	73.53±13.62
Ck -MB U/L	27.85±3.68	39.89±5.12(*)
Troponin I ng/mL	0.55±0.02	0.67±0.04(*)

Table 2. Type of dysrhythmias in high and low yielding Holstein cows.

Type of dysrhythmias	High yielding cows%	Low yielding cows%
Sinus Arrhythmia	86.95	34.7
Wandering Pacemaker	13.05	22.45
Bradycardia	0	18.37
Sinus tachycardia	0	10.20
Atrial Premature Complex	0	2.04
Atrial Fibrilation	0	8.16
SA Block	0	2.04
Atrial tachycardia	0	2.04

dogs, pigs, horses, cats, cattle, non- human primates, hamsters, and sheep (Gunes et al., 2010). The peak sensitivity of troponin I was at 12 to 24 h after onset of cardiac damage (Adams et al., 1993).

Gunes et al. (2008) used the cardiac troponin kits for the qualitative determination of myocardial cell damage due to traumatic reticuloperitonitis in twenty cattle. They observed that the mean serum concentrations of total protein, globulin, glucose, and calcium and the mean activities of creatine kinase Mb, aspartate aminotransferase, lactate dehydrogenase, and gamma-glutamyl transferase were higher in the cattle with TRP than in the control group (Gunes et al., 2008).

Tunca et al. (2008) determined the changes of the cardiac troponin I (cTnI) expression in blood and tissue during the myocardial degeneration in calves with foot-and-mouth disease (FMD). A biochemistry panel and immunohistochemistry were performed on 17 diseased calves, and 7 calves were used as controls. Creatine kinase (CK), CK-myocardial band (CK-MB), aspartate aminotransferase (AST), and lactate dehydrogenase (LDH) activities were measured for both groups. Mean cTnI (14.8 6 1.9 ng/mL) concentration and CK (573 6 407 U/L), CK-MB (238 6 37 U/L), AST (84 6 7), and LDH (298 6 29 U/L) activities were higher in FMD cases compared with controls (Tunca et al., 2008) .

Varga et al. (2009) investigated the correlation of serum cardiac troponin I and myocardial damage in cattle with monensin toxicosis. Their study confirmed that cTnI is a specific and sensitive biomarker for the detection of myocardial cell damage in cattle. A serum concentration of cTnI 1.04 ng/mL is an indicator of histopathologically detectable myocardial necrosis in cattle after monensin administration (Varga et al., 2009).

Karapinar et al. (2010) reported the high cardiac troponin I plasma concentration in a calf with myocarditis. They concluded that the cTnI assay may be useful in diagnosis of myocarditis in cattle (Karapinar et al., 2010).

Schober et al. (2002) indicated that serum cardiac troponin concentrations are associated with severity of ECG abnormalities and outcome (Schober et al., 2002).

Jesty et al. (2005) analyzed cardiac troponin I concentration in a cow with idiopathic pericarditis. They reported its value as 0.89 ng/mL (Jesty et al., 2005).

Buczinski and Bélanger (2010) reported an increase of Serum cardiac troponin I at 3.52 ng/mL in bovine tricuspid endocarditis (Buczinski et al., 2010).

In this study, in both high and low yielding Holstein cows, the serum concentration of CK- MB was 27.85±3.68 U/L and 39.89±5.12 U/L, respectively. Thus, the serum concentration of CK-MB in the low yielding Holstein cows was significantly higher than that of the high yielding Holstein cows ($p<0.05$). Therefore, according to the normal range of CK -MB, 105-409 U/L, it can be concluded that the increase of cardiac dysrhythmias in low yielding Holstein cows may be resulted from metabolic and electrolyte disorders. The peak sensitivity of CK -MB occurred at 8 to 12 h after onset of cardiac damage (Adams et al., 1993). Also, the serum concentration of CK was 57.23±11.96 U/L and 73.53±13.62 U/L in high and low yielding Holstein cows, respectively. This finding is in accordance with previous studies which have shown that CK lacks specificity for myocardial cell injury and that the measurement of CK is not sensitive enough to detect micropathology of the heart in cattle. In contrast, CK-

MB, an isoenzyme of CK, which is more specific to the cardiac muscle, has a higher specificity for myocardial cell injury (Varga et al., 2009).

In this study, the serum concentration of AST in high and low yielding Holstein cows was 67.25 U/L and 127.89 U/L, respectively. As a result, the serum concentration of AST in the low yielding Holstein cows was significantly higher than that of the high yielding Holstein cows ($p<0.05$). Therefore, according to the normal range of AST, 78-132 U/L, it can be concluded that the increase of cardiac dysrhythmias in the low yielding Holstein cows may be resulted from metabolic and electrolyte disorders.

AST enzyme is found in almost all cells including red blood cells; however, it is considered a diagnostic enzyme for liver and muscle disease because of its high activity in these tissues. Plasma half life of AST is above. AST is not an organ specific enzyme (Smith, 2009). Al-Habsi et al. reported that the reference levels of AST are 48 - 132 U/L in cattle (Al-Habsi et al., 2007).

In this study, the serum concentration of LDH in high and low yielding Holstein cows was 1005.9± 117.167 U/L and 1402.96±153.14 U/L, respectively. Hence, the serum concentration of LDH in the low yielding Holstein cows was significantly higher than that of the high yielding Holstein cows ($p<0.05$). Therefore, according to the normal range of LDH, less than 692-1449 U/L, it can be concluded that the increase of cardiac dysrhythmias in the low yielding Holstein cows may be resulted from metabolic and electrolyte disorders. LDH enzyme is found in most tissue such as heart, liver, erythrocyte, leukocytes, and kidney. LDH enzyme has 5 isoenzymes, namely LDH1 (H4), LDH2 (H3M1), LDH3 (H2M2), LDH4 (H1M3), and LDH5 (M4). LDH1 is the principal isoenzyme in cardiac muscle and kidney. In cattle and sheep, LDH1 also is found in the liver. LDH5 is the principal isoenzyme in skeletal muscle and erythrocyte (Smith, 2009).

Consequently, it can be concluded that despite significant differences in cardiac biomarkers and based on the normal range of cardiac biomarkers in the both groups, the increase in cardiac dysrhythmias in low- yielding Holstein dairy cows may be metabolic and electrolyte disorders.

Acknowledgments

This research was founded by Shahrekord University, Shahrekord, Iran.

References

1. Adams, J.E., Abendschein, D.R., Jaffe, A.S. (1993) Biochemical markers of myocardial injury. Is MB creatine kinase the choice for the 1990s? Circulation. 88: 750-763.
2. Al-Habsi, K., Johnson, E.H., Kadim, I.T., Srikandakumar, A., Annamalai, K., Al-Busaidy, R., Mahgoub, O. (2007) Effects of low concentrations of dietary cobalt on live weight gains, haematology, serum vitamin B12 and biochemistry of Omani goats. Vet J. 173: 131-137.
3. Aldous, S.J. (2012) Cardiac biomarkers in acute myocardial infarction. Int J Cardiol In Press. 16: 282-294.
4. Antman, E.M., Tanasijevic, M.J., Thompson, B., Schactman, M., McCabe, C.H., Cannon, C.P., Fischer, G.A., Fung, A.Y., Thompson, C., Wybenga, D. (1996) Cardiac-specific troponin I levels to predict the risk of mortality in patients with acute coronary syndromes. New Engl J Med. 335: 1342-1349.
5. Apple, F.S., Sharkey, S.W., Falahati, A., Murakami, M., Mitha, N., Christensen, D. (1998) Assessment of left ventricular function using serum cardiac troponin I measurements following myocardial infarction. Clin Chim Acta. 272: 59-67.
6. Buczinski, S., Rezakhani, A., Boerboom, D. (2010) Heart disease in cattle: diagnosis, therapeutic approaches and prognosis. Vet J. 184: 258-263.
7. Edwards, N.J. (1993) ECG Manual for the Veterinary Technician. W. B. Saunders. London, UK.
8. Fredericks, S., Merton, G.K., Lerena, M.J., Heining, P., Carter, N.D., Holt, D.W. (2001) Cardiac troponins and creatine kinase content of striated muscle in common laboratory animals. Clin Chim Acta. 304: 65-74.
9. Gunes, V., Atalan, G., Citil, M., Erdogan, H.M. (2008) Use of cardiac troponin kits for the qualitative determination of myocardial cell damage due to traumatic reticuloperitonitis in cattle. Vet Record. 162: 514-517.
10. Gunes, V., Ozcan, K., Citil, M., Onmaz, A.C., Erdogan, H.M. (2010) Detection of myocardial

degeneration with point-of-care cardiac troponin assays and histopathology in lambs with white muscle disease. Vet J. 184: 376-378.

11. Jesty, S.A., Sweeney, R.W., Dolente, B.A., Reef, V.B. (2005) Idiopathic pericarditis and cardiac tamponade in two cows. J Am Vet Med Assoc. 226: 1555-1558.

12. Karapinar, T., Dabak, D.O., Kuloglu, T., Bulut, H. (2010) High cardiac troponin I plasma concentration in a calf with myocarditis. Can Vet J. 51: 397-399.

13. Laterza, O.F., Modur, V.R., Ladenson, J.H. (2008) Biomarkers of tissue injury. Biomarkers. 2: 81-92.

14. Leonardi, F., Passeri, B., Fusari, A., De Razza, P., Beghi, C., Lorusso, R., Corradi, A., Botti, P. (2008) Cardiac troponin I (cTnI) concentration in an ovine model of myocardial ischemia. Res Vet Sci. 85: 141-144.

15. McLaurin, M.D., Apple, F.S., Voss, E.M., Herzog, C.A., Sharkey, S.W. (1997) Cardiac troponin I, cardiac troponin T, and creatine kinase MB in dialysis patients without ischemic heart disease: evidence of cardiac troponin T expression in skeletal muscle. Clin Chem. 43: 976-982.

16. O Brien, P.J. (2008) Cardiac troponin is the most effective translational safety biomarker for myocardial injury in cardiotoxicity. Toxicology. 245: 206-218.

17. Radostits, O.M., Gay, C.C., Hinchcliff, K.W., Constable, P.D. (2007) Veterinary Medicine: A Textbook of the Diseases of Cattle, Sheep, Pigs, Goats and Horses. (10th ed.) WB Saunders Company. London, UK.

18. Reimers, B., Lachin, M., Cacciavillani, L., Secchiero, S., Ramondo, A., Isabella, G., Marzari, A., Zaninotto, M., Plebani, M., Chioin, R. (1997) Troponin T, creatine kinase MB mass, and creatine kinase MB isoform ratio in the detection of myocardial damage during non-surgical coronary revascularization. Int J Cardiol. 60: 7-13.

19. Rezakhani, A., Paphan, A.A., Shekarfroush, S. (2004) Analysis of base apex lead electrocardiograms of normal dairy cows. Vet Arhiv. 74: 351-358.

20. Rezakhani, A., Paphan, A.A., Zarifi, M. (2010) Evaluation of cardiac disorders in cliniclally healthy cattle. J Vet Pathol. 1: 1-4.

21. Roberts, R. (1998) Early diagnosis of myocardial infarction with MB CK isoforms. Clin Chim Acta 272: 33-45.

22. Schober, K.E., Cornand, C., Kirbach, B., Aupperle, H., Oechtering, G. (2002) Serum cardiac troponin I and cardiac troponin T concentrations in dogs with gastric dilatation-volvulus. J Am Vet Med Assoc. 221: 381-388.

23. Serra, M., Papakonstantinou, S., Adamcova, M., O'Brien, P.J. (2010) Veterinary and toxicological applications for the detection of cardiac injury using cardiac troponin. Vet J. 185: 50.

24. Smith, B.P. (2009) Large Animal Internal Medicine. (4th ed.) Mosby. Missouri, USA.

25. Tunca, R., Sozmen, M., Erdogan, H., Citil, M., Uzlu, E., Ozen, H., Gokce, E. (2008) Determination of cardiac troponin I in the blood and heart of calves with foot-and-mouth disease. J Vet Diagn Invest. 20: 598-605.

26. Varga, A., Schober, K.E., Holloman, C.H., Stromberg, P.C., Lakritz, J., Rings, D.M. (2009) Correlation of serum cardiac troponin I and myocardial damage in cattle with monensin toxicosis. J Vet Int Med. 23: 1108-1116.

27. Wells, S.M., Sleeper, M. (2008) Cardiac troponins. J Vet Emerg Crit Care. 18: 235-245.

28. Willis, M.S., Snyder, J.A., Poppenga, R.H., Grenache, D.G. (2007) Bovine cardiac troponin T is not accurately quantified with a common human clinical immunoassay. J Vet Diagn Invest. 19: 106-108.

Evaluation of haematological and biochemical changes after short term tramadol usage in healthy dogs

Akhtardanesh, B.[1*], Sharifi, H.[2], Rasooli, R.[3], Aghazamani, M.[3]

[1] *Department of Clinical Sciences, Faculty of Veterinary Medicine, Shahid-Bahonar University of Kerman, Kerman, Iran*

[2] *Department of Food Hygiene, Faculty of Veterinary Medicine, Shahid-Bahonar University of Kerman, Kerman, Iran*

[3] *Graduated from the Faculty of Veterinary Medicine, Shahid Bahonar University of Kerman, Kerman, Iran*

Key words:
dog, kidney, liver, tramadol

Correspondence
Akhtardanesh, B.
Department of Clinical Sciences,
Faculty of Veterinary Medicine,
Shahid-Bahonar University of
Kerman, Kerman, Iran

Email: akhtardanesh@uk.ac.ir

Abstract:

BACKGROUND: Tramadol is a synthetic, centrally acting opioid analgesic that has the best analgesic efficacy without excessive sedation and significant side effects in the postoperative pain relief in dogs. **OBJECTIVES:** In this study, hematological and biochemical changes due to short usage of tramadol were assessed in clinically healthy dogs. **METHODS:** For this purpose, eighteen male mongrel dogs aged 14 to 22 months were used in three equal groups. In the first and second groups respectively (2 and 5 mg/kg) intramuscular tramadol and in control group distillate water was given once a day for five consecutive days. Complete cell blood count (CBC) and biochemical evaluation were done to measure aspartate amino-transferase (AST), alanine aminotransferase (ALT), lactate dehydrogenase (LDH), creatinin (Cr), and blood urea nitrogen (BUN) levels, before the intervention (day 0) and on days 6 and 13, post-treatment. **RESULTS:** Thirteen days post treatment, Red blood cell (RBC) and white blood cell (WBC) count and ALT, AST, ALP, Cr, BUN and packed cell volume (PCV) level was measured as 6.75±0.03, 3.86±0.13, 40.00±7.98, 43.67±8.62, 57.00±17.03, 0.90±0.27, 25.00±5.48 and 40.13±2.88 respectively which showed that short-term injection of even high doses of tramadol creates no significant change on hematological, liver, and kidney parameters in dogs. **CONCLUSIONS:** The present study suggests that tramadol could be a safe postoperative analgesic for control of acute pain in dogs referred for routine surgical procedures.

Introduction

The recognition of animal pain as a medical entity and ethical problem has attracted increasing scientific attention, leading to better animal welfare laws. Tramadol, a synthetic racemic mixture of the 4-phenyl-piperidine analogue of codeine, has received widespread acceptance in human medicine since it was first introduced in 1977 in Germany (Schenck and Arend, 1978; Osterloh et al., 1978; Scott and Perry, 2000). Tramadol plays an important role in the management of pain with its dual mechanism of action (opioid agonist; weak noradrenaline and serotonin reuptake inhibitor). Besides its proven clinical efficacy, tramadol is a safe drug with no respiratory depression, cardiovascular side effects, drug abuse, and minor clinical relevance of dependency, unlike some other opioids (Quang -

Cantagrel et al., 2000). Elimination is primarily by the hepatic route (metabolism by CYP2D6 to an active metabolite and by CYP3A4 and CYP2B6) and partly by the renal route (up to 30% of dose). Elimination half-lives of the active agents range between 4.5 and 9.5 hours, and the total plasma clearance of tramadol is moderately high (600 ml/min) (Klotz, 2003). The metabolism of tramadol has been investigated in a number of animal species (rats, mice, Syrian hamsters, guinea pigs, rabbits and dogs) as well as in humans (Lintz et al., 1981; KuKanich and Papich, 2004). The central role of liver and kidney in drug metabolism predisposes them to toxic injury. Tramadol is converted in the liver to O-desmethyl-tramadol, which is an active substance and 2 to 4 times more potent than tramadol (Wu et al., 2001; Tao et al., 2002). Furthermore, biotransformation results in inactive metabolites, which are excreted by kidneys (Lee et al., 1993; Matthiessen et al., 1998, Atici et al., 2005). Likewise, if kidney or liver function is severely impaired, some dosage reduction (approximately by 50%) or extension of the dosage interval should be considered (Klotz, 2003). The efficacy of tramadol in pain relief in small animal medicine was confirmed in previous studies (Cagnardi et al., 2011; Vettorato et al., 2010). However, in this study, haematological and biochemical changes in liver and kidneys due to short usage of tramadol were assessed in healthy dogs.

Materials and Methods

Animals: In this study, eighteen healthy male mongrel dogs were used, with body weight ranging between 20 to 30 kg, and ages between 14 and 22 months. The dogs were considered healthy based on physical examination, complete blood count, serum biochemistry, and urine analysis before the initiation of the study. All animals were kept in an approved animal care facility in separate cages with ad libitum access to food and water. They were divided to three equal (two treatments and one control) groups.

Drug administration: Two treatment groups were given intramuscular tramadol (Aboraihan company, Iran), once a day 2 and 5 mg/kg, respectively, and the control group was given distilled water for five consecutive days.

Blood sampling protocol: Blood samples were taken from the brachiocephalus vein from the control and treatment groups, prior to the experiment (day 0), at the end of treatment period (day 6), and one week later (day 13). Five-milliliter (5mL) blood samples were divided in two tubes, 1 mL used with anticoagulant, ethylenediamine tetra-acetic acid (EDTA) for haematological evaluation and 4 mL without anticoagulant, for serum collection and biochemical assay.

Haematological studies: Complete blood counts were performed by cell counter instrument (EXW Shenzhen, China) for all dogs.

Biochemical studies: Serum samples were separated by centrifugation for measurement of serum alanine aminotransferase (ALT), aspartate aminotransferase (AST), alkaline phosphatase (ALP), and creatinine level using an autoanalyzer (Autolab, AMS -18A, China) and commercial kits (Mans company, Iran) according to the manufacturer's instructions.

Statistical analysis: Statistical analyses were performed using repeated-measures analysis of variance. For WBC and RBC, analysis was done on log 10 of measures. Data were presented as mean ± SD and $p<0.05$ was considered statistically significant. All calculations were made using SPSS version 18.

Results

There were no significant differences in the studied parameters between different groups. Although significant differences were seen in hepatic enzymes level during different times in some animals in treatment groups, all kidney and liver enzymes and haematological parameters (mean levels) were in the normal range in the studied dogs on days 6 and 13 post-treatment in two treatment groups, suggesting that tramadol is a safe post-operative analgesic for control of acute pain in dogs (Table 1).

Discussion

Opioids are used in veterinary and human medicine. It has been proven that liver and kidney are responsible for the metabolism and excretion of all opioids (coughtvie et al.,1989; Milne et al., 1997; Bannwarth, 1999). Based on author's knowledge,

Table1. Mean± SD level of haematological and biochemical parameters in studied dogs. (*) Before intervention (Day 0). (**) Day 6. (***) Day 13.

Parameter	Control	Tramadol(2mg/kg)	Tramadol (5 mg/kg)
	Mean±SD	Mean±SD	Mean±SD
Log-RBC/μL (Red Blood Cell)			
T0(*)	6.74±0.03	6.75±0.03	6.75±0.03
T1(**)	6.74±0.03	6.73±0.03	6.92±0.41
T2(***)	6.76±0.03	6.92±0.40	6.75±0.03
Log-WBC/μL (White Blood Cell)			
T0	3.97±0.07	3.96±0.06	3.97±0.08
T1	3.87±0.06	3.90±0.06	3.94±0.07
T2	3.92±0.07	3.92±0.04	3.86±0.13
ALT (IU/l)			
T0	23.50±5.92	25.50±7.39	28.33±4.63
T1	34.67±9.20	37.00±6.07	38.00±13.47
T2	34.00±10.37	39.17±8.57	40.00±7.98
AST (IU/l)			
T0	26.17±7.90	32.00±8.76	38.33±9.85
T1	28.67±15.59	35.67±6.89	42.67±9.56
T2	28.17±15.63	36.33±9.73	43.67±8.62
ALP(IU/l)			
T0	57.67±17.44	57.83±16.65	44.83±14.27
T1	63.50±18.27	61.33±12.74	54.50±17.48
T2	66.67±18.62	71.83±17.11	57.00±17.03
Cr(IU/l)			
T0	0.83±0.29	0.75±0.22	0.57±0.12
T1	0.88±0.29	1.00±0.28	0.72±0.28
T2	0.91±0.28	0.97±0.24	0.90±0.27
BUN (mg/dl)			
T0	21.50±6.31	19.33±5.78	18.67±5.56
T1	25.33±7.94	34.50±6.66	24.00±6.63
T2	23.83±7.17	25.83±8.64	25.00±5.48
PCV (%)Packed Cell Volume			
T0	40.50±1.97	40.50±2.67	38.83±3.13
T1	41.35±2.59	38.15±4.30	39.13±2.68
T2	39.67±1.97	42.58±2.88	40.13±2.88

there is no investigation about the side effects of short or long term tramadol administration on hematological and biochemical factors in dogs, whereas results of the present study showed that short term tramadol administration to dogs does not induce any significant hematological, renal and hepatic disorders.

Hepatotoxic effects of both morphine and tramadol were confirmed after long-term administration in rats; however, the toxic effects of tramadol were less severe compared to morphine. On the other hand, no significant changes were seen in BUN and creatinin levels after chronic usage of tramadol, indicating that tramadol may be a safer drug in terms of renal side effects compared to morphine (Atici et al., 2005). Renal damage like focal corticomedullary mineralization, focal regeneration in tubular epithelium, and mineral crystal deposition in intertubular region in kidneys has been reported after long-term use of morphine like agent, levo-alpha acetyl methadol hydrochloride (Borzelleca et al., 1994). Nevertheless, tramadol caused minimal histopathological changes in kidneys limited only to tubular cells in rats (Atici et al., 2005). A significant increase in the level of ALT, which has been reported among long term heroin users, were also indicated after long term usage of tramadol (Panchenko et al., 1999; Atici et al., 2005). In another study that was performed by Habibian-Dehkordi et al. (2010), short term intravenous administration of tramadol had no effect on ALT, AST, and ALP levels in sheep, which is in agreement with our study. On the other hand, no significant changes were observed in BUN and Cr levels in blood serum by these researchers, the same as what we found in the present study (Habinian-Dehkordi et al., 2010).

Total number of WBC did not show any significant changes during present experiment, which is against Tsai's (2001) findings which showed that tramadol administration causes an increase in number of lymphocytes in rats. Other M opioid agonists like morphine were reported to cause decrease in the number of lymphocytes (Tsai and Won, 2001).

The number of blood RBC and packed cell volume were the other hematological parameters that were considered in normal range, and tramadol did not affect them in our study. In a study by Verde et al. (2003), it was shown that Hb, hematocrit, RBC, and WBC counts in blood samples of opiate addicts of both sexes were higher than those levels found in control groups. On the contrary, a significant decrease in RBC count and PCV was indicated after short-term tramadol administration in sheep (Habibian-Dehcordi et al., 2010; Verde et al., 2003).

In conclusion, results of the present study showed that short-term injection of various doses of tramadol has no significant effect on hematological, liver, and kidney parameters in dogs, suggesting that tramadol may be an effective postoperative analgesic for control of acute pain in dogs referred for routine surgical procedures. Further investigation about the side effects of long term tramadol administration in dogs must be performed.

Acknowledgments

The authors are grateful to Research Council of Shahid Bahonar University for the financial support and chief of teaching and research veterinary hospital," Dr. Omid Azari" for his technical support.

References

1. Atici, S., Cinel, I., Cinel, L., Doruk, N., Eskandari, G., Oral, U. (2005) Liver and kidney toxicity in chronic use of opioids: an experimental long term treatment model. J Biosci. 30: 245-252.
2. Bannwarth, B. (1999) Risk-benefit assessment of opioids in chronic non-cancer pain. Drug Saf. 21: 283-296.
3. Borzelleca, J.F., Egle, J.L., Harris, L.S., Johnson, D.N., Terrill, J.B., Belleville, J.A. (1994) Toxicological evaluation of mu-agonists. Part I: assessment of toxicity following 30days of repeated oraldosing of male and female rats with levo-alpha-acetylmethadolHCl (LAAM). J Appl Toxicol. 14: 435-446.
4. Cagnardi, P., Villa, R., Zonca, A., Gallo, M., Beccaglia, M., Luvoni, G.C., Vettorato, E., Carli, S., Fonda, D., Ravasio, G. (2011) Pharmacokinetics, intraoperative effect and postoperative analgesia of tramadol in cats. Res Vet Sci. 6: 503-509.
5. Collet, B.J. (2001) Chronic opioid therapy for non-cancer pain. Br J Anaesth. 87: 133-143.
6. Coughtrie, M.W, Ask, B., Rane, A., Burchell, B., Hume, R. (1989) The enantioselective glucuronidation of morphine in rats and humans. Evidence for the involvement of more than one UDP glucuronosyl transferase isoenzyme. Biochem Pharmacol. 38: 3273-3280.
7. Habibian- Dehkordi, S., Bigham-Sadegh, A., Abaspour, A., Beigi Brojeni, N., Aali, E., Sadeghi, E. (2010) Intravenous administration of tramadol hydrochloride in sheep. J Comp Clin Pathol. 21: 289-293.
8. Klotz, U. (2003) Tramadol-the impact of its pharmacokinetic and pharmacodynamic properties on the clinical management of pain. Azneimittelforschung. 53: 681-7.
9. KuKanich, B., Papich, M.G. (2004) Pharmacokinetics of tramadol and the metabolite O-desmethyltramadol in dogs. J Vet Pharmacol Therap. 27: 239-246.
10. Lee, R.C., Tavish, M.C., Sorkin, E.M. (1993) Tramadol: a preliminary review of its pharmacodynamic and pharmacokinetic properties, and therapeutic potential in acute and chronic pain states. Drugs. 46: 313-340.
11. Lintz, W., Erlacin, S., Frankus, E., Uragg, H. (1981) Biotransformation of tramadol in man and animal. Arzneimittelforschung Drug Res. 31: 1932-1943.
12. Matthiessen, T., Wöhrmann, T., Coogan, T.P., Uragg, H. (1998) The experimental toxicology of tramadol: an overview. Toxicol Lett. 95: 63-71.
13. Milne, R.W., McLean, C.F., Mather, L.E., Nation, R.L., Runciman, W.B., Rutten, A.J., Somogyi, A.A. (1997) Influence of renal failure on the disposition ofmorphine-3-glucuronide and morphine glucuronide in sheep during intravenous infusion with morphine. J Vet Pharmacol Ther. 282: 779-786.
14. Osterloh, G., Friderichs, E., Felgenhauer, F., Günzler, W.A., Henmi, Z., Kitano, T., Nakamura, M., Hayashi, H., Ishii, I. (1978) General pharmacological studies on tramadol, a potent analgesic agent. Arzneimittelforschung. 28: 135- 151.
15. Panchenko, L.F., Pirozhkov, S.V., Nadezhdin, A.V., Baronets, V.I., Usmanova, N.N. (1999) Lipid peroxidation, peroxyl radical-scavenging system of

plasma and liver and heart pathology in adolescence heroin users. Vopr Med Khim. 45: 501-506.
16. Quang-Cantagrel, N.D., Wallace, M.S., Magnuson, S.K. (2000) Opioid substitution to improve the effectiveness of chronic non cancer pain control a chart review. Anesth Analg. 90: 933-937.
17. Schenck, E.G., Arend, I. (1978) The effect of tramadol in an open clinical trial. Arzneimittelforschung. 28: 209-212.
18. Scott, L.J., Perry, M.P. (2000) Tramadol: a review of its use in perioperative pain. Drugs. 60: 139-176.
19. Tao, Q., Stone, D.J., Borenstein, M.R., Cod, E.E.D., Coogan, T.P. (2002) Differential tramadol and O-desmethyl metabolite levels in brain vs plasma of mice and rats administered tramadol hydrochloride orally. J Clin Pharm Therap. 27: 99-106.
20. Tsai, Y.C., Won, S.J. (2001) Effects of tramadol on T lymphocyte proliferation and natural killer cell activity in rats with sciatic constriction injury. Pain. 92: 63-69.
21. Verde, M., Diaz-Flores, J.F., Sanudo, R.I., Rodriguez, E.M., Diaz, R.C. (2003) Haematologic parameters in opiate addicts. Nutr Hosp. 8: 358-365.
22. Vettorato, E., Zonca, A., Isola, M., Villa, R., Gallo, M., Ravasio, G., Beccaglia, M., Montesissa, C., Cagnardi, P. (2010) Pharmacokinetics and efficacy of intravenous and extradural tramadol in dogs. Vet J. 183: 310-315.
23. Wu, W., McKown, L., Gauthier, A., Jones W., Raffa, R. (2001) Metabolism of the analgesic drug, tramadol hydrochloride in rat and dog. Xenobiotica. 31: 423- 441.

Heavy metals content of canned tuna fish marketed in Tabriz, Iran

Pourjafar, H.[1*], Ghasemnejad, R.[2], Noori, N.[1], Mohammadi, Kh.[3]

[1] *Department of Food Hygiene and Quality Control, Faculty of Veterinary Medicine, University of Tehran, Tehran, Iran*

[2] *Department of Food Hygiene and Quality Control, Science and Research Campus, Islamic Azad University, Tehran, Iran*

[3] *Department of Food Hygiene and Quality Control, Faculty of Veterinary Medicine, Tabriz Branch, Islamic Azad University, Tabriz, Iran*

Key words:
atomic absorption spectrophotometry, canned tuna, heavy metals

Correspondence
Pourjafar, H.
Department of Food Hygiene and Quality Control, Faculty of Veterinary Medicine, Tehran University, Tehran, Iran

Email: pourjafarhadi59@ut.ac.ir

Abstract:

BACKGROUND: Some heavy metals are dangerous to health and there is rising concern about the quality of foodstuffs in some parts of the world. Fish, particularly Tuna fish, can concentrate huge quantities of several metals from water and they even play a significant role in human nourishment. **OBJECTIVES:** In this study, the concentrations of mercury and four trace metals in five brands of canned tuna samples purchased within the Tabriz city (Iran) were determined after digestion via the Association of Official Analytical Chemists techniques. **METHODS:** A total of 40 samples were collected. Lead and cadmium levels were determined via graphite tube atomic absorption spectrophotometry, whereas nickel and tin levels were determined via flame atomic absorption spectrophotometry, and mercury levels were determined via hydride generation atomic absorption spectrophotometry. **RESULTS:** The ranges obtained for the elements were Pb (0.01-0.242), Ca (0.0-1.05), Ni (0.113-0.589), Sn (0.05-0.9), and Hg (0.1-0.205) mg/kg wet weight. **CONCLUSIONS:** The results showed that tuna fabricated and marketed in Tabriz (Iran) had safe level of heavy metals that were lower than the averages of EC/FAO/WHO levels for these toxic metals.

Introduction

The topic of heavy metals is receiving growing popularity in food manufacturing because of elevated occurrence of contamination in agricultural and seafood products. Some heavy metals are very dangerous to health and there is rising concern about the quality of foodstuffs in some parts of the world. Small quantities of these elements are ordinary in our environment and diet and are really essential for physical wellbeing; however, large quantities of any of them will result in acute or chronic poisoning (Ikem and Egiebor, 2005; Inskip and Piotrowsiki, 1985; Rauf et al., 2009; FDA, 2001). The poisonous effects of heavy metals, mostly mercury, lead, cadmium, nickel, and tin have been largely investigated (Inskip and Piotrowsiki, 1985; Mergler et al., 2007; Yi et al., 2011). Heavy metals can enter the human being body throughout foodstuff, atmosphere, water, and absorption through the skin; nevertheless, ingestion is the most probable method of exposure (Ikem and Egiebor, 2005; Rauf et al., 2009). The aquatic environment is one of the major places contaminated by heavy metals. Moreover, several factors including season, physical and chemical quality of water are able to play an important role in metal gathering in different fish tissues (Ashraf et al., 2006; Ikem and Egiebor, 2005; Olowu et al., 2010; Rauf et al., 2009; Vinodhini and Narayanan, 2008). Aside from the hazard from contaminated environment, canned foodstuff is exposed to heavy metal contamination for the duration of the canning procedure (Ashraf et al., 2006; Malakootian et al., 2011; Mol, 2011; Voegborlo et al., 1999).

Accumulation of heavy metals in aquatic creatures can cause a long-term effect on biogeochemical cycling in the ecosphere (Rauf et al., 2009). Fish is frequently at the top of aquatic foodstuff succession and possibly will concentrate huge quantities of several metals from the water and they even play a significant role in human being nourishment (FDA, 2001; Mansour and Sidky, 2002; Rauf et al., 2009). They should be carefully monitored to make sure that unnecessary high level of several toxic trace metals are not being transmitted to human being by fish consumption (Emami Khansari et al., 2005; Ikem and Egiebor, 2005; Malakootian et al., 2011; Schmitt and Brumbaugh, 1990).

Canned fish in particular are well consumed in developed and developing countries, and metal contamination particularly in canned fish and other marine products have been largely investigated (Burgera and Gochfeld, 2005; Castro-Gonzalez and Mendez-Armenta, 2008; Dural et al., 2007; Emami Khansari et al., 2005; Hutcheson et al., 2008; Qiao-qiao et al., 2007; Sivaperumal et al., 2007; Türkmen et al., 2005; Tüzen, 2003; Yilmaz et al., 2007).

Fish, particularly Tuna fish can concentrate a large amount of heavy metals. Most importantly, it is recognized for gathering large amount of mercury (Castro-Gonzalez and Mendez-Armenta, 2008; Emami Khansari et al., 2005; Ikem and Egiebor, 2005; Malakootian et al., 2011; Mansour and Sidky, 2002; Voegborlo et al., 1999). Once heavy metals are consumed, several health-related problems will occur; especially pregnant women and children are exposed to them (Ikem and Egiebor, 2005). Eating a lot of tuna would result in serious health problems because of inorganic mercury and methyl mercury and other heavy metals effects (Ashraf et al., 2006; Ikem and Egiebor, 2005; Mol, 2011; Mergler et al., 2007). The aim of this study was to evaluate heavy metals content of canned tuna fish in Tabriz city (Iran), spectrometrically.

Materials and Methods

Instruments: All the glassware employed in the procedures were soaked in 10% (v/v) nitric acid for 20 min, followed by washing with 10% (v/v) hydrochloric acid, and washed with deionized water before utilization. A Varian Model 240 atomic absorption spectrophotometer prepared with a deuterium setting corrector was employed for the determination of heavy metals.

Reagents and materials: All reagents employed in this study were analytical reagent grade, Merck, Germany. Twice distilled water was employed for the preparation of solutions. Standard stock solutions of mercury, lead, cadmium, nickel, and tin were prepared from Titrasol (1000 mg/L) and were diluted to the related metal solution. The operational solution was prepared by diluting a suitable aliquot of the stock solutions via 1 M HCl and 5% H2SO4 for diluting mercury solution, 10% HNO3 for diluting lead and cadmium solutions, and 5% HCl for diluting nickel and tin solution (Emami Khansari et al., 2005).

Sample collection and digestion: Canned tuna samples were collected from random popular supermarkets in Tabriz (Iran) between January 2011 and October 2011. Forty canned tuna were employed. In this study, digestion procedure was performed as described earlier by Emami Khansari, Ghazi-Khansari and Abdollahi (2005). After unbolting of each can (180 ± 3g), its content was homogenized via food blender. Then, the homogenized sample (2±0.001g) was weighed into a 0.51 glass digestion tube, and for mercury 10 ml of concentrated HNO3 and 5 ml of concentrated H2SO4 were little by little added. Next, the tube was put on top of a steam bath item to be completely dissolved. After the tube had cooled, the solution was cautiously moved into a 50 mL volumetric flagon. For the reduction of mercury, 5mL SnCl2 was employed. For the determination of lead and cadmium, 2±0.001g of homogenized sample was weighed into a 200 mL beaker and 10 mL of concentrated HNO3 were added. A glass coated the beaker and the majority of the sample had dissolved via resting during the night then warmed on a hot plate with boiling until any dynamic reaction settled. The solution was left to cold, and then moved into a 50 mL volumetric flagon and diluted to the mark by means of distilled water. For the determination of nickel and tin, 10±0.001g of homogenized sample were weighed into a beaker and 10mL of concentrated HNO3 were added. After boiling the quantity was decreased to 5mL, concentrated HCl was added and warmed smoothly until the sample bumping finished. Afterward solution was left to cold, and then moved in a 25mL volumetric flagon and diluted to the mark by means of distilled water.

Chemical examination: Mercury was determined via the hydride generation method. The produce process method involves regular adding up of reductant, consisting of 0.3%NaBH4 and 0.5% NaOH. The level of Nickel and Tin was determined via straight aspiration of the sample solution into the NO2/acetylene flame. The blanks and calibration standard solutions were as well examined using a similar technique to the sample solutions. Lead and Cadmium were determined via graphite heating system atomic absorption spectro-photometry, using pyrolytic podium graphite tubes, ascorbic acid, and palladium for medium adjustment and using the process of adding up for quantification (Emami Khansari et al., 2005; Malakootian et al., 2011).

Statistical analyses: The conduct tests were triplicate (n=3). Data were analyzed via one-way analysis of variance (ANOVA). All statistical analyses of data were performed by SPSS 16.0 (SPSS Inc., Chicago, IL, USA) software.

Results

Recoveries of mercury, lead, cadmium, nickel, and tin from canned tuna samples in five brands (A, B, C, D and E) are presented in Table 1.

The accumulation of mercury, lead, cadmium, nickel, and tin in five brands in canned tuna marketed in Tabriz city of Iran were analyzed at the end of the investigational era, which were exposed to the chosen heavy metals (Table 2). In this study; the highest average of Hg was found in the A brand (0.203±0.136 mg/kg $\mu g/g$) and the lowest average was in the D one (0.187±0.125 mg/kg), the highest average of Pb was found in the B brand (0.125±0.087 mg/kg) and the lowest average was in the C one (0.055±0.041 mg/kg), the highest average of Cd was found in the B brand (0.391±0.389 mg/kg) and the lowest average was in the E one (0.076±0.061 mg/kg), the highest average of Ni was found in the B brand (0.348±0.198 mg/kg) and the lowest average was in the C one (0.262±0.152 mg/kg) and the highest average of Sn was found in the A brand (0.47±0.487 mg/kg) and the lowest average was in the D one (0.086±0.353 mg/kg). Statistical analysis of results via ANOVA demonstrated no major variations among all samples.

Table 1. Recoveries of mercury, lead, cadmium, nickel and tin from canned tuna samples in five brands (A, B, C, D and E).

Tuna fish	%Recovery				
	Hg	Pb	Cd	Ni	Sn
A	95	100	95	99	100
B	95	103	96	100	102
C	95	100	95	99.5	99.6
D	93	98	90	97	100
E	95	101	95	100	99.8

Discussion

Data of heavy metal concentrations in fish is significant with regard to the nature of managing and human being consumption of fish. Fish is regularly at the top of the foodstuff chain and has the affinity to concentrate heavy metals from water (Mansour and Sidky, 2002; Rauf et al., 2009). Consequently, bio-accumulation of metals in fish can be considered as an index of metal contamination in the aquatic bodies that possibly will be a practical implement to study the natural function of metals present at upper concentrations in fish (Ikem and Egiebor, 2005; Rauf et al., 2009).

Mercury (Hg): Mercury in fish fleshy tissue can signify an ecological and human health risk to those ingesting the fish (Hutcheson et al., 2008). Mercury possibly will make changes in the regular growth of the brain of children and at higher levels might make neurological changes in adults (Commission of the European Communities, 2001; Ikem and Egiebor, 2005). Furthermore, Mercury has toxicity result on the kidney, and it is probably a carcinogen (Occupational Safety and Health Administration, 2004; Inskip and Piotrowsiki, 1985; Mergler et al., 2007). Tuna can accumulate a large amount of mercury and methyl mercury (Castro-Gonzalez and Mendez-Armenta, 2008; Emami Khansari et al., 2005; Ikem and Egiebor, 2005; Malakootian et al., 2011; Mansour and Sidky, 2002; Voegborlo et al., 1999). In this study, the average Hg concentration was investigated in five brands; A, B, C, D, and E which were 0.203±0.136, 0.195±0.13, 0.154±0.101, 0.102±0.136 and 0.187±0.125 mg/kg, respectively. All the samples were below the acceptable limits

Table 2. Range and mean values (±SD) of mercury, lead, cadmium, nickel and tin (mg/kg)in five brands (A, B, C, D and E) in canned tuna fish (n=3).

Tuna fish	Heavy metals									
	Hg		Pb		Cd		Ni		Sn	
	Range	Mean ± SD	Range	Mean ± SD	Range	Mean ± SD	Range	Mean ± SD	Range	Mean ± SD
A	0.109-0.298	0.203±0.136	0.002-0.109	0.090±0.048	0.151-0.359	0.236±0.134	0.005-0.988	0.312±0.211	0.102-1.099	0.470±0.487
B	0.100-1.335	0.195±0.130	0.055-0.653	0.125±0.087	0.099-0.854	0.391±0.389	0.001-0.775	0.348±0.198	0.004-0.652	0.303±0.340
C	0.010-0.333	0.154±0.101	0.000-0.259	0.055±0.041	0.012-0.895	0.266±0.143	0.008-0.951	0.262±0.152	0.040-0.299	0.144±0.412
D	0.000-0.319	0.102±0.136	0.006-0.851	0.076±0.057	0.001-0.557	0.106±0.063	0.018-1.000	0.327±0.243	0.000-0.991	0.086±0.353
E	0.095-0.326	0.187±0.125	0.017-0.451	0.098±0.064	0.031-0.099	0.076±0.061	0.000-0.394	0.297±0.234	0.008-1.014	0.403±0.430

recommended as 0.5 mg/kg (EU, 2005; FAO, 1983; FAO/WHO, 1972; Mergler et al., 2007). In a similar study, Emami Khansari, Ghazi-Khansari and Abdollahi (2005) determined the average concentration of Hg in canned tuna in Iran. They reported the average Hg contents as 0.117 mg/kg.

Lead (Pb): Lead is broadly distributed in environment and solder employed in the produce of cans is an important resource of contamination of food via Pb (Mol, 2011). Lead can reduce cognitive growth and intellectual performance in kids and cause high blood pressure and cardiovascular syndrome in adults (Commission of the European Communities, 2001; Ikem and Egiebor, 2005; Malakootian et al., 2011). Consequently, monitoring lead concentration becomes very important. In accordance with European commission (EC) 2001 instruction and FAO/WHO (1972), the highest lead level acceptable for canned fish are 0.4 and 0.5 mg/kg, respectively. In this study, all the samples were lower than the acceptable limits recommended as 0.2 mg/kg (EC) and 0.5 mg/kg (FAO/WHO). In a similar study, Malakootian et al. (2011) determined Pb concentration in sixteen brands of canned tuna in southern Iran. They reported the greatest average concentration of lead in four brands (Sahel, Jonob, Bartar and Darya) was 0.3 mg/kg and the lowest average of lead concentration in one brand (Bist) was 0.11 mg/kg. In another study, Emami Khansari, Ghazi-Khansari and Abdollahi (2005) reported the average Pb concentration as 0.0366 mg/kg in canned tuna in Iran. Ashraf (2006) studied the concentration of lead in some samples of tuna in Saudi Arabia. He reported the quantity of lead in tuna 0.002, 0.21, 0.23, and 0.84 mg/kg in every sample.

Cadmium (Cd): Large amounts of cadmium can cause chronic toxicity, including impaired renal function, poor reproductive ability, skeletal damage, hepatic dysfunction, hypertension, and cancers (Commission of the European Communities, 2001; Ikem and Egiebor, 2005; Mol, 2011). FAO (1983) recommended the highest limit for this metal in fish as 0.5 mg/kg. Moreover, in accordance with EC 2001 highest limit of cadmium in fish is 0.05 mg/kg (Malakootian et al., 2011; Sivaperumal et al., 2007). In this study, all the samples were lower than the acceptable limits recommended as 0.5 mg/kg (FAO). Malakootian et al., (2011), and Emami Khansari, Ghazi-Khansari and Abdollahi (2005), reported the average concentration of Cd, 0.019 and 0.022 mg/kg in canned tuna in Iran.

Nickel (Ni): Nickel is also one of the important heavy metals that tuna can accumulate in its tissue. Ni can cause respiratory difficulties, nervous and digestive disorders, psychological problems, and also it is carcinogenic (Ashraf et al., 2006; Ikem and Egiebor, 2005). In the studied tuna, the quantity of Ni was below the US-EPA standards (Joyeux et al., 2004; Malakootian et al., 2011). In a similar study, Malakootian et al., (2011) reported the average concentration of Ni, 0.24 mg/kg in canned tuna fish in southern Iran.

Tin (Sn): Too much consumption of Sn possibly will cause gastrointestinal irritation, nausea, vomiting, diarrhea, anemia, kidney and liver difficulties, and skin and eye irritation (Ikem and Egiebor, 2005). Estimation of tin in canned foodstuff is significant for the quality evaluation. For the reason that, Sn content shows the level of corrosion of the container, consequently influences the acceptability of foodstuff (Mol, 2011). As a matter of fact, a chief resource of Sn contamination in canned foodstuffs is poor lacquering of canned containers. Other reasons that can speed up the leaching of Sn from metal containers into seafood comprise the pH of the food in the can, temperature of the canned foods, storage time, and exposure to atmosphere of opened canned fish (Ikem and Egiebor, 2005; Mol, 2011). In this study, Sn concentrations were under the acceptable limit of 250 mg/kg (Mol, 2011) in every one of the samples. Emami Khansari, Ghazi-Khansari and Abdollahi (2005) reported the average concentration of Sn as non-detectable. In another study, the middling of 0.140 mg/kg and 0.023 mg/kg were attained for canned anchovies and for canned rainbow trout, respectively (Mol, 2011).

The results of this study showed that tuna fish (in five brands; A, B, C, D and E fore examples) fabricated and marketed in Tabriz (Iran) had safe level of heavy metals that were lower than the averages of EC/FAO/WHO levels for these toxic metals.

Acknowledgments

The authors would like to express their gratitude to Mr. Jamal Jafari Sarai for his beneficial comments about the grammaticality of the manuscript.

References

1. Ashraf, W., Seddigi, Z., Abulkibash, A., Khalid M. (2006) Levels of selected metals in canned fish consumed in kingdom of Saudi Arabia. Environ Monit Assess. 117: 271-279.
2. Burgera, J., Gochfeld, M. (2005) Heavy metals in commercial fish in New Jersey. Environ Res. 99: 403-412.
3. Castro-Gonzalez, M. I., Mendez-Armenta M. (2008) Heavy metals: Implications associated to fish consumption. Environ Toxicol Pharmacol. 26: 263-271.
4. Commission of the European Communities (2001) Commission Regulation (EC), No. 221/2002 of 6 February 2002 amending regulation (EC) No. 466/2002 setting maximum levels for certain contaminations in foodstuffs. Official J Eur Uni. Brussels, Belgium.
5. Dural, M., Lugal GÖksu, M. Z., Akif Özak, A. (2007) Investigation of heavy metal levels in economically important fish species captured from the Tuzla lagoon. Food Chem. 102: 415-421.
6. Emami Khansari, F., Ghazi-Khansari, M., Abdollahi, M. (2005) Heavy metals content of canned tuna fish. Food Chem. 93: 293-296.
7. EU. (2005) Commission regulation as regards heavy metals. Amending Regulation, 466/2001, No. 78/2005.
8. FAO. (1983) Compilation of legal limits for hazardous substances in fish and fishery products. In: FAO Fishery Circular, Inland Water Resources and Aquaculture Service, No. 464. Rome, Italy. p. 5-100.
9. FAO/WHO. (1972) Evaluation of certain food additives and the contaminants mercury, cadmium and lead. WHO Technical Report Series. No. 505. Geneva: WHO. Geneva, Switzerland.
10. FDA. (2011) Fish and fishers products hazards and controls guidance. In: U.S. Food and Drug Administration center for food safety and applied nutrition chapter 9, Environmental Chemical Contaminants and Pesticides. (4rd ed.) New Hampshire, USA. p. 155-180.
11. Hutcheson, M.S., Smith, C.M., Wallace, G.T., Rose, J., Eddy, B., Sullivan, J., Pancorbo, O., west, C.R. (2008) Freshwater fish mercury concentrations in a regionally high mercury deposition area. Water Air Soil Pollut. 191: 15-31.
12. Ikem, A., Egiebor, N.O. (2005) Assessment of trace elements in canned fishes (mackerel, tuna, salmon, sardines and herrings) marketed in Georgia and Alabama (United States of America). J Food Comp Anal. 18: 771-787.
13. Inskip, M. J., Piotrowsiki, J. K. (1985) Review of the health effects of methyl mercury. J Appl Toxicol. 5: 113-133.
14. Joyeux, J.C., Campanha Filho, E.A., Jesus, H.C. (2004) Trace metal contamination in estuarient ria

fishest Bay, ES, Brazil. Braz Arch Biol Technol. 47: 8509-8515.

15. Malakootian, M., Tahergorabi, M., Daneshpajooh, M., Amirtaheri, K. (2011) Determination of Pb, Cd, Ni, and Zn concentrations in canned fish in southern Iran. Sacha J Environ Stud. 1: 94-100.
16. Mansour, S.A., Sidky, M.M. (2002) Ecotoxicological studies. 3: Heavy metals contaminating water and fish from Fayoum Governorate, Egypt. Food Chem. 78: 15-22.
17. Mergler, D., Anderson, H.A., Chan, L.H.M., Mahaffey, K.R., Murray, M., Sakamoto, M., Stern, H. (2007) Methylmercury exposure and health effects in humans: A worldwide concern. Ambio. 36: 3-11.
18. Mol, S. (2011) Determination of trace metals in canned anchovies and canned rainbow trouts. Food Chem Toxicol. 49: 348-351.
19. Occupational Safety and Health Administration (2004) Toxic metals, Occupational Safety and Health Administration. US department of labor, 200 constitution avenue, NW, Washington DC, USA.
20. Olowu, R.A., Ayejuyo, O.O., Adewuyi, G.O., Adejoro, I.A., Denloye, A.A.B., Babatunde, A.O., Ogundajo, A.L. (2010) Determination of heavy metals in fish tissues, water and sediment from Epe and Badagry Lagoons, Lagos, Nigeria. E-J Chem. 7: 215-221.
21. Qiao-qiao, C., Guang-wei, Z., Langdon, A. (2007) Bioaccumulation of heavy metals in fishes from Taihu Lake, China. J Environ Sci. 19: 1500-1504.
22. Rauf, A., Javed, M., Ubaidullah, M. (2009) Heavy metal levels in three major Carps (Catla Catla, Labeo Rohita and Cirrhina Mrigala) from the river Ravi, Pakistan. Pak Vet J. 29: 24-26.
23. Schmitt, C.J., Brumbaugh, W.G. (1990) National contamination biomonitoring program: Concentrations of arsenic, cadmium, copper, lead, mercury, selenium and zinc in US fresh water fish, 1976-1984. Arch Environ Contam Toxicol. 19: 731-747.
24. Sivaperumal, P., Sankar, T.V., Viswanthan Nair, P.G. (2007) Heavy metal concentrations in fish, shellfish and fish products from internal markets of India vis-à-vis international standards. Food Chem. 102: 612-620.
25. Türkmen, A., Türkmen, M., Tepe, T., Akyurt, I. (2005) Heavy metals in three commercially valuable fish species from Iskenderun Bay, Northern East Mediterranean Sea, Turkey. Food Chem. 91: 167-172.
26. Tüzen, M. (2003) Determination of heavy metals in fish samples of the middle Black Sea (Turkey) by graphite furnace atomic absorption spectrometry. Food Chem. 80: 119-123.
27. Vinodhini, R., Narayanan, M. (2008) Bioaccumulation of heavy metals in organs of fresh water fish Cyprinus carpio (Common carp). Int J Environ Sci Technol. 5: 179-182.
28. Voegborlo, R.B., El-Methnani, A.M., Abedin, M.Z. (1999) Mercury, cadmium and lead content of canned tuna fish. Food Chem. 67: 341-345.
29. Yi, Y., Yang, Z., Zhang, S. (2011) Ecological risk assessment of heavy metals in sediment and human health risk assessment of heavy metals in fishes in the middle and lower reaches of the Yangtze River basin. Environ Pollut. 159: 2575-2585.
30. Yilmaz, F., Özdemir, N., Demirak, A., Tuna, A.L. (2007) Heavy metal levels in two fish spices Leucisus cephalus and Lepomis gibbosus. Food Chem. 100: 830-835.

12

Ghrelin improves rat sperm kinematic parameters during abdominal position of the testis

Kheradmand, A.*

Department of Clinical Sciences, School of Veterinary Medicine, Lorestan University, Khorram Abad, Iran

Key words:
cryptorchidism, ghrelin, rat, sperm quality

Correspondence
Kheradmand, A.*
Department of Clinical Sciences,
School of Veterinary Medicine,
Lorestan University, Khorram Abad,
Iran

Email: arashkheradmand@yahoo.com

Abstract:

BACKGROUND: Disruption of testicular function and arrest of spermatogenesis are the consequence of cryptorchidism in response to elevated temperature. **OBJECTIVES:** This investigation was set to clarify the possible ghrelin efficacy in altering some sperm quality parameters upon experimentally-induced cryptorchidism. **METHODS:** Thirty male adult rats were scheduled for the study and were divided into three groups: group 1 was served as control-saline (CS), group 2 was designed as cryptorchidism-saline (CrS), and group 3 was defined as cryptorchidism-ghrelin (CrG). After surgically inducing cryptorchidism in groups 2 and 3, the researchers gave 10 nmol of ghrelin to CrG rats for 7 consecutive days. Five animals in each group were equally killed on days 3 and 7 after operation and their testes were taken for sperm evaluation. **RESULTS:** Testicular weight, sperm forward progressive motility (FPM), functional membrane integrity (assessed by HOS-test), and sperm concentration displayed slight changes after heating on day 3. However, abdominal position of the testes for 7 days caused a significant reduction in the percentages of HOS-positive cells ($p<0.0001$), FPM ($p<0.0001$), and sperm concentration ($p<0.01$). Although a 30% decrease occurred in the testicular weight at this point, however, this reduction was not statistically significant. Interestingly, HOS-test and FPM percentages were significantly higher in the ghrelin-exposed animals compared to the CrS group on day 7 ($p<0.05$). However, ghrelin treatment had not considerable influence on sperm parameters by day 3. Moreover, sperm concentration and testicular weight did not exhibit any changes either on day 3 or at day 7 upon ghrelin injection ($p>0.05$). **CONCLUSIONS:** Indeed, this function of ghrelin could be attributed to its antioxidant properties and it may be implicated as a potential agent in attenuation of impaired spermatogenesis after cryptorchidism.

Introduction

It has been established that in mammals, lower scrotal temperature is require for normal spermatogenesis (Shikone et al., 1994). Failure in testicular descending into the scrotum or cryptorchidism induced by surgery in rats results in disruption of spermatogenesis (Jegou et al., 1983). The spermatogenesis disorder and subsequent male infertility is due to the germ cell loss in response to abdominal elevated temperature (Liu et al., 2012). It has been well shown that an increased level of reactive oxygen species (ROS) and lipid peroxidation, as sign of oxidative stress, are associated with cryptorchid testes which cause impaired spermatogenesis (Peltola et al., 1995; Kumagai et al., 2002). Changes in the lipids containing polyunsaturated fatty acids have also been indicated (Furland et al., 2007).

Therefore, it seems that antioxidant therapy may attenuate the adverse effects of ROS on the spermatogenesis and inhibit the changes in spermatozoa membrane lipids during cryptorchidism.

It has been recently proposed that ghrelin is an endogenous antioxidant and functions as a free radical scavenger (Dong and Kaunitz, 2006). The antioxidative properties of ghrelin via increasing the antioxidant enzymes activities and reducing lipid peroxidation have been newly reported in our laboratory in the normal rat testis (Kheradmand et al., 2009a,b) and ovary (Kheradmand et al., 2010), as well as in other tissues such as preadipocyte cell culture (Zwirska-Korczala et al., 2007) and gastric injuries (Iseri et al., 2005; El Eter et al., 2007). The ghrelin gene is expressed in stomach, small intestine, brain, pituitary, salivary gland, adrenal, ovary, and testis (Ghelardoni et al., 2006). Within the testis, expression of ghrelin has been demonstrated in mature Leydig cells of rats and humans. In addition, expression of the functional ghrelin receptor, the GHS-R type 1a, has been shown in Sertoli and Leydig cells (Tena-Sempere, 2005; Barreiro and Tena-Sempere, 2004). The expression of GHS-R 1a in the seminiferous tubules strongly suggests that the seminiferous epithelium might be a target for ghrelin action and directly regulates seminiferous tubules function (Barreiro and Tena-Sempere, 2004).

Thus, with regard to these literatures, this study attempted to examine the possible ghrelin protective effects on rat sperm quality and membrane integrity following experimentally induced cryptorchidism.

Materials and Methods

Animals: Thirty male Wistar rats weighing 200 to 220 gr were used for the experiment. The animals were maintained under constant conditions of light (12 h of light, from 07:00 h) in an animal room in groups of five rats per cage and controlled temperature (21-24°C) with free access to pelleted food and tap water. Rat lyophilised acylated ghrelin (n-octanoylated research grade) were purchased from Tocris Cookson Ltd. (Bristol, UK).

Surgical technique: The animals were randomly divided into three equal groups (each containing 10 rats): group 1 was served as sham-operated or control-saline (CS), group 2 was defined as cryptorchidism-saline (CrS), and group 3 was assumed as cryptorchidism-ghrelin (CrG) animals. Surgical procedure for induction of bilateral cryptorchidism was performed according to the method of inguinoscrotal approach as previously described by Dundar et al. (2001). General anesthesia was achieved intraperitonealy by a combination of 70 mg kg_{-1} of ketamin and 5 mg kg_{-1} of xylazine hydrocholoride. After anesthesia, the scrotal area was shaved and prepared by povidone iodine solution. In groups 2 and 3, inguinoscrotal region was incised and gubernaculum was separated where it protruded from the abdominal wall, and then the external inguinal ring was revealed. After pushing the gubernaculum into the abdominal cavity, the external inguinal ring and inguinoscrotal wall was closed by 2.0 simple silk suture. During the sham operation, both testes were brought through the incision and then replaced after a few manipulations. Immediately after surgery, CrG rats were given ghrelin subcutaneously (10 nmol/100 μL saline) for 7 consecutive days. Five rats from each group were killed upon diethyl ether anesthesia by decapitation on days 3 and 7 after surgery for sperm evaluation parameters.

Sperm collection and evaluation: Immediately after rats were killed and the weight of each testicle was measured, the right epididymis of three groups were removed and trimmed of fat. Rat spermatozoa were obtained using Cancel et al.'s (2000) method. Briefly, 5 mm of right cauda epididymis was minced in 2-ml of physiological saline and incubated at 37°C for 30 min to allow dispersion of spermatozoa. The obtained spermatozoa from all groups were assessed for forward progressive movement, plasma membrane integrity, and sperm concentration.

The FPM percentage (of the motile spermatozoa showing progressive movement) was assessed according to the method as previously described by Sonmez et al. (2005). The fluid obtained from cauda epididymis was diluted to 2 mL of PBS and an aliquot of this suspension was placed on the microscope slide covered with a coverslip and examined visually under a light microscope at the magnification of 400. Motility estimations were performed from four different fields in each sample and the mean of the four estimations was used as the final motility score. Samples for motility evaluation were kept at 37°C.

To evaluate the membrane integrity, hypoosmotic

swelling (HOS) test was applied. Assessment of functional integrity of sperm membrane was determined by HOS-water test according to the method as described previously by Sliwa and Macura (2005). In short, 10 μL of sperm was added into 0.4 mL of distilled water and incubated for 5 minutes at 37°C. The swelling reaction was measured by counting of spermatozoa with curled tail using a light microscope at magnification of 400. All of the examinations above were performed by the same person, counting at least 100 sperms.

The concentration of spermatozoa was determined after adding 50 μL of sperm into the 1 mL of formalin-saline to achieve the dilution rate of 1:20. Approximately, 10 μL of the diluted sperm suspension was transferred to each counting chamber of the haemocytometer and the total number of spermatozoa per mL was counted with the help of light microscope.

Statistical analysis: Results were analyzed using the SPSS/PC program. All data were tested for normality and thereafter by Levene static test for homogeneity of variance. When the variance was homogenous, testicular weight, FPM, HOS-positive percentage, and sperm concentration among the CS, CrS, and CrG rats at different days were separately analyzed using one-way ANOVA and Tukey test as post hoc, in order to determine the difference among groups (Petrie and Watson, 1999). Data are presented as mean ± SEM.

Results

Testicular weight: Abdominal position of the testes was associated with not significant decrease in testicular weight particularly on day 7. However, the changes were negligible after 3 days of exposure to heat. As indicated in figure 1, ghrelin treatment was not able to enhance testicular weight to its normal value up to day 7 ($p>0.05$).

Assessment of sperm motility: The results of the FPM analysis are depicted in Figure 2. Testicular hyperthermia resulted in a drastic decrease in the percentages of FPM in both CrS and CrG animals on day 7 ($p<0.0001$). Notably, ghrelin administration significantly promoted FPM rate compared to the CrS rats (19.80 ± 1.85% versus 4.40 ± 2.11%) on day 7 ($p<0.01$). However, it was still lower than that of the control group at this point ($p<0.001$).

Plasma membrane integrity: Exposure to abdominal heat for three days did not affect the mean values of HOS-reactive spermatozoa among groups. In contrast, examining the data revealed that the spermatozoa with functionally intact membrane were reduced by day 7 after surgery in both CrS and CrG animals ($p<0.01$, Figure 3). Ghrelin exposure could enhance the percentage of HOS-positive cells compared to the CrS group at day 7 (38.80 ± 3.78% versus 22.40 ± 4.38%, $p<0.05$).

Sperm concentration: Abdominal testicular temperature caused a marked reduction in the number of spermatozoa on day 7 ($p<0.01$). However, the comparison of the data on day 3 did not exhibit significant differences among groups. In addition, ghrelin failed to alter the sperm number compared to the CrS rats on day 7 ($p>0.05$, Figure 4.).

Discussion

The results of the present study are probably the first which clearly demonstrated the ghrelin ability in promotion of main sperm quality parameters, progressive motility, and functional membrane integrity following experimentally-induced cryptorchidsm in the rat testis. However, it failed to change the sperm concentration and testicular weight upon treatment.

The expression of functional ghrelin receptor in the seminiferous tubules strongly suggests that the seminiferous epithelium might be a target for ghrelin action and might directly regulate seminiferous tubules functions (Barreiro and Tena-Sempere, 2004). In human, a positive correlation between the percentage of swollen sperm and that of motile sperm was seen (Chan et al., 1985). Likewise, the high correlation ($r=0.90$) between the percentage of sperm in semen sample that were capable of swelling and the percentage of zona-free hamster oocytes that were penetrated by sperms from the same semen samples were found (Jeyendran et al., 1984). This may be the reason of why the sperm motility rate is greater in the treated animals when the HOS percentage was high. Because in the current work, the increase in the HOS-positive cells in the ghrelin-exposed animals was associated with the simultaneous and significant improvement in the FPM rate by day 7.

The sperm plasma membrane contains a high

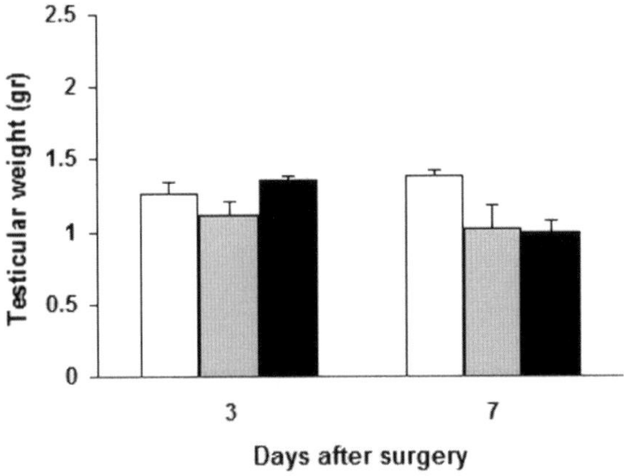

Figure 1. Mean ± SEM of testicular weight on 3th and 7th days after induction of cryptorchidism in three experimental groups. The data did not represent significant differences among groups. □ Control-saline ▩ Cryptorchidism-saline ■ Cryptorchidism-ghrelin

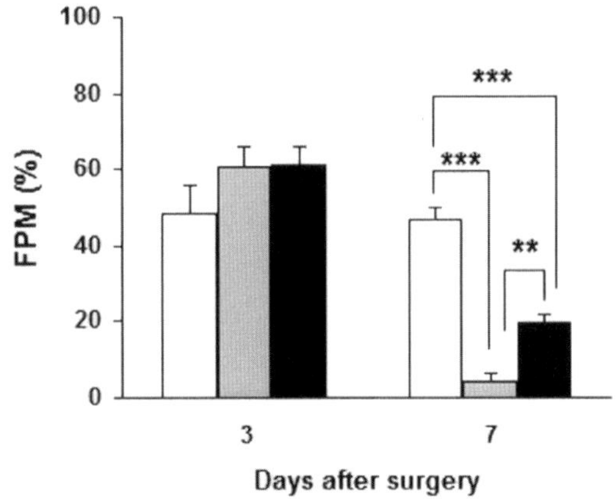

Figure 2. Mean ± SEM of FPM percentages on 3th and 7th days after induction of cryptorchidism in three experimental groups. All means marked with *($p<0.05$), **($p<0.01$) and ***($p<0.001$) are significantly different from each other. □Control-saline ▩Cryptorchidism-saline ■Cryptorchidism-ghrelin

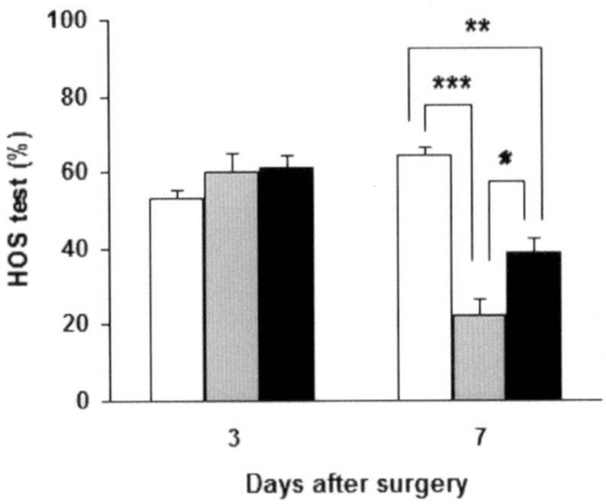

Figure 3. Mean ± SEM of HOS test percentages on 3th and 7th days after induction of cryptorchidism in three experimental groups. All means marked with *($p<0.05$), **($p<0.01$) and ***($p<0.001$) are significantly different from each other. □Control-saline ▩Cryptorchidism-saline ■Cryptorchidism-ghrelin

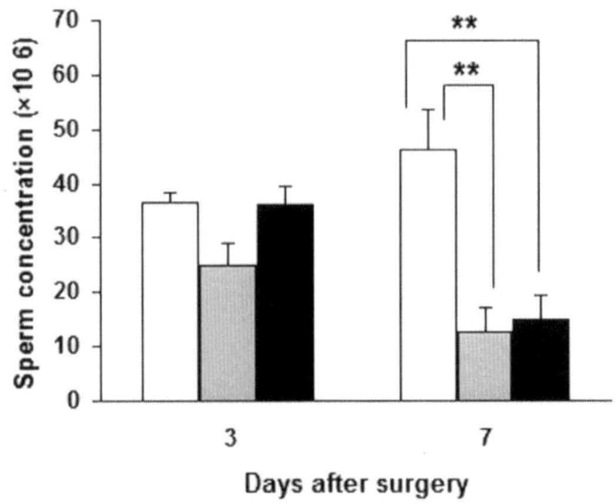

Figure 4. Mean ± SEM of sperm concentration on 3th and 7th days after induction of cryptorchidism in three experimental groups. All means marked with **($p<0.01$) are significantly different from each other. □Control-saline ▩Cryptorchidism-saline ■Cryptorchidism-ghrelin

amount of unsaturated fatty acids which can be attacked by ROS and therefore is particularly susceptible to peroxidative damages with subsequent loss of membrane integrity, impaired cell function and decreased motility of spermatozoa. This oxidative stress is one of the factors associated with decline in fertility of spermatozoa (Aitken et al., 1989; Tramer et al., 1998). Furthermore, the high level of polyunsaturated fatty acids in mammalian testes previously reported (Aitken et al., 1989; Robinson et al., 1992) suggests that the plasma membranes of most testicular cells may be greatly susceptible to free radical attack. In this sense, it has been well documented that impaired detoxification of ROS results in the oxidative stress and increased peroxidation of cellular lipids in abdominal position of the testes (Ahotupa and Huhtaniemi, 1992; Peltola et al., 1995; Furland et al., 2007).

It is believed that ghrelin is one of the endogenous antioxidants that attenuate the oxidative stress responses (Dong and Kaunitz, 2006). Therefore, enhancement of the HOS-reactive spermatozoa following ghrelin administration is possibly due to the antioxidant properties of this hormone which resulted in higher motility index 7 day after operation. This may be the reason for greater sperm motility in the treated animals simultaneous with increment in the HOS percentage.

In most mammalian species, the testis is kept approximately 4-5°C below body temperature. It is well established that cryptorchidism induced by surgery results in disruption of spermatogenesis (Liu et al., 2012; Barqawi et al., 2004). Cryptorchidism induces complete arrest of spermatogenesis by 2 days (Kumar et al., 2012) or 4 days (Barqawi et al., 2004) of post operation. In cryptorchid rats, spermatogenic arrest is associated with the formation of multinuclear giant cells leading to large scale apoptosis and elimination of germ cells from the seminiferous epithelium. Subsequently, many large and small giant cells populate the affected tubules (Kumar et al., 2012; Barqawi et al., 2004). It was indicated that the percentage of motile spermatozoa started to decrease not significantly 1 day after surgery; however, it decreased significantly and reached to 50% of the control group level on day 5 of post operation (Ren et al., 2006). In the present study, the percentages of FPM were unchanged among groups until day 3; however, there was a drastic reduction in the spermatozoa showing progressive movement on day 7. However, the most surprising finding in the current study was the beneficial effects of ghrelin on sperm kinematic parameter,to a point that it could significantly elevate the sperm motility in CrG animals on day 7. In fact, it seems that the improvement in the functional membrane integrity (HOS reaction) on 7 days after ghrelin administration resulted in the greater sperm motility at this point. This action of ghrelin is probably mediated through its antioxidant properties. We have demonstrated that ghrelin significantly increases antioxidant enzyme activities and reduces MDA level, as lipid peroxidation marker, in the rat normal testis (Kheradmand et al., 2009a). Likewise, very recently, we have shown that ghrelin acts as a suppressor of testicular histopathological damage following experimentally induced cryptorchidism in the rat (Kheradmand et al., 2014).

The sperm concentration was another parameter that was investigated in our study. It was shown that testicular sperm count begins to decline rapidly at day 7 after cryptorchidism induction (Barqawi et al., 2004). Abdominal temperature caused a marked drop in the number of spermatozoa in both CrS and CrG groups on day 7. However, ghrelin was not able to enhance sperm concentration prominently. The action of ghrelin upon testicular stem cell factor (SCF) mRNA expression may have implications not only in Leydig cell proliferation, but also in the control of spermatogenesis. SCF has been pointed out as the major paracrine stimulator of germ cell development, and it also acts as a survival factor for spermatogonia, spermatocytes and spermatids in the adult rat seminiferous epithelium (Budak et al., 2006; Hakovitra et al., 1999). In this sense, intratesticular injection of ghrelin (15 μg for 2 day) in adult rats inhibited expression of the gene encoding stem cell factor (SCF), a key signal in spermatogenesis and putative regulator of Leydig cell development. Thus it was logical for ghrelin not to be able to alter sperm count remarkably. A similar result was also obtained in our earlier report in which the sperm concentration was unchanged during ghrelin therapy in the normal healthy rats (Kheradmand et al., 2009b).

In conclusion, this study indicated the ghrelin efficacy in improvement of rat sperm quality, forward progressive movement and functional membrane integrity, following exposure to abdominal temperature induced by experimental cryptorchidism. This may have potential implication that ghrelin could be used as a promising agent for spermatogenesis recovery in the heat-induced infertility.

Acknowledgments

This study was financially supported by research project (No. 906021) of Research Vice-Chancellery of Lorestan University in common to Lorestan University of Medical Sciences, Iran.

References

1. Ahotupa, M., Huhtaniemi, I. (1992) Impaired detoxification of reactive oxygen and consequent oxidative stress in experimentally cryporchid rat testis. Biol Reprod. 46: 1114-1118.
2. Aitken, R.J., Clarkson, J.S., Fishel, S. (1989) Generation of reactive oxygen species, lipid peroxidation and human sperm function. Biol Reprod. 41: 183-197.
3. Barqawi, A., Tummer, H., Meacham, R. (2004)

Effect of prolonged cryptorchidism on germ cell apoptosis and testicular sperm count. Asian J Androl. 6: 47-51.

4. Barreiro, M.L., Tena-Sempere, M. (2004) Ghrelin and reproduction: a novel signal linking energy status and fertility? Mol Cell Endocrinol. 226: 1-9.
5. Budak, E., Fernandez-Sanchez, M., Bellver, J., Cervero, A., Simon, C., Pellicer, A. (2006) Intractions of the hormones leptin, ghrelin, adiponectin, resistin and PYY3-36 with the reproductive system. Fertil Steril. 85: 1563-1581.
6. Cancel, A.M., Lobdell, D., Mendola, P., Perreault, S.D. (2000) Objective evaluation of hyperactivated motility in rat spermatozoa using computer-assisted sperm analysis. Hum Reprod. 15: 1322-1328.
7. Chan, S.Y., Fox, E.J., Chan, M.M.C. (1985) The relationship between the human sperm hypoosmotic swelling test, routine semen analysis, and the human sperm zona-free hamster ovum penetration assay. Hum Reprod. 44: 668-672.
8. Dong, M.H., Kaunitz, J.D. (2006) Gastroduodenal mucosal defense. Curr Opin Gastroentrol. 22: 599-606.
9. Dundar, M., Kocak, I., Culhaci, N. (2001) A new experimental model for cryptorchidism: inguino-scrotal approach. Urol Res. 29: 178-181.
10. El Eter, E., Al Tuwarijiri, A., Hagar, H., Arafa, M. (2007) In vitro and in vivo antioxidant activity of ghrelin: attenuation of gastric ischemic injury in the rat. J Gastroen Hepatol. 22: 1791-1799.
11. Furland, N.E., Maldonado, E.N., Aresti, P.A., Aveldano, M.I. (2007) Changes in lipids containing long-and very long chain polyunsaturated fatty acids in cryptorchid rat testes. Biol Reprod. 77: 181-188.
12. Ghelardoni, S., Carnicelli, V., Frascarelli, S., Ronca-Testoni, S., Zucchi, R. (2006) Ghrelin tissue distribution: comparison between gene and protein expression. J Endocrinol Invest. 29: 115-121.
13. Hakovitra, H., Yan, W., Kaleva, M., Zhang, F., Vanttinen, K., Morris, P.L., Soder, M., Parvinen, M., Toppari, J. (1999) Function of stem cell factor as a survival factor of spermatogonia and localization of messenger ribonucleic acid in the rat seminiferous epithelium. Endocrinology. 140: 1492-1498.
14. Jegou, B., Laws, A.O., Kretser, D.M. (1983) The effect of cryptorchidism and subsequent orchidopexy on testicular function in adult rats. J Reprod Fertil. 69: 137-145.
15. Jeyendran, R.S., Van Der Ven, H.H., Perez-Pelaez, M., Crabo, B.G., Zaneveld, L.J.D. (1984) Development of an assay to assess the functional integrity of the human sperm membrane and its relationship to other semen chracteristics. J Reprod Fertil. 70: 219-228.
16. Kheradmand, A., Alirezaei, M., Asadian, P., Rafiei Alavi, E., Joorabi, S. (2009a) Antioxidant enzyme activity and MDA level in the rat testis following chronic administration of ghrelin. Andrologia. 41: 335-340.
17. Kheradmand, A., Taati, M., Babaei, H. (2009b) The effects of chronic administration of ghrelin on rat sperm quality and membrane integrity. Anim Biol. 59: 159-168.
18. Kheradmand, A., Dezfoulian, O., Alirezaei, M., Hadian, B. (2014) Ghrelin is a suppressor of testicular damage following experimentally induced cryptorchidism in the rat. J Pediatr Surg. 49: 593-98.
19. Kheradmand, A., Alirezaei, M., Birjandi, M. (2010) Ghrelin promotes antioxidant enzyme activity and reduces lipid peroxidation in the rat ovary. Regul Pept. 162: 84-89.
20. Kumar, V., Misro, M.M., Datta, K. (2012) Simultaneous accumulation of hyaluronan binding protein 1 (HABP1/p32/gC1qR) and apoptotic induction of germ cells in cryptorchid testis. J Androl. 33: 114-121.
21. Iseri, S.O., Sener, G., Yuksel, M., Contuk, G., Cetinel, S., Gedik, N., Yegen, B.C. (2005) Ghrelin against alendronate-induced gastric damage in rats. J Endocrinol. 187: 399-406.
22. Liu, F., Huang, H., Xu, Z., Qian, X.J., Qiu, W.Y. (2012) Germ cell removal after induction of cryptorchidism in adult rats. Tissue Cell. 44: 281-287.
23. Peltola, V., Huhtaniemi, I., Ahotupa, M. (1995) Abdominal position of the rat testis is associated with high level of lipid peroxidation. Biol Reprod. 53: 1146-1150.
24. Petrie, A., Watson, P. (1999) Statistics for Veterinary and Animal Science. (1st ed.) Blackwell Science, London, UK.
25. Robinson, B.S., Johnson, D.W., Poulos, A. (1992) Novel molecular species of sphingomyelin containing 2-hydroxylated polyenoic very-long-chain fatty acids in mammalian testes and spermatozoa. J Biol Chem. 267: 1746-1751.

26. Shikone, T., Billig, H., Hsueh, A.J.W. (1994) Experimentally induced cryptorchidism increases apoptosis in rat testis. Biol Reprod. 51: 865-872.
27. Sliwa, L., Macura, B. (2005) Evaluation of cell membrane integrity of spermatozoa by hypoosmotic swelling test-water test in mice after intraperitoneal daidzein administration. Arch Androl. 51: 443-448.
28. Sonmez, M., Turk, G., Yuce, A. (2005) The effect of ascorbic acid supplementation on sperm quality, lipid peroxidation and testosterone levels of male Wistar rats. Theriogenology. 63: 2063-2072.
29. Tena-Sempere, M. (2005) Ghrelin: novel regulator of gonadal function. J Endocrinol Invest. 28: 26-29.
30. Tramer, F., Rocco, F., Micali, F., Sandri, G., Panfili, E. (1998) Antioxidant systems in rat epididymal spermatozoa. Biol Reprod. 59: 753-758.
31. Zwirska-Korczala, K., Adamczyk-Sowa, M., Sowa, P., Pilc, K., Suchanek, R., Pierzchala, K., Namyslowski, G., Misiolek, M., Sodowski, K., Kato, I., Kuwahara, A., Zabielski, R. (2007) Role of leptin, ghrelin, angiotensin II and orexins in 3T3 L1 preadipocyte cells proliferation and oxidative metabolism. J Physiol Pharmacol. 58: 53-64.

The effects of herbal plants on *Mucin 2* gene expression and performance in ascetic broilers

Kamali Sangani, A.[1], Masoudi, A.A.[2*], Hosseini, S.A.[3]

[1] *Graduated from the Faculty of Agriculture, University of Tarbiat Modares, Tehran, Iran*

[2] *Department of Animal Sciences, University of Tarbiat Modares, Tehran, Iran*

[3] *Department of Animal and Poultry Nutrition, Animal Sciences Research Institute, Karaj, Iran*

Key words:
broiler chicken, cinnamon, *mucin* 2 gene expression, thyme, turmeric

Correspondence
Masoudi, A.A.
Department of Animal Sciences,
University of Tarbiat Modares,
Tehran, Iran

Email: masoudia@modares.ac.ir

Abstract:

BACKGROUND: The mucus layer plays an important role as an intermediate for the protection of the gut against acidic chyme, digestive enzymes, and pathogens; in addition, it acts as a lubricant and facilitator of nutrient transportation. Phytogenic compounds seem to promote intestinal mucus production. **OBJECTIVES:** The current study was conducted to investigate the effects of low and high levels of energy and amino acids in combination with turmeric, thyme, and cinnamon on chicken performance and expression of *mucin* 2 gene. **METHODS:** The eight experimental groups consisted of diluted and condensed diet with and without the addition of 5g/kg of each turmeric, thyme, and cinnamon to the diet. Chicken performance was recorded. Expression analysis of the *mucin* 2 gene was carried out by quantitative RT-PCR. **RESULTS:** Body weight gain, feed intake, FCR, and mortality rate were not affected by diets ($p>0.05$). A significant ($p<0.05$) reduction of the *mucin* 2 gene expression was observed in chickens fed by condensed diet; however, the expression increased by supplementation of turmeric, thyme, and cinnamon. **CONCLUSIONS:** These results, in addition to the function of herbs in increasing the activity of some enzymes which is possibly related to the mucin biological pathways, showed that the application of turmeric, thyme, and cinnamon could be useful in poultry diets. It appears that supplementation of turmeric, thyme, and cinnamon could increase *mucin* 2 gene expression in the small intestine, and this can improve intestinal digestive function and defense.

Introduction

Over the last decade, the importance of gastrointestinal tract health in broiler chicken was increasingly studied due to its contribution to their overall health and performance (Mountzouris et al., 2007; Rehman et al., 2007). The use of antibiotics at sub-therapeutic levels have been a basis of the poultry industry for the control of subclinical diseases, maintenance of gut health, and growth promotion for a number of decades (Mathew et al., 2007). The emergences of antibiotic resistant strains of pathogens have raised some restrictions on antibiotic use in food animals. In Europe, sub-therapeutic use of antibiotics in poultry rearing has been phased out since 2006. In accordance with these restrictions, the use of phytogenic feed additives, which comprise a wide variety of herbs, has recently gained increasing interest, especially for use in poultry.

Numerous studies have demonstrated anti-oxidative and anti-microbial efficacy of phytogenic compounds in vitro; however, in vivo experimental evidences are still quite limited (Denli et al., 2004). In addition, it was hypothesized that phytogenic compounds may specifically enhance the activities of digestive enzymes and promote intestinal mucus production (Moghaddam et al., 2011).

The epithelium of the intestinal tract is covered mainly by a layer of mucus composed of mucin glycoproteins that are synthesized and secreted by goblet cells. The mucus layer plays an important role in protecting the gut against acidic chyme, digestive enzymes, and pathogens; mucin also acts as lubricant and facilitated nutrition transport between the luminal contents and the epithelial cells (Montagne et al., 2004). In humans, mucins are now categorized into three distinct families according to the structure of the protein product which are gel-forming (*Mucin* 2, *Mucin* 5AC, *Mucin* 5B and *Mucin* 6), soluble (Mucin 7), and membrane-bound (*Mucin* 1, *Mucin* 3, *Mucin* 4 and *Mucin* 12) (Moniax et al., 2001). *Mucin* 2 is the major intestinal *mucin* gene that was initially isolated from a human jejunum cDNA library (Sadasivan et al., 2011).

In the current study, we investigate the effects of two different kinds of diets (lower and higher levels of energy and protein according to the Arian strain recommendation) and three kinds of herbal plants (turmeric, thyme, and cinnamon) on performance traits and *mucin* 2 gene expression.

Materials and Methods

Broiler management: 960 one day old Arian chickens were randomly divided into eight groups of 120 chicks; with four replicates of 30 chicks assigned to each replicate. The chicks were reared for 42 days on wood shavings under standard conditions and provided adlibitum access to feed and water. Formulation of diluted and condensed diets is shown in table 1. Treatment groups were as follows:1) diluted diet 2) condensed diet; 3) diluted diet + 5 g/kg turmeric; 4) condensed diet + 5 g/kg turmeric; 5) diluted diet + 5 g/kg thyme; 6) condensed diet + 5 g/kg thyme; 7) diluted diet + 5 g/kg cinnamon; and 8) condensed diet + 5 g/kg cinnamon (Table 2). Herbal plants used in this experiment were obtained from a commercial source as dry powder.

Traits measured and tissue sampling: Body weights were measured weekly. Total feed intake was measured per pen weekly and mortality rate was recorded daily. FCR was measured and adjusted for mortality. On day 42, six birds from each treatment were slaughtered and their intestine (jejunum) segments were removed and immediately were frozen at -80°C.

Real-time RT-PCR: Total RNA was isolated from the jejunum samples using the RNXTM (Plus) (RN7713C, Cinnagen Inc., Tehran, Iran) according to the manufacturer's instructions. The RNA samples were aliquoted into four replicates and stored at -80°C until analysis.

RNA was reverse transcribed to cDNA using a RevertAidTM first strand cDNA synthesis kit (K1622, Fermentas). All RNA samples were reverse transcribed simultaneously for minimizing the variations. The cDNA samples were stored at -80°C until analysis. Real-time PCR was performed using universal SYBER Green PCR master mix (RR350Q, Takara) in Corbett Science Rotor-Gene 3000 sequence detection system (Qiagen). The PCR was performed in a reaction volume of 25 µL containing the reagents at the following final concentrations: 1X Universal SYBER Green PCR master mix (2X), forward primer 10 µM, reverse primer 10 µM and 2µL of cDNA sample. The cycling profiles used for three genes were: 1 cycle at 95°C for 5 min, 40 cycles PCR (denaturation at 95°C for 30s; annealing at 63°C for 30s and extension at 72°C for 30s) followed by a final extension at 72°C for 5 min. The specific primers for intestinal *mucin* 2 are shown in table 3. This primer was designed by using the reference sequence of the gene in Gallus gallus.

In each run, a negative control, a calibrator sample, cDNA samples, and endogenous control (GAPDH) were included. GAPDH samples were analyzed in duplicate and the target genes were analyzed in triplicate. The relative gene expression was quantified by the $\Delta\Delta C_t$ method. ΔC_t was calculated by subtracting the Ct amount of *mucin* 2 gene from Ct of GAPDH for each sample, then $\Delta\Delta C_t$ was calculated from subtract ΔC_t of each treatment of ΔC_t control. We selected the diluted diet as control and then 2-$\Delta\Delta C_t$ was calculated.

Statistical analysis: Data were analyzed using GLM procedures of SAS software (SAS, 2006).

Results

Performance measurements: Performance traits

Table 1. Composition of basal diet fed to broilers. [1]Premix provided the following per kilogram of diet: vitamin A(vitamin A acetate) 9000 U; vitamin B1, 1.8 mg; vitamin B2, 6.6 mg; niacin, 30 mg; vitamin B6, 3 mg; Calcium pantothenate, 10 mg; Folic Acid, 1 mg; B12, 0.015 mg; 0.1 mg D-biotin, vitamin D3 2000 U; vitamin E 18 U; vitamin K2, 2 mg; Choline chloride, 500 mg; manganese (Manganese oxide), 100 mg; zinc, 100 mg; iron (Iron sulfate, 7H2O), 50 mg; copper (copper sulfate, 5H2O), 10 mg; iodine (Calcium iodine), 1 mg; selenium (Sodium selenite), 0.2 mg.

Ingredients	1 to 21 days age		21 to 42 days age	
	Condensed diet	Diluted diet	Condensed diet	Diluted diet
Corn	55.09	49.9	60.31	54.53
Soybean meal	38	36.5	34	34.7
Fish meal	1	5	-	1.9
Soybean oil	1.5	4.83	1.45	5
Dicalcium phosphate	1.9	1.63	1.78	1.63
Oyster shell	1.19	0.94	1.11	1.01
Baking soda	0.04	0.05	0.09	0.05
Salt	0.33	0.33	0.33	0.33
L - Met	0.28	0.22	0.26	0.22
L - Lys	0.07	-	0.07	0.03
Vitamins and minerals[1]	0.6	0.6	0.6	0.6

Table 2. Nutrient analysis of diets.

Chemical composition of diets	1 to 21 days age		21 to 42 days age	
	Diluted diet	Condensed diet	Diluted diet	Condensed diet
Crude protein, %	22	23.5	20	21.07
MEn, (kcal/kg)	2850	3050	2910	3100
Calcium, %	1	1	0.9	0.9
Threonine, %	0.85	0.92	0.76	0.81
Methionine + cysteine, %	0.99	1	0.9	0.91
Lysine, %	1.27	1.37	1.13	1.20
Available phosphorus, %	0.5	0.5	0.45	0.45
Sodium %	0.17	0.18	0.17	0.17
Anion Cation Balance	241	243	230	230

of broilers are presented in table 4. Chickens fed condensed diet showed more body weight gain than those fed by diluted diet. Body weight gain had no differences in chickens fed by various herbal plants. Supplementation of diluted diet with turmeric, thyme, and cinnamon had no effect on body weight gain as well as condensed diet with turmeric. Feed intake, FCR, and the rate of mortality were not significantly affected by diet concentration and adding the herbs to each diet ($p>0.05$).

***Mucin* 2 mRNA expression:** The expression of *mucin* 2 gene in the chicken jejunum, was significantly reduced in chickens fed condensed diet compared with those fed diluted diet. Addition of turmeric, thyme, and cinnamon to both basal diets increased the expression of *mucin* 2 mRNA in jejunum of chickens (Table 4).

Discussion

The prohibition of antibiotic use in poultry feed has forced investigators to research growth promoting alternatives (Marcincák et al., 2011). These alternatives are greatly favored in the poultry industry. Turmeric (*Curcuma Longa*) thyme (*Thymus vulgaris*) and cinnamon (Cinnamomum verum) are among alternatives for growth promoting antibiotics. The major components of turmeric, thyme, and cinnamon are curcumin, thymol, and carvacrol and trans-cinnamyl acetate and β-caryophyllene, respectively. It has been demonstrated that all of these components have antioxidative properties (Toghyani et al., 2010).

In this study we observed that the application of condensed diet increased body weight gain in comparison to the diluted diet. Supplementation of turmeric, thyme, and cinnamon to each of the diluted and turmeric to the condensed diet (interaction effect) had no effect on body weight gain ($p>0.05$). It was expected that supplementation of diets with herbs would stimulate the growth performance of broilers (Al-Kassie, 2009; Toghyani et al., 2011). The bio-active substances of these herbs may improve feed digestibility, the gut microbial balance, and excitation of digestive enzymes and thus improve growth performance in broilers without affecting FCR (Sadeghi et al., 2012). These herbs also may improve safety in host animals and increase availability of nutrients in the intestine for absorption; thereby resulting in animals to grow better and decreasing incidences of disease and mortality. Some unknown parameters may have interacted with the herbs such as basal diet, age, strain, and environmental conditions that affect the herbal plant.

The results of the present study are in agreement with the previous observations that indicated no effect of these herbs ($p<0.05$) on body weight gain, feed intake, or feed conversion ratio in broilers (Mehala and Moorthy, 2008; Toghyani et al., 2010).

Table 3. Primers used for RT-PCR analysis of chicken mRNAs.

Target (Accession No.)	Primer	Sequence (5'→ 3')	Size of PCR product (bp)	T_m °C
GAPDH	Forward	TGAAGGGTGGTGCTAAGCGTG	288	66
(NM_204305.1)	Reverse	GGATGATGTTCTGGGCAGCAC		
MUC2	Forward	CTGTTGTGGATGGGCGGATTG	157	66
(XM_421035.2)	Reverse	CCAAACTTGCTGTCCAGCTCC		

Table 4. Measured parameters for performance of broiler chickens from 1 to 42 days of age. (a, b and c) Means with no common superscripts differ significantly ($p<0.05$). MSE is mean squared error.

Dietary treatment	Body weight gain, (g/bird)	Feed intake, (g/bird)	Feed conversion ratio, (g/g)	Mortality %
Diluted diet	57.20[b]	106.60	1.90	3.80
Condense diet	60.00[a]	107.10	1.80	3.90
None herbs	58.50	109.40	1.90	3.90
Turmeric	57.90	105.80	1.80	3.50
Thyme	59.10	106.00	1.80	4.30
Cinnamon	58.90	106.10	1.80	3.80
Diluted diet without any herbs	56.57	107.61	1.90	3.25
Condense diet without any herbs	60.40	111.20	1.84	4.50
Diluted diet + 5 g/kg diet turmeric	56.70	107.57	1.90	4.00
Condensed diet + 5 g/ kg diet turmeric	59.11	104.00	1.76	3.11
Diluted diet + 5 g/ kg diet thyme	57.85	104.44	1.80	4.25
Condensed diet + 5 g/ kg diet thyme	60.31	107.50	1.78	4.25
Diluted diet + 5 g/ kg diet cinnamon	57.50	106.77	1.86	3.75
Condensed diet+ 5 g/ kg diet cinnamon	60.31	105.52	1.74	3.75
MSE	4.77	36.78	0.01	0.53

Table 5. Relative quantification using the comparative CT method. (a, b and c) Means with no common superscripts differ significantly ($p<0.05$). MSE is mean squared error.

Dietary treatment	*Mucin* 2 (Average C_T)	GAPDH (Average C_T)	ΔC_T (MUC2- GAPDH)	$\Delta\Delta C_T$ (ΔC_T- ΔC_T^0)	Fold change in *mucin* 2 gene
Diluted diet	15.50	12.48	3.02	0	1.00[a]
Condense diet	21.02	12.95	8.08	5.52	0.03[b]
Diluted diet + 5 g/kg diet turmeric	14.97	12.54	2.43	-0.17	1.50[c]
Condensed diet + 5 g/ kg diet turmeric	17.35	14.43	2.92	-0.03	1.07[a]
Diluted diet + 5 g/ kg diet thyme	16.15	13.74	2.41	-0.18	1.52[c]
Condensed diet + 5 g/ kg diet thyme	16.76	14.58	2.18	-0.25	1.78[d]
Diluted diet + 5 g/ kg diet cinnamon	16.87	14.73	2.14	-0.26	1.84[d]
Condensed diet+ 5 g/ kg diet cinnamon	15.98	13.85	2.13	-0.26	1.85[d]
MSE					0.028

However, extracted oil from thyme and cinnamon improved body weight gain, feed intake, and feed conversion ratio in broiler diets (Al-Kassie, 2009). Supplementing of thyme and cinnamon to each of the diets increased body weight of broilers ($p<0.05$), which was in agreement with some studies (Ocak et al., 2008; Toghyani et al., 2010) but is not concordant with the others (Tekeli et al., 2009; Rahimi et al., 2011).

Carbohydrates, proteins, and specific amino acids such as threonine have been demonstrated to alter mucin secretion and may interact directly with goblet cells or with the enteric nervous system to elicit changes in mucin secretion (Smirnov et al., 2005; Smirnov et al., 2006; Horn et al., 2009; Moghaddam et al., 2011). *Mucin* 2 gene expression enhanced after starvation in chickens (Smirnov et al., 2004). There was no effect of threonine on intestinal goblet cell density or *mucin* 2 mRNA abundance for broilers (Horn et al., 2009; Moghaddam et al., 2011). The expression 5 pattern of the *mucin* 2 gene in chickens fed antibiotic growth promoter (AGP) or a probiotic product were greater than the observation in controls (Smirnov et al., 2005).

Thus, changes of the mucus layer would be expected to influence nutrient digestion processes. Supplementation of turmeric, thyme and cinnamon to both basal diets increased the expression of *mucin* 2 mRNA in jejunum of chickens. Any component, dietary or environmental, that induces changes in *mucin* gene expression has the potential to affect the integrity of the mucus layer and nutrient absorption. Reduction of the *mucin* 2 gene expression in jejunum of broiler chickens fed condensed diet may be related to the decrease of the mRNA stability. Several lines of evidence indicated that the regulation of mRNA stability, in response to external stimuli, changes the gene expression (Cheadle et al., 2005; Barnett et al., 2007). Stability of *mucin* 2 mRNA can be influenced by the initiation factor 5A, which affects the turnover of mRNA. Cytokines, growth factors, and bacterial products or any conditions that affect differentiation of goblet cells can also affect *mucin* 2 gene expression. It is possible that bioactive substances of these herbs may influence the HapA concentration that is an extracellular proteinase and increases secretion and accumulation of *mucin* 2 gene in the gastrointestinal tract. The bioactive substances also may alter the activity of transcription factors such as GATA4 and Fox1 that regulates *mucin* 2 gene expression in broiler chickens (Van der Sluis et al., 2004; Van der Sluis et al., 2008). Supplementation herbs to broiler chickens' diets could change the mucin expression and nutrient utilization.

Our results showed that supplementation of turmeric, thyme, and cinnamon enhanced the *mucin* 2 gene expression in jejunum of broiler chickens, and thus it may influence its protective properties and nutrient absorption. Application of these herbs that could promote *mucin* 2 gene expression can be useful for poultry.

Acknowledgements

This study was supported by a grant of Tarbiat Modares University, Iran. The authors would like to thank all the colleagues who contributed to the collection and analysis of the data.

References

1. Al-Kassie, G. A. M. (2009) Influence of two plant extracts derived from thyme and cinnamon on broiler performance. Pak Vet J. 29: 169-173.
2. Barnett, T.C., Bugrysheva, J., V.Scott, J.R. (2007) Role of mRNA stability in growth phase regulation of gene expression in the group A streptococcus. J Bacteriol. 189: 1866-1873.
3. Cheadle, C., Fan, J., Cho-Chung, Y.S., Werner, T., Ray, J., Do, L., Gorospe, M., Becker, K.G. (2005) Stability regulation of mRNA and the control of gene expression. Ann N Y Acad Sci. 1058: 196-204.
4. Denli, M., Okan, F., Uluocak, A.N. (2004) Effect of dietary supplementation of herb essential oils on the growth performance, carcass and intestinal characteristics of quail (*Coturnix coturnix japonica*). S Afr J Anim Sci. 34: 174-179.
5. Horn, N.L., Donkin, S.S., Applegate, T.J., Adeola, O. (2009) Intestinal mucin dynamics: Response of broiler chicks and White Pekin ducklings to dietary threonine. Poult Sci J. 88: 1906-1914.
6. Marcincák, S., Popelka, P., Zdolec, N., Mártonová, M., Šimková, J., Marcincáková, D. (2011) Effect of supplementation of phytogenic feed additives on performance parameters and meat quality of broiler chickens. Slov Vet Res. 48: 27-34.
7. Mathew, A.G., Cissell, R., Liamthong, S. (2007) Antibiotic resistance in bacteria associated with food animals: a United States perspective of livestock production. Foodborne Pathog Dis. 4: 115-133.
8. Mehala, C., Moorthy, M. (2008) Production performance of broilers fed with aloevera Curcuma longa (turmeric). Int J Poult Sci. 7: 852-856.
9. Moghaddam, H.S., Moghaddam, H.N., Kermanshahi, H., Mosavi, A.H., Raji, A. (2011) The effect of threonine on *mucin* 2 gene expression, intestinal histology and performance of broiler chicken. Ital J Anim Sci. 10: e14.
10. Moniax, N., Escande, F., Porchet, N., Aubert, J.P., Batra, S.K. (2001) Structural organization and classification of the human *mucin* genes. Front Biosci. 6: D1192-1206.
11. Montagne, L., Piel, C., Lalles, J.P. (2004) Effect of Diet on mucin kinetics and composition: nutrition

and health implications. Nutr Rev. 62: 105-114.

12. Mountzouris, K.C., Tsirtsikos, P., Kalamara, E., Nitsch, S., Schatzmayr, G., Fegeros, K. (2007) Evaluation of the efficacy of a probiotic containing lactobacillus, bifidobacterium, enterococcus, and pediococcus strains in promoting broiler performance and modulating cecal microflora composition and metabolic activities. Poult Sci J. 86: 309-317.

13. Ocak, N., Erener, G., Burak Ak, F., Sungu, M., Altop, A.A., Ozmen, A. (2008) Performance of broilers fed diets supplemented with dry peppermint (*Mentha piperita* L.) or thyme (*Tymus vulgaris* L.) leaves as growth promoter source. J Anim Sci. 53: 169-175.

14. Rahimi, S., Teymouri Zadeh, Z., Karimi Torshizi, M. A., Omidbaigi, R., Rokni, H. (2011) Effect of the three herbal extracts on growth performance, immune system, blood factors and intestinal selected bacterial population in broiler chickens. J Agric Sci Technol. 13: 527-539.

15. Rehman, H., Rosenkranz, C., Böhm, J., Zentek, J. (2007) Dietary inulin affects the morphology but not the sodium-dependent glucose and glutamine transport in the jejunum of broilers. Poult Sci J. 86: 118-122.

16. Sadasivan, V., Narpala, S., Budil, D., Sacco, A., Carrier, R. (2011) Modeling the human intestinal Mucin (MUC2) C-terminal cystine knot dimer. J Mol Model. 17: 2953-2963.

17. Sadeghi, G., Karimi, A., Padidar Jahromi, S., Azizi, T., Daneshmand, A. (2012) Effects of cinnamon, thyme and turmeric infusions on the performance and immune response in of 1- to 21-day-old male broilers. Rev Bras Ciênc Avíc. 14: 15-20.

18. Smirnov, A., Perez, R., Romach, E.A., Sklan, D., Uni, Z. (2005) Mucin dynamics and microbial populations in chicken small intestine are changed by dietary probiotic and antibiotic growth promoter supplementation. J Nutr. 135: 187-192.

19. Smirnov, A., Sklan, D., Uni, Z. (2004) Mucin dynamics in the chick small intestine are altered by starvation. J Nutr. 134: 736-742.

20. Smirnov, A., Tako, E., Ferket, P.R., Uni, Z. (2006) *Mucin* gene expression and mucin content in the chicken intestinal goblet cells are affected by in ovo feeding of carbohydrates. Poult Sci J. 85: 669-673.

21. Toghyani, M., Toghyani, M., Gheisari, A.A., Ghalamkari, G., Eghbalsaied, S. (2011) Evaluation of cinnamon and garlic as antibiotic growth promoter substitutions on performance, immune responses, serum biochemical and haematological parameters in broiler chicks. Livest Sci. 138: 167-173.

22. Toghyani, M., Tohidi, M., Gheisari, A.A., Tabeidian, S.A. (2010) Performance, immunity, serum biochemical and hematological parameters in broiler chicks fed dietary thyme as alternative for an antibiotic growth promoter. Afr J Biotechnol. 9: 6819-6825.

23. Van Der Sluis, M., Melis, H.M., Jonckheerec, N., Marie-Paule, D.A., Bullera, H.A., Renes, I., Einerhand, A.W.C., Van Seuningen, I. (2004) The murine Muc2 *mucin* gene is transcriptionally regulated by the zinc-finger GATA-4 transcription factor in intestinal cells. Biochem Biophys Res Commun. 325: 952-960.

24. Van Der Sluis, M., Vincent, A., Bouma, J., Korteland-Van Male, A.B., Van Goudoever, J.B., Renes, I., Van Seuningen, I. (2008) Forkhead box transcription factors Foxa1 and Foxa2 are important regulators of Muc2 mucin expression in intestinal epithelial cells. Biochem Biophys Res Commun. 369: 1108-1113.

14

Radiographic measurements of front feet of the sound Akhal-Teke horses

Masoudifard, M.[1*], Vajhi, A.R.[1], Mansouri, Sh.[2], Molazem, M.[1], Bahonar, A.R.[3], Zehtabvar, O.[4]

[1] *Department of Surgery and Radiology, Faculty of Veterinary Medicine, University of Tehran, Tehran, Iran*

[2] *Private Veterinary Practitioner, Tehran, Iran*

[3] *Department of Food Hygiene and Quality Control, Faculty of Veterinary Medicine, University of Tehran, Tehran, Iran*

[4] *Department of Basic Sciences, Faculty of Veterinary Medicine, University of Tehran, Tehran, Iran*

Key words:
Akhal-Teke horse, front feet, measurement, radiography

Correspondence
Masoudifard, M.
Department of Surgery and Radiology, Faculty of Veterinary Medicine, University of Tehran, Tehran, Iran

Email: mmfard@ut.ac.ir

Abstract:

BACKGROUND: The Akhal-Teke is an ancient horse originating from Asia where it was used by nomadic tribes and used as a warhorse. Lameness examinations require proper interpretation of clinical and radiographic findings. Therefore, understanding of normal radiographic findings of the foot is necessary. Although the radiographic appearance of the normal foot must be understood to recognize abnormalities ,there are no studies examining the normal hoof and digital soft tissues in Akhal-Teke horses. **OBJECTIVES:** The purpose of the study reported here was to determine a normal radiographic appearance and morphometry of the distal phalanx and its related soft tissue in mature Akhal-Teke racehorses without any clinical signs of lameness and foot problems. **METHODS:** Radiography of the distal phalanx and associated soft-tissue structures of the front feet of 10 healthy pure Akhal-Teke horses were performed to determine normal radiographic appearance and morphometry. Lateromedial radiographic views of each front distal phalanx were used to measure important distances, angles and ratios of the hoof wall. All the measurements from lateromedial radiographs were multiplied by the magnification correction factor to gain the actual distances. **RESULTS:** Mean ± SD thickness of the soft tissues dorsal to the middle aspect of distal phalanx was 18.3 ± 1.22 mm. There was not any significant difference between left and right digits for any radiographic determination. **CONCLUSIONS:** This study introduced S-Founder and CF-Founder as important criteria in evaluating laminitis and sinking of P3.

Introduction

The Akhal-Teke is an ancient horse originating from Asia where it was used by nomadic tribes and used as a warhorse. The Akhal-Teke is among the most elegant of the world's horses. The conformation of The Akhal-Teke can be favorably compared to the Persian Arab, another breed of ancient origin.

Lameness and prepurchase examination require proper interpretation of clinical and radiographic findings. Therefore, understanding the normal radiographic findings of the foot is necessary. The most important disease of horses' limbs is laminitis which needs rapid diagnosis on the early taken radiographs. Radiography of the distal phalanx (DP) is necessary, so one must know the normal radio-graphic findings.

Although the radiographic appearance of the normal foot must be understood to recognize subtle abnormalities (Rendano and Grant, 1978), no study has examined the normal hoof and digital soft tissues in Akhal-Teke horses. However, these findings were previously studied in Thoroughbred, Hanoverian, Pony, and Arab breeds horses. Bushe et al. (1988) have mentioned the relation between the third phalanx angle and coffin angle in sound horses. Qualitative and morphometric radiographic findings in the distal phalanx and digital soft tissue for sound and footsore thoroughbreds were compared by Linford (1987). The mean thickness of the soft tissue dorsal to the distal phalanx was measured and compared between the two groups. Linford et al. (1993) have also qualified distal phalanx and digital soft tissue findings of sound Thoroughbred racehorses and matched the data with their racing performance. Cripps and Eustace (1999) have measured the normal radiographic findings of the feet in normal horses with relevance to laminitis.

The purpose of the study reported here was to determine a normal radiographic appearance and morphometry of the distal phalanx and its related soft tissue in mature Akhal-Teke racehorses without any clinical signs of lameness and foot problems.

Materials and Methods

Case selection: A total of 10 healthy pure Akhal-Teke horses were selected from one of the stables in the east of Tehran. All the horses had their own history and certificates and they were approximately similar in size and weight. They included 5 males and 5 females and were 7.7± 3.3 (mean± SD) years old with the same diet and training management and also a same farrier. There was no history of lameness and limb abnormality for at least one year prior to the study. Each horse was observed trotting in circles to the left and right, and walking and trotting in a straight line.

Radiography: Radiographs were made using a portable 10 mAmp; 80 kVolt X-ray generator with variable timer. Care was taken to ensure straight lateromedial projections without obliquity by aligning the radiographic beam so that it passed perpendicularly to the sagittal plane through the foot while being centered in the middle of the hoof 3Cm proximal to the bearing surface. The hoof also was placed on a 7Cm thick wooden block so that the distance of the center of the beam to ground surface was 10 Cm. To differentiate the bearing surface from the block a metal bar was placed on the block surface. The focus-film distance for each projection was 75Cm.

All horseshoes were removed and the frog sulci and the sole surface of the digits were cleaned prior to radiography. A layer of Barium Sulfate contrast agent with proper concentration was robbed on the dorsal surface of hoof wall, sole surface, and frog sulci for better visualization of these parts on the radiographs. A metal marker was used to determine the amount of radiographic magnification as well as to delineate the coronary band at the lateromedial radiographs (Figure 1).

All the measurements from lateromedial radiographs were multiplied using the magnification correction factor (MCF) to gain the actual distances. The MCF was determined by dividing the actual metal marker length to the length of the radiographic image of the marker.

Morphometric analysis of the radiographs: In each obtained radiograph, 7 distances, 7 angles, and 3 ratios of the distal phalanx and the hoof wall were measured. The morphometric assessments were made as follows:

1. The hoof wall and its soft tissue thickness included 3 regions:

a) Total soft tissue thickness dorsal to the distal aspect of the DP (STTD) (Figure 2 A),

b) Total soft tissue thickness dorsal to the middle aspect of the DP (STTM) (Figure 2 B),

c) Total soft tissue thickness dorsal to the proximal aspect of the DP (STTP) (Figure 2 C).

They were the shortest distance between the dorsal surface of the hoof wall and the dorsal cortex of DP.

2. Palmarocortical length (PCL) of the DP: The distance from the tip of the solar margin to the middle of the articulation between the phalanx and the navicular bone (Figure 2).

3. The ratios of the wall thickness to the PCL: These ratios assessed by proper thickness of STTD, STTM, and STTP expressed as a percentage.

4. Hoof wall axis (S-angle): The caudal angle formed between a line along the dorsal surface of the hoof wall and a line along the bearing surface of the hoof (Figure 2).

5. Distal phalanx axis (T-angle): The caudal angle

formed between a line along the dorsal cortex of the phalanx and a line along the bearing surface of the hoof wall (Figure 2).

6. The difference between S and T-angles (H-angle).

7. Middle phalanx axis (U-angle): The caudal angle formed between a line through the central axis of the middle phalanx and a line along the bearing surface of the hoof wall (Figure 2).

8. The difference between U and T-angle (R-angle).

9. D-Founder: The perpendicular distance from the horizontal line through the extensor process to the horizontal line through the coronary band (Figure 2).

10. S-Founder: The perpendicular distance from the horizontal line through the highest point of the sole surface which was robbed by contrast agent (Barium Sulfate) in front of the frog to the tip of the DP (Figure 2).

11. CF-Founder: The perpendicular distance from the horizontal line through the top point of the frog corium to the extensor process (Figure 2).

12. P-angle: A caudal angle formed between a line through the palmarocortical and a line through dorsal surface of the DP (Figure 2).

13. J-angle: A caudal angle formed between a line through the solar margin of the distal phalanx and a line along the bearing surface of the hoof.

Statistical evaluation: All the obtained data were analyzed by SPSS software (Ver. 11.5). The average, standard deviation, and minimum and maximum data were determined as standard measurements in Akhal-Teke horses. The paired T-test was also used to compare the measurements between males and females, right and left front feet.

Results

The result of the measurements of the distances, ratios, and angles of morphometric variables of distal phalanx and hoof in lateral radiographs of total, left and right front feet, and male and female Akhal-Teke horses are shown in tables 1 and 2.

In this research, there was no statistically significant difference ($p>0.10$) in measured parameters between the left and right fore limb radiographs. Data comparison of the distal phalanx and hoof box in male and female horses showed significant differences in STTP ($p<0.01$), PCL ($p<0.05$), J-angle ($p<0.05$), D-Founder ($p<0.05$), and CF-Founder ($p<0.01$).

Table 1. Mean ± Standard Deviation (SD) measurements of the distances and ratios of morphometric variables of distal phalanx and hoof in lateral radiographs of front feet of total, left and right front feet, and male and female Akhal-Teke horses.

Variables	Mean (SD) of total	Mean (SD) of Left & Right	Mean (SD) of Male & Female
STTD (mm)	18.0 (1.04)	**L:** 17.9 (1.16) **R:** 18.1 (0.97)	**M:** 17.5 (1.14) **F:** 18.4 (0.78)
STTM (mm)	18.3 (1.22)	**L:** 18.5 (1.39) **R:** 18.2 (1.08)	**M:** 17.9 (1.31) **F:** 18.8 (0.99)
STTP (mm)	18.5 (1.23)	**L:** 18.6 (1.41) **R:** 18.5 (1.09)	**M:** 17.8 (1.23) **F:** 19.3 (0.63)
PCL (mm)	64.3 (3.37)	**L:** 64.1 (3.75) **R:** 64.5 (3.15)	**M:** 62.5 (2.38) **F:** 66.1 (3.31)
STTD/PCL (%)	28.0 (1.80)	**L:** 27.9 (2.12) **R:** 28.1 (1.52)	**M:** 28.1 (1.23) **F:** 27.9 (2.30)
STTM/PCL (%)	28.5 (1.86)	**L:** 28.9 (1.98) **R:** 28.2 (1.77)	**M:** 28.6 (1.40) **F:** 28.5 (2.31)
STTP/PCL (%)	28.9 (1.51)	**L:** 29.0 (1.57) **R:** 28.7 (1.51)	**M:** 28.5 (1.07) **F:** 29.3 (1.82)
D-Founder (mm)	6.2 (2.93)	**L:** 6.8 (3.05) **R:** 5.6 (2.82)	**M:** 4.9 (3.42) **F:** 7.5 (1.62)
S-Founder (mm)	10.7 (3.65)	**L:** 10.6 (3.62) **R:** 10.8 (3.87)	**M:** 10.8 (4.38) **F:** 10.6 (2.98)
CF-Founder (mm)	48.6 (5.96)	**L:** 49.0 (7.54) **R:** 48.2 (4.20)	**M:** 45.2 (1.73) **F:** 52.0 (6.80)

Table 2. Mean ± Standard Deviation (SD) measurements of the angles of morphometric variables of distal phalanx and hoof in lateral radiographs of front feet of total, left and right front feet, and male and female Akhal-Teke horses.

Variables	Mean (SD) of total	Mean (SD) of Left & Right	Mean (SD) of Male & Female
S-angle (Degree)	49.6 (7.33)	**L:** 51.5 (9.70) **R:** 47.6 (3.31)	**M:** 47.5 (2.99) **F:** 51.7 (9.73)
T-angle (Degree)	48.5 (2.47)	**L:** 48.7 (1.79) **R:** 48.3 (3.10)	**M:** 48.6 (2.02) **F:** 48.4 (2.97)
H-angle (Degree)	0.4 (2.58)	**L:** 0.2 (2.91) **R:** 0.6 (2.33)	**M:** 1.1 (2.66) **F:** -0.25 (2.44)
U-angle (Degree)	49.2 (6.23)	**L:** 47.0 (5.44) **R:** 51.4 (6.47)	**M:** 46.8 (6.31) **F:** 51.6 (5.40)
R-angle (Degree)	-0.2 (5.36)	**L:** 1.7 (5.21) **R:** -2.1 (5.05)	**M:** 1.8 (6.54) **F:** -2.2 (3.00)
P-angle (Degree)	36.8 (2.48)	**L:** 36.5 (2.17) **R:** 37.2 (2.83)	**M:** 37.2 (2.51) **F:** 36.5 (2.52)
J-angle (Degree)	3.6 (2.77)	**L:** 4.6 (1.42) **R:** 2.7 (3.49)	**M:** 2.4 (2.34) **F:** 4.9 (2.70)

Discussion

Since it is very important to reduce failure in measuring the DP and the middle phalanx for

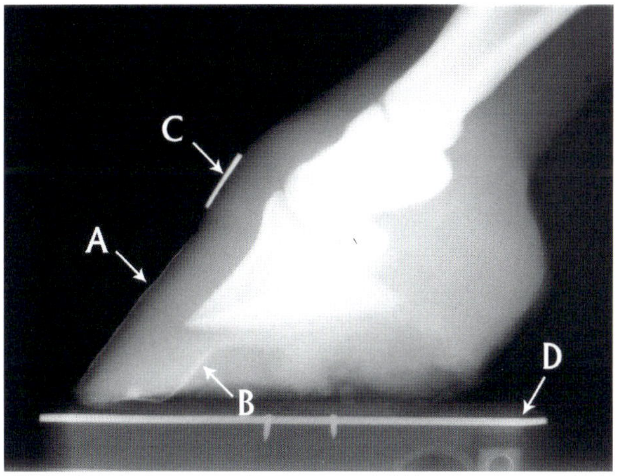

Figure 1. Lateromedial radiograph of the foot of an Akhal-Teke horse. A. Hoof wall, B. Sole surface, C. Metal marker, D. Metal bar was placed on the wooden block surface.

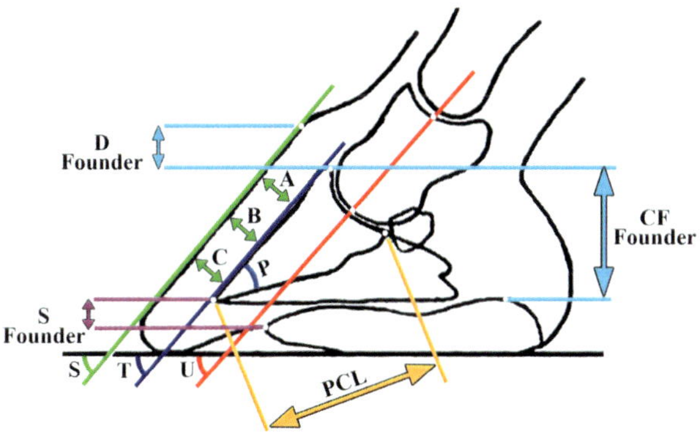

Figure 2. Schematic drawing of the foot illustrating measured distances and angles on lateromedial radiographs. PCL: Palmarocortical length, S-angle: Hoof wall, T-angle: Distal phalanx axis, U-angle: Middle phalanx axis, D-Founder: The perpendicular distance from the horizontal line through the extensor process to the horizontal line through the coronary band, S-Founder: The perpendicular distance from the horizontal line through the highest point of the sole surface which was robbed by contrast agent (Barium Sulfate) in front of the frog to the tip of the DP, CF-Founder: The perpendicular distance from the horizontal line through the top point of the frog corium to the extensor process, P-angle: A caudal angle formed between a line through the palmarocortical and a line through dorsal surface of the DP.

laminitis detection, the limb must be in an exact perpendicular position, and weight bearing is necessary too.

Linford et al. (1993) reported that the widest thickness at the hoof wall and its soft tissue was 18 mm. O'Brien and Baker (1986) stated that increasing in the hoof wall thickness and its related soft tissue to more than 20 mm is the first radiographic sign of laminitis. This increase is due to the inflammation of the laminea and will be seen on lateromedial radiographs almost 48 to 72 hours after laminitis start to grow. None of the hoof wall and its related soft tissue thickness was more that 20 mm in the present study. There are some differences between hoof wall thickness and soft tissue measurements in this study and other studies, especially the Linford et al. (1993), Cripps and Eustace (1999) and Golshani (2000), which can be due to the differences in breeds, ages, hoof cares, sport activities, or the nutrition of the examined horses.

Linford et al. (1993) and Peloso et al. (1996) have reported the thickness of the hoof wall and its related soft tissue less than 30% of the palmarocortical length of the DP in sound horses, and they stated that a higher percent will be a sign for laminitis. In this study, the mean of this criterion was less than 30% in all three levels, although there were sporadic cases with a percent of more than 30% without evident of laminitis.

Cripps and Eustace (1999) and Baxter (1996) stated that measuring the D-Founder, which is the horizontal line through the extensor process to the coronary band, is a sinking diagnostic criterion in Laminitis. Since finding the coronary band location will be almost difficult when it is inflamed or sinker, in this study the CF-Founder and S-Founder criteria were introduced to measure the sinking occurrence more accurately. The average of D-Founder in this study was 6.2mm which seems to be more than the amount of the previous reports in other horse breeds (Baxter 1996, Cripps and Eustace 1999). It may be because of the larger hoof box size, the longer hoof wall, and more penetration of the distal phalanx into the hoof box in Akhal-Teke horses.

Significant differences in STTP, PCL, J-angle, D-Founder, and CF-Founder between female and male horses may be due to varieties in their amount of sport activities and pregnancy periods in females.

Linford et al. (1993) propounded that existence of palmarocortical resorption, which cause an obvious convexity on the palmarocortical region on the lateral radiographs, is a sign for laminitis and founder. In this relation, Golshani (2000) assessed a new creation called P-angle. This criterion may be useful as an indicator of laminitis.

The results of the present study can be used as a reference in further laminitis investigations on Akhal-Teke horses.

Acknowledgements

The authors gratefully acknowledge the contributions and help of Dr. F. Adibhashemi and D. Faskhoodi.

References

1. Baxter, GM. (1996) Diagnosing and treating acute laminitis. Vet Med. 91: 940-952.
2. Bushe, T., Turner, T.A., Poulos, P.W., Harwell, N.M. (1988) The effect of hoof angle on coffin, pastern and fetlock joint angles. Proc Am Assoc Equine Practnrs. 33: 729-738.
3. Cripps, P.J., Eustace, R.A. (1999) Radiological measurements from the feet of normal horses with relevance to laminitis. Equine Vet J. 31: 427-432.
4. Eliashar, E., McGuigan, M.P.,Wilson, A.M. (2004) Relationship of foot conformation and force applied to the navicular bone of sound horses at the trot. Equine Vet J. 36: 431-435.
5. Linford, R.L., O'Brien, T.R., Trout, D.R. (1993) Qualitative and morphometric radiographic findings in the distal phalanx and digital soft tissue of sound thoroughbred racehorses. Am J Vet Res. 54: 38-51.
6. Peloso, J.G., Cohen, N.D., Walker, M.A., Watkins, J.P., Gayle, J.M., Moyer, W. (1996) Case-control study of risk factors for the development of laminitis in the contralateral limb in Equidae with unilateral lameness. J Am Vet Med Assoc. 209: 1746-1749.
7. Rendano, V.T., Grant, B. (1978) The equine third phalanx: its radiographic appearance. J Am Vet Radiol. 19: 125-135.
8. Riggs, C.M. (2006) Osteochondral injury and joint disease in the athletic horse. Equine Vet Educ. 18: 100-112.
9. Van Eps, A.W., Pollitt, C.C. (2006) Equine laminitis induced with oligofructose. Equine Vet J. 38: 203-208.
10. Van Eps, A.W., Pollitt, C.C. (2009) Equine laminitis model: Lamellar histopathology seven days after induction with oligofructose. Equine Vet J. 41: 735-740.

Prevalence of *Linguatula serrata* nymphs in slaughtered goats in Isfahan province

Pirali Kheirabadi, Kh.[1*], Fallah, A.[2], Abolghasemi, A.[3]

[1] *Department of Pathobiology, Faculty of Veterinary Medicine, Shahrekord University, Shahrekord, Iran*

[2] *Department of Food Hygiene and Quality Control, Faculty of Veterinary Medicine, Shahrekord University, Shahrekord, Iran*

[3] *Graduated from the Faculty of Veterinary Medicine, Shahrekord University, Shahrekord, Iran*

Key words:
goat, human, *Linguatula serrata*

Correspondence
Pirali Kheirabadi, Kh.
Department of Pathobiology, Faculty of Veterinary Medicine, Shahrekord University, Shahrekord, Iran

Email: Pirali_k@vet.sku.ac.ir

Abstract:

BACKGROUND: *Linguatula serrata*, a tongue worm, is an aberrant cosmopolitan parasite, which inhabits the canine respiratory system (final host). The discharged eggs infect many plant feeder, including ruminants and human being, that produce visceral and nasopharyngeal linguatulosis which is known as Marrara syndrome in man. **OBJECTIVES:** In the current study, the prevalence rate of infection with *L. serrata* nymphs in mesenteric and mediastinal lymph nodes (MLNs) of slaughtered goats was investigated by cutting in MLNs and observing them in Isfahan Province, Iran. **METHODS:** The MLNs of 620 slaughtered goats, including 197 females and 423 males, after the preparation of the lymph nodes, were examined for *L. serrata* nymphs by cutting them longitudinally and testing them by using a dissecting microscope for *L. serrata* nymphs. Then, in the suspected cases, the samples were digested by pepsin and hydrochloric acid and were examined for presence of *L. serrata* nymphs. Goats were categorized into four age groups, including < 1.5 year, 1.5 to 2.5 years, 2.5 to 3.5 years, and > 3.5 years. **RESULTS:** The results showed that 54.35% of the examined goats were infected with *L. serrata*. Sex had no significant effect on the prevalence rate of this parasite in goats. **CONCLUSIONS:** A high prevalence rate of infection in goats suggests a possible similar high rate of infection in other animals and man in the investigated area, which emphasizes undertaking strict control measures to reduce the risk of zoonotic outbreaks.

Introduction

Linguatula serrata Frohlic 1789, a cosmopolitan parasite, is a member of small group of parasites which from phylum Pentastomida (Gosling, 2005; Muller 2002). Adult infects the nasal sinuses and nasopharynx of carnivorous mammal, especially Canidae and probably Hyaenidae and Felidae (Khalil, 1970; Riley, 1986). A wide range of mammals are intermediate hosts for *L. serrate*; however, herbivores such as cattle, goats, sheep, camels, and other ruminants are the best hosts for the development of parasite's nymphal stages (Alcala-Canto et al., 2007). Eggs containing fully developed larvae are discharged into the environment by nasal secretion and ingested by intermediate hosts in which they develop to nymphal stage in various organs, particularly in Mesenteric Lymph Nodes (Berger and Marr, 2006; Khalil and Schacher, 1965; Soulsby, 1982). Man occasionally infected with both adult and nymphal stages of *L. serrata* (Oryan et al., 2008). Linguatulosis in humans has been reported from various parts of the world, particularly in countries of the Middle East, Africa, America, and Southeast Asia (Gardiner et al., 1984; Acha and Szyfres, 2003; Baird et al., 1988; El-Hassan et al., 1991; Yagi et al., 1996; Lazo et al., 1999). Nasopharyngeal linguatulosis, which is known as Halzoun or Marrara syndrome, is the common form of infection in man and is often produced following consumption of raw or undercooked infected viscera (liver, lung and lymph nodes) of infected animals (El-Hassan et al., 1991; Beaver et al., 1984; Drabick, 1987). This parasite has been reported in humans in Iran (Hodjati and naghili, 1987; Fata et al., 1994, Sadjjadi et al., 1998; Maleky, 2001). Several studies have shown the prevalence of *L. serrata* infection in animals including dogs, camels, buffaloes (Sisakumar et al., 2005), sheep (Esmail-Nia et al., 2000; Shekarforoush et al., 2004; Tavassoli et al., 2007; Ravindran et al., 2008; Nourollahi-Fard et al., 2011), cattle (Nourollahi-Fard et al., 2010a), and goats (Saiyari et al., 1996; Razavi et al., 2004; Nourollahi-Fard et al., 2010b).

This study aimed to determine the prevalence of *L. serrata* nymphs in MLNs of goats slaughtered in Isfahan Province, Central Iran.

Materials and Methods

Lymph nodes of 620 slaughtered goats at slaughterhouses of Isfahan province located in central part of Iran were examined for *L. serrata* nymphs from January 2010 to December 2011. After determining the sex, goats were divided into four age groups (including < 1.5 year, 1.5 to 2.5 years, 2.5 to 3.5 years, and > 3.5 years) using the eruption of permanent incisor teeth criteria, as described previously. At least, 4 mesenteric and mediastinal lymph nodes (MLNs) form each animal were collected, and totally 2480 lymph nodes were collected in PBS and transferred to the Parasitology Laboratory of Veterinary Faculty of Shahrekord University. Then, each lymph node was cut longitudinally and tested using a dissecting microscope for *L. serrata* nymphs. The number of collected nymphs from each node was recorded, and then nymphs were stored in PBS at 4 °C for further studies. The digestive method was carried out for detection of more nymphs which were not clear in the first method. For this purpose, 6 g pepsin was solved in 10 mL hydrochloric acid, and then 600 mL of distilled water was added. The Samples were placed at 37 °C for 24 h and then examined.

Statistical analysis: The Chi-Square test (SPSS version 17.0) was used to compare the relative frequency of infection among different ages, sexes, and seasons. A value of $p<0.05$ was considered significant.

Results

The results showed that MLNs in 337 goats (54.35%) were infected with *L. serrata* nymphs. The number of collected nymphs from each infected lymph node varied from 1 to 29. The infection rate in mesenteric lymph nodes was significantly higher than the infection rate in mediastinal lymph nodes (Table 1). The infection rate had no significant difference between male and female goats (Table 2). There was a significant difference between the groups with different ages (Table 3). The infection rate in winter was significantly lower than the infection rate in spring; however, there were no significant differences in the other seasons (Table 4).

Discussion

The prevalence of linguatulosis in dogs have been determined in different parts of Iran, which were found to be 76.2% in Shiraz (Oryan et al., 2008), 65.5% in Shahre-Kord (Meshgi and Asgarian, 2003), and 76.47% in Fars province (Oryan et al., 1997). In Bursa, Turkey, 20% of dogs have been found infected (Akyol et al., 1995). Many studies were carried out on the prevalence of *L. serrata* in various domestic ruminants in Iran and other parts of the world (Tavassoli et al., 2007; Tajik et al., 2006; Razavi et al.,

Table 1. Infection rate by *Linguatula serrata* nymphs in mesenteric and mediastinal lymph nodes in slaughtered goats. (a,b,c,d) The infection rate in a column with different superscript letters are significantly different ($p<0.05$).

Mesentric lymph nodes	Goats	620
	Infected	254
	Infection Rate(%)	40.56 a
Mediastinal lymph nodes	Goats	620
	Infected	83
	Infection Rate(%)	13.25 b
Mesentric and Mediastinal lymph nodes together	Goats	620
	Infected	287
	Infection Rate(%)	46.19

Table 2. Infection rate by *Linguatula serrata* nymphs in mesenteric and mediastinal lymph nodes in slaughtered goats in different sex. [a,b,c,d] The infection rate in a row with different superscript letters are significantly different (p<0.05).

		Sex	
		Male	**Female**
Mesentric lymph nodes	Goats	423	197
	Infected	167	87
	Infection Rate(%)	39.5[a]	44.2[a]
Mediastinal lymph nodes	Goats	423	197
	Infected	54	29
	Infection Rate(%)	12.8[a]	14.7[a]
Mesentric and Mediastinal lymph nodes together	Goats	423	197
	Infected	184	103
	Infection Rate(%)	43.5[a]	52.3[a]

Table 3. Infection rate by *Linguatula serrata* nymphs in mesenteric and mediastinal lymph nodes in slaughtered goats in different age. [a,b,c,d] The infection rate in a row with different superscript letters are significantly different (p<0.05).

		Age (Year)			
		<1.5	**1.5-2.5**	**2.5-3.5**	**>3.5**
Mesentric lymph nodes	Goats	460	91	40	29
	Infected	178	35	25	16
	Infection Rate(%)	38.7[a]	35.5[a]	62.5[b]	55.2[c]
Mediastinal lymph nodes	Goats	460	91	40	29
	Infected	54	14	6	9
	Infection Rate(%)	11.8[a]	15.4[a]	15[a]	31[b]
Mesentric and Mediastinal lymph nodes together	Goats	460	91	40	29
	Infected	200	42	27	18
	Infection Rate(%)	43.5[a]	46.15[a]	67.5[b]	62.1[b]

Table 4. Infection rate by *Linguatula serrata* nymphs in mesenteric and mediastinal lymph nodes in slaughtered goats in different seasons. [a,b,c,d] The infection rate in a row with different superscript letters are significantly different (p<0.05).

		Season			
		Spring	**Summer**	**Autumn**	**winter**
Mesentric lymph nodes	Goats	100	210	210	100
	Infected	42	90	90	32
	Infection Rate (%)	42[a]	42.85[a]	42.85[a]	32[b]
Mediastinal lymph nodes	Goats	100	210	210	100
	Infected	18	26	27	12
	Infection Rate (%)	18[a]	12.4[b]	12.85[b]	12[b]
Mesentric and Mediastinal lymph nodes together	Goats	100	210	210	100
	Infected	52	98	98	39
	Infection Rate (%)	52[a]	46.7[a]	46.7[a]	39[b]

2004). The infected nymphs were obtained from different visceral organs, and in most studies MLNs were evaluated because the nodes are the first place to be infected with *L. serrata* nymph. Therefore, the possibility of infection in MLNs is higher than other visceral organs (Shakerian et al., 2008). A few studies on the prevalence of *L. serrata* nymphs in goats were conducted in some areas of Iran, e.g., in Mashhad (Tajik et al., 2007) and in Najaf-Abad (Pourjafar et al., 2007; Shakerian et al., 2008). In Egypt, 4.9% of MLNs from the examined camels were infected (Razavi et al., 2004). In a recent study, from the 232 examined goats, the parasite was reported in MLNs of goats, that was higher than the reports of Oryan et al. (1993) and Wahba et al. (1997) with infection rates of 7.5% and 4.9%, respectively. The above-mentioned data were less than those reported by Tajik et al. (2007) and Pourjafar et al. (2007) with the infection rates of 75% and 35%, respectively. Therefore, our results showed that Isfahan province is an endemic area for linguatulosis in goats, and probably in other ruminants and dogs. In less than 1-year-old group of the examined goats, *L. serrata* nymphs were only observed in one sample (4%). There was not significant difference among different age groups. Similarly, there was no significant difference in the rate of infection of the male and female goats. Due to the fact that goat meat is one of the common foods in Iran, particularly in central part of Iran such as Isfahan Province, the high rate of infection with the *L. serrata* nymphs in goats in this area clearly indicates a high risk of transmission of the disease from consumption of raw or undercooked goat viscera to human beings. Also, these results show that the infection rate in goats is very high. Furthermore, goats' viscera can transmit the infection to final hosts and cause the maintenance of life cycle of parasite in this area. Based on the high prevalence of infection in goats, we supposed that the rate of problems associated with linguatulosis in humans is higher than mentioned before.

Based on the results obtained from this research, suggesting that presence of such gross changes in the color and consistency of the MLNs could be considered as an indication of infection with nymphs of *L. serrate*, the exact inspection and elimination of infected organs is necessary to interrupt the life cycle of parasites.

References

1. Acha, P.N., Szyfres, B. (2003) Pentastomosis. In: Zoonosis and Communicable Diseases Common to Man and Animals (Parasitosis). Acha, P.N., Szyfres, B. (eds.). Scientific and technical publication. Pan American Health Organization, Washington, DC, USA. p. 345-380.
2. Akyol, C.U., Coskun, S.Z., Omez, G. (1995) *Linguatula serrata* in Bursa stray dogs and its importance from the point of public health. Turkiye Parazitoloji Dergissi. 19: 261-271.
3. Alcala-Canto, Y., Alberti-Navarro, A., Ibbara-Velarde, F. (2007) Serin protease activity demonstrated in larval stage of the Pentastomid *Linguatula serrata*. Parasitol Res. 100: 1011-1014.
4. Baird, J.K., Kassebaum, L.J., Ludwig, G.K. (1988) Hepatic granuloma in a man from the North of America caused by a nymph of *Linguatula serrata*. Pathology. 20: 198-199.
5. Beaver, P.C., Jung, R.O.C., Cup, E.W. (1984) Crustacea, linguatulid, millipeds, centipeds, scorpions, spiders, ticks and mites. In: Clinical Parasitology. Beaver, P.C., Jung, R.O.C., Cup, E.W. (eds.). (9th ed.) Lea and Febiger, Philadelphia, USA. p.572-573.
6. Berger, S.A., Marr, J.S. (2006) Human Parasitic Diseases Source Book. Jones and Bartlett Publishers: Sudbury, Massachusetts, USA. p. 294.
7. Drabick, J.J. (1987) Pentastomiasis. Rev Infect Dis. 9: 1087-1094.
8. El-Hassan, A.M., Eltoum, I.A., El-Asha, B.M.A. (1991) The Marara syndrome: isolation of *Linguatula serrata* nymph from a patient and the viscera of goats. Trans R Soc Trop Med Hyg. 85: 309.
9. Esmail-Nia, K., Hadizadeh-Moalem, S., Derakhshanfa, A. (2000) A study on the prevalence of *Linguatula serrata* infestation in small ruminants of Mazandaran Province in babol abattoir. Pajouhesh and Sazandegi. (In persian). 54: 94-95.
10. Fata, A., Elahi, M.R., Berenji, F. (1994) Pentastomiasis and report of the first case of Halazoun syndrome in Khorasan Province. Med J Mashhad Uni Med Sci. 37: 137-142.
11. Gardiner, C.H., Dyke, J.W., Shirley, S.F. (1984) Hepatic granuloma due to a nymph of *Linguatula serrata* in a woman from Michigan: a case report and review of the literature. Am J Trop Med Hyg. 33: 187-189.
12. Gosling, P.Y. (2005) Dictionary of Parasitology. CRC pres. Boca Raton, USA.
13. Hodjati, M.H., Naghili, B. (1987) Report of a case with nasopharyngeal pentastomiasis from West Azarbaijan. Med J Tabriz Uni Med Sci. 23: 42-50.
14. Khalil, G.M., Schacher, J.F. (1965) *Linguatula serrata*-in relation to halzoun and the marrara syndrome. Am J Trop Med Hyg. 15: 736-746.
15. Khalil, G.M. (1970) Incidence of *Linguatula serrata* infection in Cairo mongrel dogs. J Parasitol. 56: 458.
16. Lazo, R.F., Hidalgo, E., Lazo, J.E. (1999) Ocular linguatulosis in Ecuador: A case report and morphometric study of the larva of *L. serrata*. Am J Trop Med Hyg. 60: 405-406.
17. Maleky, F. (2001) A case report of *Linguatula serrata* in human throat from Tehran, Central Iran. Ind J Med Sci. 55: 439-441.
18. Meshgi, B., Asgarian, O. (2003) Prevalence of *Linguatula serrata* infestation in stray dogs of Shahrekord, Iran. J Vet Med. B 50: 466-467.
19. Muller, R. (2002) Worm and Human Diseases. CABI Publishing Co. Wallingford, UK. p. 240-242.
20. Nourollahi-Fard, S.R., Kheirandish, R., Nourouzi-Asl, E. (2010 a) The prevalence of *Linguatula serrata* nymphs in mesenteric lymph nodes in cattle. Am J Anim Vet Sci. 5: 155-158.
21. Nourollahi-Fard, S.R., Kheirandish, R., Nourouzi-Asl, E. (2010 b) The prevalence of *Linguatula serrata* nymphs in goats slaughtered in Kerman slaughterhouse, Kerman, Iran. Vet Parasitol. 171: 176-178.
22. Nourollahi-Fard, S.R., Kheirandish, R., Nourouzi-Asl, E. (2011) Mesenteric and mediastinal lymph node infection with *Linguatula serrata* nymphs in sheep slaughtered in Kerman slaughterhouse, Southeast Iran. Trop Anim Health Prod. 43: 1-3.
23. Oryan, A., Moghadar, N., Hanifepour, M.R. (1993) Arthropods recovered from the visceral organs of camel with special reference to their incidence and pathogenesis in Fars Provinces of Iran. Indian J Anim Sci. 63: 290-293.
24. Oryan, A., Sadjjadi, S.M., Mehrabani, D. (2008) The status of *Linguatula serrata* infection of stray dogs in Shiraz, Iran. Comp Clin Pathol. 17: 55-60.
25. Pourjafar, M., Azizi, H., Darabi, S. (2007) The prevalence of nymphal stage of Lingautula serrata in camels (Camelus dromedaries) in Najaf-Abad, Iran. J

Camel Pract Res. 14: 171-173.
26. Ravindran, R., Lakshmanan, B., Ravishankar, C. (2008) Prevalence of *Linguatula serrata* in domestic ruminants in South India, Southeast Asia. J Trop Med Public Health. 39: 808-812.
27. Razavi, S.M., Shekarforoush, S.S., Izadi, M. (2004) Prevalence of *Linguatula serrata* nymph in goats in Shiraz, Iran. Small Rumin Res. 54: 213-217.
28. Riley, J. (1986) The biology of Pentastomids. Adv Parasitol. 25: 45-128.
29. Sadjjadi, S.M., Ardehali, S.M., Shojaei, A.A. (1998) case report of *Linguatula serrata* in human pharynx from Shiraz, Southern Iran. Med J Islamic Rep Iran. 12: 193-194.
30. Saiyari, M., Mohammadian, B., Sharma, R.N. (1996) *Linguatula serrata* (Forlich 1789) nymphs in lungs of goats in Iran. Trop Anim Health Prod. 28: 312-314.
31. Shakerian, A., Shekarforoush, S.S., Ghafari-Rad, H. (2008) Prevalence of *Linguatula serrata* nymphs in Najaf-Abad, Iran. Res Vet Sci. 44: 243-245.
32. Shekarforoush, S.S., Razavi, S.M., Izadi, M. (2004) Prevalence of *Linguatula serrata* nymph in sheep in Shiraz, Iran. Small Rumin Res. 52: 99-101.
33. Sisakumar, P., Sankar, M., Nambi, P.A. (2005) The occurrence of nymphal stage of *Linguatula serrata* in water buffaloes (*Bubalus bubalis*): Nymphal morphology and lymph node pathology. J Vet Med. A52: 506-509.
34. Soulsby, E.J.L. (1982) Helminths Arthropods and Protozoa of Demestocated Animals, (7th ed.) Bailliere Tindall. London, UK.
35. Tajik, H., Tavassoli, M., Dalir-Naghadeh, B. (2006) Mesentric lymph nodes in infection with *Linguatula serrata* nymphs in cattle. Iran J Vet Res. 7: 82-85.
36. Tajik, H., Tavassoli, M., Khani, H. (2007) Prevalence of *Linguatula serrata* nymphs in slaughtered camels of Iran. J Camel Pract Res. 14: 69-71.
37. Tavassoli, M., Tajik, H., Dalir-Naghadeh, B. (2007) prevalence of *Linguatula serrata* nymphs and gross changes of infected mesenteric lymph nodes in sheep in Urmia, Iran. Smal Rumin Res. 72: 73-76.
38. Wahba, A.A., Shehab, G.J., El-Refaii, M.A.H. (1997) Some parasitological and pathological studies on two camel parasites, *Dicrocoelium dendriticum* (rudolphi, 1819) and *Linguatula serrata* (Frohlich, 1789) in Egypt. Assiut Vet Med J. 36: 153-156.
39. Yagi, H., El-Bahari, S., Mohamed, H.A. (1996) The Marrara syndrome: a hypersensitivity reaction of the upper respiratory tract and buccopharyngeal mucosa to nymphs of *Linguatula serrata*. Acta Trop. 62: 127-134.

The first study of bovine immunodeficiency virus (BIV) and bovine viral diarrhea virus (BVDV) co- infection in industrial herds of cattle in two provinces of Iran

Mokhtari, A.*, Mahzounieh, M.R.

Department of Pathobiology, Faculty of Veterinary Medicine, University of Shahrekord, Shahrekord, Iran

Key words:
BIV, BVDV, co- infection

Correspondence
Mokhtari, A.
Department of Pathobiology, Faculty of Veterinary Medicine, University of Shahrekord, Shahrekord, Iran

Email: a.mokhtari@alumni.ut.ac.ir

Abstract:

BACKGROUND: BIV is a well-known bovine immunosuppressive cause, but its pathogenesis has not been well characterized. It seems that it is possible that cofactors such as co- infection with other bovine viral pathogens may play a role in enhancing the pathogenesis of BIV infection; BVDV also has immunosuppressive effects. **OBJECTIVE:** The aim of this study was determination of possible correlation between BIV and BVDV infections. **METHODS:** Blood samples were randomly collected from a total of 1800 cattle in dairy industrial farms in Isfahan and Chaharmahal va Bakhtiari provinces of Iran. First BIV or BVDV positive sera were screened by ELISA, and then samples were analyzed to detect BIV proviral DNA or BVDV RNA, using PCR. **RESULTS:** Out of 1800 blood samples, 19 (1.06%) samples were BVDV positive, while BIV positive samples were 10 (0.55%). Nine (0.5%) samples contained both BIV and BVDV genomes and were positive in ELISA, while one of the samples (0.05%) was only BIV positive. **CONCLUSIONS:** In this study, there was a statistically significant relationship between BIV status and BVDV infection using Chi square and Pearson's correlation coefficient test (p=0, r=0.65).

Introduction

Bovine immunodeficiency virus (BIV) is an infectious pathogenic lentivirus in the family Retroviridae. BIV infections are lifelong and generally subclinical (Amborski et al., 1989; Belloc et al., 1996). There are some evidences that BIV can cause immunosuppression with increased incidences of secondary bacterial infections in herds with high seroprevalences (Burkala et al., 1999; Carpenter et al., 1992; Cyrcoats et al., 1994; Evermann et al., 1997; Gonda et al., 1987; Gonda et al., 1994; McNab et al., 1994; Fakur et al., 2008) or following experimental infections (Yilmaz et al., 2008). It has also been suspected that the stress of parturition in BIV infected cows is associated with the progression of other bovine viral and bacterial infections (Cyrcoats et al., 1994; Gonzalez et al., 2001a,b).

Bovine viral diarrhea virus (BVDV) is one of the most important viral pathogens of cattle, affecting herds worldwide and causing significant economic impacts. Many production losses from BVDV occur (e.g. reduced milk production and conception rate, respiratory disorders, and increased susceptibility to other disease) (Lambeth et al., 2007).

While pathogenic and economic effects of BVDV are known clearly, the role of BIV in animal disease remains controversial. Since both these viruses have suppressor effects in the bovine immune system, existence of a synergism between BVDV and BIV is possible in the co- infected cases. Therefore, we proposed that each virus may predispose cattle to other infection. In this study, we tried to determine a correlation between these active infections without focusing on how this synergism occurs.

Materials and Methods

Herd management and size: The samples were obtained from dairy industrial provinces in Isfahan and Chaharmahal va Bakhtiari provinces of Iran from 2008 to 2009 from 1800 cattle. These industrial herds use more advanced technology with average milk production from about 4300 to 7900 Kg/cow/year. The populations of these industrial farms were between 100 and 7500. The total 20 herds for sampling were categorized by density such as: 8 small (100-500), 9 medium (500-2000), and 3 large herds (≥2000). We eliminated the effect of cows' age on BVDV or BIV prevalence by selecting the cattle in the same age (2 <age < 3 years). The cow population of the tested herds included was 1800. We collected samples from all of these farms so that one-tenth of the population between 2 and 3 years old from each farm to be sampled. All of the cows were Holstein breed. They were housed in an intensive system. About 95% of the herds had free-stall system. The calves were kept in individual boxes. All of the female cows were vaccinated against brucellosis. The animals were immunized against foot and mouth disease and clostridial diseases according to routine schedule in Iran. All of the herds used artificial insemination.

Blood sampling and DNA/RNA extraction: The samples were obtained from dairy industrial provinces in Isfahan and Chaharmahal va Bakhtiari provinces of Iran during the period of 2008-2009 from 1800 cattle and then were centrifuged (2000 rpm/ 50 min) to obtain serum samples. Blood samples were randomly collected from cows that were between 2 and 3 years old (We gave a number to each cow, then using SPSS v. 16, from the transform menu-->random number generator-->under the Active Generator Initialization, clicking on random, we selected a random number). The sera were stored at -20°C until further use. All serum samples were analyzed to detect anti BIV and BVDV antibodies applying Lab-ELISA and I-ELISA respectively. For PCR assay confirming the BIV serology results, blood samples with EDTA were obtained from seropositives and seronegatives dairy cows, and Genomic DNA was extracted from peripheral PBMC using the DNA isolation kit for mammalian whole blood (Roche Applied Science) according to the manufacturer's directions within 48h. For RT-PCR assay confirming the BVDV results in ELISA, blood samples with Heparin Sodium were obtained from seropositives. Seronegatives dairy cows and total RNA was extracted from sera using the Qiagen RNA extraction kit (Qiagen RNeasy Mini kit, catalogue number: 52906) according to the manufacturer's directions within 24 h. Then cDNAs were made using Fermentas cDNA synthesis kit (catalogue number: K1622) according to the manufacturer's instructions.

Detection of anti- BIV antibodies by labeled avidin- biotin enzyme-linked immunosorbent sssay (Lab- ELISA): Serological analysis was performed on 1800 serum samples using a synthetic peptide derived from the available sequence of the transmembrane (TM) glycoprotein of BIV-FL112, produced at the Veterinary Laboratories Agency, Weybridge, Surrey, UK (Scobie et al., 1999). The results were expressed as the absorbance at 405 nm. A sample to positive ratio was calculated based on the positive and negative control sera included (Generous donations from Jean Pierre Frossard - Veterinary Laboratories Agency, UK) in each plate (Scobie et al., 1999).

Detection of anti- BVDV antibodies by I-ELISA: Samples were tested with an indirect ELISA (SVANOVIR™ BVDV-Ab ELISA, Svanova Biotech AB, Sweden, cat. no: P06029) according to the manufacturer's instructions.

Sample and reference optical density (OD) values were corrected before interpretation by subtracting the OD values of the corresponding wells containing the control antigen. The antibody titer was interpreted on the basis of the percentage positivity (PP) by dividing the sample OD values by positive reference sample OD values. According to the kit's instructional manual, the criteria for a sample to be assessed as positive was PP≥14.

Detection of BIV by PCR assay: The presence of BIV was detected using the Gene Pak DNA PCR test kit specific for the gag gene of BIV (catalogue number 12134 and from Isogene Lab Ltd, Moscow). The assay was performed according to the manufacturer's instructions. The PCR products were visualized after electrophoresis in 1.3% agarose by staining with ethidium bromide and compared to DNA markers (50 base pair ladder, Fermentas).

Briefly, in PCR test for detection of BIV proviral DNA, each PCR microtube contained 10 μL PCR diluents, 5 μL Master mix and 5 μL DNA sample. The thermal cycling conditions for the amplification were 1 cycle for 2 min at 95°C, 30 cycles of 45s at 95°C, 45s at 58°C and 60s at 74°C, with a final extension step of 2 min at 74°C. Positive and negative controls (Generous donations from Jean Pierre Frossard - Veterinary Laboratories Agency, UK) were included in each analysis. Six microliters of the amplified products were loaded on a 1.3% agarose gel and were visualized by staining with ethidium bromide and compared to DNA markers (50 base pair ladder, Fermentas).

Detection of BVDV by RT-PCR assay: The optimized RT-PCR assay was used to screen pooled sera under diagnostic laboratory conditions. A volume of 100 μL of serum from each cow was pooled in groups of 10 samples, and RNA was extracted according to the manufacturer's instructions (refer to the Qiagen RNeasy Mini Kit protocol available online). For RT-PCR, a BVDV specific PCR was used as Pfe¡er et al. described (Pfe¡er et al., 2000). The BVDV reactive 324 (5´- ATG CCC TTA GTA GGA CTA GCA -3´) and 326 (5´- TCA ACT CCA TGT GCC ATG TAC-3´) primers (17) flank a 288bp DNA fragment were selected. The amplification mixtures (50μL) consisted of 5μL 10 x reaction PCR buffer (Promega), 5μL of 25 mM MgCl2, 1mμL of 2mM each dNTP (Pharmacia), 15pmol of each primer, 1U Taq DNA polymerase (Promega), and 3μL cDNA. Positive and negative controls were provided by the manufacturer were included in each test. In vitro, amplifications were performed in a Thermal Cycler (Corbett Research, Australia) using the following thermal profile: denaturation at 94°C for 1 min, annealing for 1 min at 56°C, extension at 72°C for 1 min. After 36 cycles, the last extension step was prolonged for 7min.

After revealing the BVDV positive pool samples in the RT-PCR test, the same test was performed on each of the 10 samples in a positive pool sample separately.

Statistical analysis: The results were analyzed using Chi square and Pearson's correlation coefficient tests by using SPSS software v.16.

Results

Co-infection and statistics: The rate of active infections of BIV and BVDV in dairy farms in Isfahan and Chaharmahal va Bakhtiari provinces were 0.55% (No. 10) and 1.06% (No. 19), respectively (Table 1 and 2). Nine samples out of 1800 bovine sera (0.5%) were positive for both BIV and BVDV at the same time. They contained both BIV proviral DNA and BVDV RNA and were also positive in ELISA test. One sample (0.05%) was only BIV positive (Table 4). Out of BIV positive samples (n=10) 9 samples (90%) were BVDV positive in ELISA and PCR tests, while among BIV negative samples (n=1790) 10 (0.55%) samples were BVDV positive. In this study, there was a statistically significant relationship between BIV status and BVDV status using Chi square and Pearson's correlation coefficient test ($p = 0$, $r = 0.65$) (table 4).

I-ELISA: Of the 1800 samples, 19 (1.06%) were BVDV seropositive using I-ELISA test, while 10 (0.55%) samples were positive in BIV Lab-ELISA test. In ELISA tests performed in this study, 9 (0.5%) sera had antibodies against both BIV and BVDV. S/P ratios of the BIV positive samples were from 0.27 to 1.86, while BVDV positive PP values were from 20 to 124. Tables 2 and 3 show the results.

PCR: The presence of BIV provirus was detected using PCR test specific for the gag gene of BIV in peripheral blood mononuclear cells (PBMCs) from the bovine samples using the Gene Pak DNA PCR test kit. The BIV-specific band with the size of 298bp was detected in DNA positive control sample. The positive PCR products were in the same size as those from the positive control sample, while as expected, a 288bp DNA fragment was amplified in BIV-positive samples using the general BVDV primers 324 and 326. This band also was detected in positive control sample for BVDV.

Discussion

In this study, we found a consistency between serological and genomic detection of BVDV and BIV results.

Seroepidemiological studies of BIV infections in cattle have been reported in many countries (Amborski et al., 1989; Baron et al., 1998; Belloc et al., 1996; Burkala et al., 1999; Carpenter et al., 1992; Cyrcoats et al., 1994; Evermann et al., 1997; Gonda et al., 1987; Gonda et al., 1994; McNab et al., 1994;

Table 1. Co-infection of BVDV and BIV with PCR and ELISA tests: Using ELISA and PCR tests. Out of 1800 cattle 9 (0.5%) samples were positive for both BIV and BVDV.

BIV seronegtive		**BIV positive**		**Total**	
Number of samples	BVDV positive samples	Number of samples	BVDV positive	Number of samples	BVDV positive
1790	10 (0.55%)	10	9 (0.5%)	1800	19 (1.06%)

Table 2. Seroprevalence of BVDV and BIV in Isfahan and Chaharmahal va Bakhtiari areas.

BIV Prevalence		**BVDV Prevalence**	
Number of samples	BIV seropositive samples	Number of samples	BVDV seropositive samples
1800	10 (0.55%)	1800	19 (1.06%)

Table 3. CODs and PP values for BVDV seropositive samples: Sample and reference optical density (OD) values were corrected before interpretation by subtracting the OD values of the corresponding wells containing the control antigen. The antibody titer was interpreted on the basis of the percentage positivity (PP) by dividing the sample OD values by positive reference sample OD values. According to the kit's instructional manual, the criteria for a sample to be assessed as positive was as PP≥14.

No	**Location of the herd**	**Sample number**	**PP**
1	Isfahan	135	124
2	Isfahan	138	24
3	Isfahan	140	20
4	Isfahan	201	25
5	Isfahan	941	20
6	Isfahan	945	30
7	Isfahan	949	25
8	Isfahan	1292	100
9	Isfahan	1293	110
10	Isfahan	1294	26
11	Isfahan	1	35
12	Isfahan	2	43
13	Isfahan	3	27
14	Isfahan	4	65
15	Isfahan	5	54
16	Chaharmahalo Bakhtiari	6	76
17	Chaharmahalo Bakhtiari	7	62
18	Chaharmahalo Bakhtiari	8	35
19	Chaharmahalo Bakhtiari	9	47

Table 4. Statistical results for co- infection of BVDV and BIV. Out of 1800 cattle 9 (0.5%) samples contained both BIV and BVDV genomes and were positive in ELISA while one of samples (0.05%) was only BIV positive.

	BVDV positive	**BVDV negative**	**p-value**
BIV negative	10	1780	0
BIV positive	9	1	0

Fakur et al., 2008; Yilmaz et al., 2008). Despite the worldwide distribution of BIV infection, whether the presence of BIV in a host leads to primarily pathologic changes or can cause secondary bacterial and/or viral infections as a predisposition factor has not been fully elucidated. Under practical conditions, infection with BIV has a different effect on the host than has been observed under experimental conditions. The presence of BIV combined with the stresses associated by parturition and a modern dairy production system was considered causal for the development of secondary diseases in immuno-compromised cattle. The frequent development of concurrent infections in BIV-infected animals suggested that persistent BIV infection had a role in reducing functional immune competence, in accordance with other studies.

It has been hypothesized that infection with BIV, and potential consequent immunosuppression, might predispose cattle to infection by other agents (Nikbakht Borujeni et al., 2010). The co-infection of BIV and BVDV in dairy cattle in Iran is not reported.

In our study, the overall BIV-seroprevalence in industrial dairy farms was 0.55%. The prevalence of BVDV active infection in industrial farms was 1.06%. Therefore, BVDV active infection is more common than BIV infection in the Iranian cattle in the studied industrial farms. Previously, the presence of antibodies against BIV in dairy cattle of non industrial farms in Iran was reported by Nikbakht Borujeni et al., (2010) and Tajbakhsh et al., (2010). The BIV seroprevalence in these studies were 20.3% and 60%, respectively, which are much more than expected in the world average (4 - 5%).

Also, in the previous studies performed by Iranian researchers (Fakur et al., 2008; Badiei et al., 2010; Morshedi et al., 2004) on BVDV seroprevalence, the rate of infection in non industrial farms in Shiraz, Urmia, and Sanandaj provinces of Iran were 37-86%, 31.38% and 27.7%, respectively. Previous studies of these viruses have done in non- industrial farms in Iran, so these findings may vary with our results. The main cause of difference was interpretation of results. We only consider active infection which showed both anti - BVDV antibodies and viral RNA, but in previous published data, the researchers recorded only seropositive which had only antibodies and it showed previous or transient infection. In the study

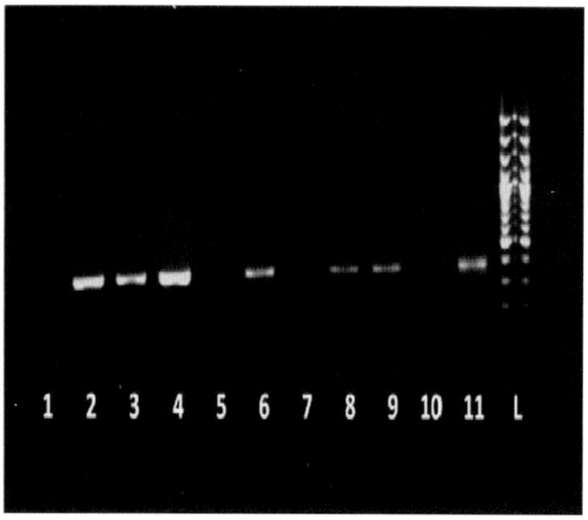

Figure 1. BIV-gag PCR amplification products following electrophoresis. L= 50bp DNA ladder, 11=positive control (BIV infected animal), 1=negative control (uninfected animal), 2 to 10 samples (Iranian animals), 7= a negative sample.

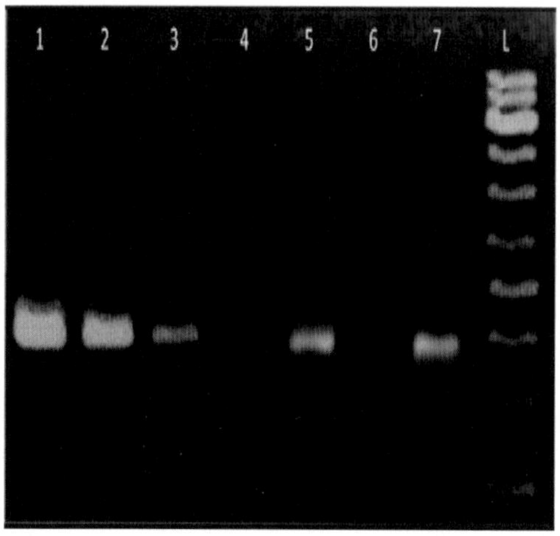

Figure 2. BVDV RT-PCR amplification products following electrophoresis. (BVDV RT-PCR test was performed on BIV positive samples). L= 100bp DNA ladder, 7= positive control (BVDV infected animal), 6= negative control (uninfected animal), 1,2,3,5 are BVDV positive samples.

performed by Badiei et al. in Shiraz, cows in semi-industrial herds were tested (the populations of the herds were between 50 and 1700). Talebkhan Garoussi et al. (Talebkhan Garoussi et al., 2009) have found higher BVDV seroprevalence among the industrial dairy cattle herds in suburb of Mashhad in Iran (72.25%). As mentioned above , the main cause of difference between our study and Talebkhan Garoussi et al.'s survey was using the method for finding positive cows. They had just used serology to find seropositive cows, while in this study we try to find active infection with BVDV. However, we have eliminated the age effect on prevalence of these two infections by selecting an age group.

The aim of this study was not to investigate the prevalence of BVDV or BIV in herds of Isfahan and Chaharmahal va Bakhtiari provinces of Iran; we were looking for a meaningful relationship between co-infection with both viruses. So far, co- infection of BVD and BIV has not been studied. Carpenter et al. for characterization of early pathogenic effects after experimental infection of calves with BIV attempted to separate the effects of BVDV and BIV in their study. The authors believed that fever and leucopenia are characteristic of acute infection with BVDV that is a common contaminant of cell culture and previous infection with this virus is causing confusion in identifying the exact symptoms of the BIV.

In fact, they were convinced that no synergism existed between these two viruses, but they saw that in the cattle which was co-infected with BIV and BVDV or cell cultures that were contaminated with BVDV, BIV has caused more changes. The pathogenesis of the BIV infection has not been well characterized. Experimentally-infected animals did not develop immunodeficiency. It is possible that co-factors may play a role in enhancing the pathogenesis of BIV infection, and one of these co-factors could be bovine viral diarrhea virus (BVDV) because of its immunosuppressive effects. (Carpenter et al., 1992)

In the present study, a seroepidemiological survey of BIV and BVDV was performed to determine a correlation between BIV and BVDV infections. We found a statistically significant relationship between these viruses infections.

Overall, among 1800 cattle tested, 19 (1.06%) were BVDV positive and 9 (0.5%) animals were positive to both BIV and BVDV. The statistical analysis shows a p value less than 0.05 ($p=0.0$) for the chi square test, and r equal to zero. These indexes demonstrated there is an association between BIV and BVDV infections.

This study had some limitations. First, it was difficult to know whether the disorders observed were due to BIV or BVDV infections alone; because of the fact that BIV-positive or BVDV positive cattle were not further analyzed for other infectious agents like viruses or bacteria that may play a role in that kind of clinical disorder. Second, it is difficult to select uniform patient and control populations in animal studies. Therefore, control animals were selected from among BIV-seronegative cattle from the same herds including BIV-positive animals, because of the fact that some factors, i.e. climate, magnitude of farm, and management, are well known to affect the health status of dairy cattle. Third, the number of lactations could have been recorded in the present study was limit.

Co -factors such as BVDV infection may enhance the pathogenesis of BIV infection, and BIV can be a risk factor for other infections such as BVD. It is difficult to distinguish in cattle co-infected with these viruses, which of them predispose the infection with the other. On the other hand, we did not determined viral cytopathogenicity. While pathogenic and economic effects of BVDV are known clearly, the role of BIV in animal disease remains controversial. Since these two viruses have suppressor effects in the bovine immune system, the existence of a synergism between BVDV and BIV is hypothetically possible in the co-infected. In this study, we tried to determine a correlation between these infections without focusing on how this synergism occurs. We found a statistically significant relationship between BIV status and BVDV status using Chi square and Pearson's correlation coefficient test ($p=0$, $r=0.65$) and high co-infection rate of these 2 viruses can support our hypothesis, but it needs further studies.

Conclusions

In this study, the statistical analysis shows $P= 0.0$ for the chi square test, and $r=0.65$ demonstrated there is a statistical association between BIV and BVDV. So, the existence of a synergism between BVDV and BIV is possible in the co-infected cases.

Acknowledgements

The authors wish to thank Y. Nikzadeh (University of Tehran, Iran) for statistical advice, F. Yektaneh (University of Shahrekord, Iran) for assistance in the laboratory techniques, and Jean Pierre. Frossard (Veterinary Laboratories Agency, Wheybridge, UK) because of his effective guidance for the BIV ELISA/PCR setting up.

References

1. Amborski, G.F., Lo, J.J., Seger, C.L. (1989) Serological detection of multiple retroviral infections in cattle: bovine leukemia virus, bovine syncytial virus and bovine visna virus. Vet Microbiol. 20: 247-253.
2. Badiei, K.H., Ghane, M., Mostaghni, K.H. (2010) Prevalence of Bovine viral diarrhea virus antibodies among the Industrial dairy cattle herds in suburb of Shiraz, Iran. MEJSR. 6: 403- 407.
3. Baron, T., Betemps, F., Mallet, F., Cheynet, V., Levy, D., Belli, P. (1998) Detection of bovine immunodeficiency-like virus infection in experimentally infected calves. Arch Virol. 143: 181-189.
4. Belloc, C., Polack, B., Schwartz, I., Brownlie, J., Levy, D. (1996) Bovine immunodeficiency virus: facts and questions. Vet Res. 27: 395-402.
5. Burkala, E.J., Ellis, T.M., Voigt, V., Wilcox, G.E. (1999) Serological evidence of an Australian bovine lentivirus. Vet Microbiol. 68: 171-177.
6. Carpenter, S., Miller, L.D., Alexardensen, S., Whetstone, C.A., Van Der Maaten, M.J., Viuff, B., Wannermuehler, Y., Miller, J.M., Roth, J.A. (1992) Characterization of early pathogenic effects after experimental infection of calves with bovine immunodeficiency-like virus. J Virol. 66: 1074-1083.
7. Cyrcoats, K.S., Pruett, S.B., Nash, J.W., Cooper, C.R. (1994) Bovine immunodeficiency virus: incidence of infection in Mississippi dairy cattle. Vet Microbiol. 42: 181-189.
8. Evermann, J., Jackson, M.K. (1997) Laboratory diagnostic tests for retroviral infections in dairy and beef cattle. Vet Clin North Am Food Anim Pract. 13: 87-106.
9. Fakur, S.H., Hemmatzadeh, F. (2008) Serological study on Bovine viral diarrhea- (BVD) in Sanandaj area. SIAU J Vet Med. 1: 1-11
10. Gonda, M.A., Braun, M.J., Carte, S.J., Kost, T.A., Bess, J.W., Arthur, T.A., Van Der Maaten, M.J. (1987) Characterization and molecular cloning of a bovine lentivirus related to human immunodeficiency virus. Nature. 330: 388-391.
11. Gonda, M.A., Gene Luther, D., Fong, S.E., Tobin, G.J. (1994) Bovine immunodeficiency virus: molecular biology and virus-host interactions. Virus Res. 32: 155-181.
12. Gonzalez, G.C., Johnston, J.B., Nickel, D.D., Jacobs, R.M., Olson, M., Power, C. (2001a) Very low prevalence of bovine immunodeficiency virus

infection in western Canadian cattle. Cancer J Vet Res. 65: 73-76.
13. Gonzalez, E.T., Oliva, G.A., Valera, A., Bonzo, E., Licursi, M., Etcheverrigaray, M.E. (2001b) Leucosis enzoo´ tica bovina: Evaluacio´n de te´cnicas diagno´ sticas (ID, ELISA-i, WB, PCR) en bovine's experimentalmente inoculados. Analecta Vet J. 21: 8-15.
14. Lambeth, L., Moore, R.J., Muralitharan, M.S, Doran, T.J. (2007) Suppression of bovine viral diarrhea virus replication by small interfering RNA and short hairpin RNA-mediated RNA interference. Vet Microbiol. 119: 132-143.
15. McNab, W.B., Jacobs, R.M., Smith, H.E. (1994) A survey for bovine immunodeficiency-like virus in Ontario dairy cattle and associations between test results production records and management practices. Can J Vet Res. 58: 36-41.
16. Morshedi, A. (2004) Serological study on Bovine viral diarrhea (BVD) in Sanandaj area. J Vet Res. 59: 23-34.
17. Nikbakht Borujeni, G.R., Taghi Poorbazargani, T., Nadin-Davis, S., Tolooie, M., Barjesteh, N. (2010) Bovine immunodeficiency virus and bovine leukemia virus and their mixed infection in Iranian Holstein cattle. J Infect Dev Ctries. 9: 576-579.
18. Pfe¡er, M., Von Freyburg, M., Kaaden, O.R. and Beer, M. (2000) A universal `one-tube' RT-PCR protocol for smplifying isolates of bovine viral diarrhoea virus. Vet Res Commun. 24: 491-503.
19. Scobie, L., Venables, C., Hughes, K., Dawson, M., Jarret, O. (1999) The antibody response of cattle infected with Bovine Immunodeficiency Virus to peptides of the viral transmembrane protein. J Gen Virol. 80: 237-243.
20. Tajbakhsh, E., Nikbakht Borujeni, G., Momtazan, H., Amirmozafari, N. (2010) Molecular prevalence for Bovine immunodeficiency virus infection in Iranian cattle population. Afr J Microbiol Res. 12: 1199-1202.
21. Talebkhan Garoussi, M., Haghparast, A., Hajenejad, M.R. (2009) Prevalence of bovine viral diarrhoea virus antibodies among the industrial dairy cattle herds in suburb of Mashhad-Iran. Trop Anim Health Prod. 41:663-667.
22. Yilmaz, Z., Yezilbag, K. (2008) Clinical and haematological findings in bovine immuno-deficiency virus (BIV) infected cattle. Turk J Vet Anim Sci. 32: 207-214.

A trace analysis of oxytetracycline and tetracycline residues in pasteurized milk supplied in Tehran: a one-year study (April 2011-March 2012)

Rassouli, A.[1*], Amani, Z.[1], Bahonar, A.[2], Shams, Gh.[1], Abdolmaleki, Z.[1]

[1] *Department of Pharmacology, Faculty of Veterinary Medicine, University of Tehran, Tehran, Iran*

[2] *Department of Food Hygiene and Quality Control, Faculty of Veterinary Medicine, University of Tehran, Tehran, Iran*

Key words:
HPLC, milk, residue, tetracyclines

Correspondence
Rassouli, A.
Department of Pharmacology,
Faculty of Veterinary Medicine,
University of Tehran, Tehran, Iran

Email: arasooli@ut.ac.ir

Abstract:

BACKGROUND: Tetracyclines (TCs) are broad-spectrum antibiotics that are widely used in veterinary medicine. The presence of TCs residues in milk is a public health concern all over the world. **OBJECTIVES:** This study aimed to determine TCs residuals in pasteurized milk marketed by some dairy companies in Tehran from April 2011 to March 2012. **METHODS:** 432 pasteurized milk samples were purchased from supermarkets supplying the milk products of 12 major dairy companies in Tehran (3 samples from each company every month), and they were stored at -20 0C until analysis. Oxytetracycline (OTC) and Tetracycline (TC) residues in each sample were extracted by a liquid - liquid phase procedure and quantitated using a high performance liquid chromatographic (HPLC) method. Chromatographic conditions included a mobile phase as oxalic acid buffer- acetonitril (80: 20) with a flow rate of 1mL/min and UV-detection at 355 nm. **RESULTS:** TCs residuals in most milk samples were lower than 100 ppb, maximum residue level (MRL); however, in seven samples (1.62%) the total residues of OTC and TC were more than MRL. In the latter milk samples, the median total TCs residue was 625 ppb, ranging between 274 and 1270 ppb. **CONCLUSIONS:** Because of the presence of TC residues above the MRL level in a limited number of milk samples, it is concluded that more studies and supervision of health authorities are needed in this field.

Introduction

Tetracyclines are broad-spectrum antibiotics with a bacteriostatic effect on a wide range of gram-negative and gram-positive bacteria and are widely used in veterinary medicine and in humans. They are used for prevention or treatment of a great number of diseases and for growth promotion in animal husbandry. These antibiotics are produced by Streptomyces spp., and the mode of action is exerted by binding to 30S ribosomal subunits of susceptible bacteria, which in turn inhibits their protein synthesis (Chopra, 1981).

The use of TCs in dairy farms may have serious adverse effects due to the potential presence of antibiotic residues in milk. Antibiotic residues are small amounts of drugs or their active metabolites that remain in milk or meat after treating the cows. Problems associated with antibiotic residues in milk include the risk of allergic reactions, increased resistance of pathogens against antibiotics, and inhibition of bacterial starter cultures used in dairy production. Low levels of these residues in milk when consumed over a period of time can lead to the development of drug-resistant microorganisms. The occurrence of drug residues mainly results from failure to implement the mandatory withdrawal periods; illegal or extra-label use of drugs and incorrect dosage levels are hazardous (Ivona et al., 2002).

In order to reduce the risks of TC residues in milk on public health, international organizations such as World Health Organization (WHO), US Food and Drug Administration (FDA), and the European Union (EU), Codex Alimentarius Commission (CAC) proposed 100ng/mL of parent drugs, separately or in combination, as MRL (Kaplan et al., 1962; WHO, 1990; Commission of EC, 1991; Rassouli et al., 2010).

The MRL level for each compound in any specified foodstuff is not a fixed value throughout the world, and it may vary in different countries according to their dietary habits as well as the policies and authorities of their public health organizations. Although the primary purpose of establishing MRLs is to ensure the food safety and to protect the health of the consumer against possible harmful effects resulting from exposure to residues, it should be uniformly established and harmonized to facilitate the marketing and free trade of foodstuffs of animal origin in national and international levels.

A number of methods including microbiological and physicochemical ones are used to determine TCs residues in biological matrices (lwaki et al., 1992; Jacques et al., 1998; Furusawa, 1999; Ding et al., 2000; Fritz and Zuo, 2007). However, HPLC method-s are the most sensitive and specific techniques in this regard. Therefore, in the present study, a rapid and easy HPLC procedure was adopted and modified for determination of TCs residue levels in milk.

This project was carried out due to the widespread use of TCs in lactating cows in Iran and occasional debates between public health and veterinary of-ficials regarding the presence and the levels of antibiotic residues in foods of animal origin as well as the lack of long-term studies (covering an entire year) in milk industry.

Materials and Methods

Milk sample collection and preparation: Four hundred and thirty two pasteurized milk samples were purchased from Tehran supermarkets supplying the products of 12 major dairy companies from April 2011 to March 2012 (three milk samples from each company every month and in total 36 samples in each month). The milk samples were collected once in the middle of each month, and then they were transferred to the laboratory of the Department of Pharmacology, Faculty of Veterinary Medicine, University of Tehran, and were stored at -20 0C until analysis.

OTC and TC residues in milk were extracted by a liquid-liquid phase procedure (described briefly below) and quantified by an HPLC method. This technique was used just after validation of the HPLC method for analysis of both antibiotics including limits of detection (LOD), limits of quantification (LOQ), recovery rates, and linearity of calibration curves.

100 μL of NaOH (0.1 g in 100 mL H2O) was added to 1.0 mL of milk and was mixed using a vortex mixer. 1.5 mL of acetonitril (HPLC grade, Merck, Germany) was added and mixed again. The whole solution was centrifuged at 3000 rpm for 5 min, and then 1.0 mL of saturated Na2SO4 solution was added. 300 μL of supernatant was transferred into another tube and 600μL of 0.01 M oxalic acid buffer (pH, 7.0) was added and mixed. Finally, it was filtered into an autoinjector vial using 0.45μm membrane filter (Millipore, USA) to make the final solution for HPLC analysis.

Determination of TCs levels: All samples were analyzed by HPLC system (Knauer, Germany) after their preparations, using the HPLC method of Fritz and Zuo (2007) with some modifications. The chromatographic conditions included a mobile phase as 0.01 M oxalic acid buffer - acetonitril (80: 20) running through a C18 column (Eurospher 100; 5μm, 4.0*300 mm) isocratically with a flow rate of 1.0 mL/min and UV- detection at 355 nm. Chromatographic data including peak areas were recorded and analyzed by Chromgate software (Knauer, Germany).

OTC and TC residue levels in milk samples were calculated using their corresponding peak areas and calibration curve formula of each antibiotic by Microsoft Office Excel 2007.

Data analysis: Descriptive statistics were used for TCs residue data analysis. Median and the range of total TCs residues in milk samples containing residues above MRL were presented. The MRL value in this study was adopted according to the MRLs established by Codex Alimentarius Commission, i.e.,

100ng/mL of total TCs in milk or 100ppb.

Results

The HPLC method validation data: The retention times for OTC and TC were 2.1 and 2.5 min, respectively, without any interference in the retention times (Figure 1). The recovery rates for the OTC and TC residues in milk were 85.5 +/- 3.4% and 77.9 +/- 5.2 %, respectively. The linearity of calibration curve and curve formula for OTC levels at 0.05 - 10 μg/mL were R2=0.999 and Y= 613327 X+ 46850, respectively. The linearity and calibration curve formula for TC levels between 0.05 and 10 μg/mL were R2=0.999 and Y = 775277 X + 47631, respectively. The limit of detection (LOD) and limit of quantification (LOQ) for OTC analysis were 5 and 16 ng/mL, respectively, and for TC analysis they were 4 and 13 ng/mL, respectively.

TCs levels in milk: In 418 milk samples out of 432, the total residue levels of OTC and TC were lower than LOQ. In seven milk samples, although the TCs levels were quantifiable, total TCs residue contents were lower than 100 ng/mL (MRL). However, in seven milk samples (1.62 %), the total TCs residue levels were more than MRL. The specifications of the milk samples in which the amounts of total TCs residues were more than MRL are shown in Table 1.

TCs residues had not been detected in the samples collected in spring and summer seasons at all and all seven samples with TC residue levels above MRL were collected in autumn and winter seasons, 2 samples in October and 5 samples in February. The other seven milk samples with quantifiable TCs levels, but lower than MRL, had been collected in November (4 samples), January (1 sample), and February (2 samples).

Table 1. The specifications and amounts of oxytetracycline and tetracycline residues in seven pasteurized milk samples in which the total TCs residues were above MRL(100 ng/mL) in a one-year study (April 2011-March 2012). OTC: Oxytetracycline; TC: Tetracycline.

Sample No.	Month	OTC level (ng/mL)	TC level (ng/mL)	Total TCs Level (ng/mL)
7-5-3	Oct	483	-	483
7-12-2	Oct	526	706	1232
11-1-2	Feb	123	151	274
11-1-3	Feb	474	151	625
11-2-1	Feb	071	290	361
11-2-2	Feb	566	593	1159
11-8-1	Feb	-	1270	1270

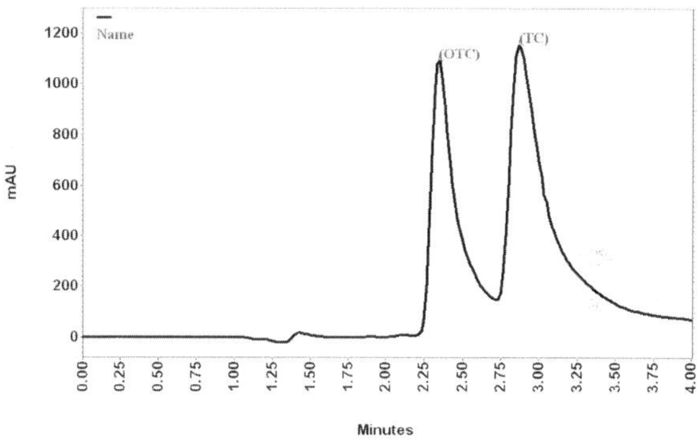

Figure 1. The chromatogram of mixed standard solution of oxyteracycline and tetracycline (1μg/mL of each).

Discussion

Public health concerns in connection with drug residues in milk are growing all over the world including Iran, in which occasional debates occur between public health sectors and veterinary officials. Recent cross-sectional studies regarding the TCs residue in milk in different parts of Iran indicate the presence of these antibiotics in marketed milk samples (Rassouli et al, 2010; Mesgari Abbasi et al., 2011). In a similar fashion, the present one-year study suggests that a limited number of milk samples (1.62%) have TCs residues above MRL. Regarding the relationship between seasonal changes and occurrence of residues in milk samples, it was notable that all milk samples with detectable TCs residues had been collected in cold seasons, autumn and winter.

Initial residue studies in milk were done in the 1950s by US-FDA. More studies on the crude and pasteurized milk supply in USA, Canada, UK, and South Africa between 1955 and 1959 revealed that approximately 3 to 5% of tested samples contained drug residues. Therefore, the US-FDA proposed plans in 1960 to prevent drug residues in milk, which included the establishment of withdrawal (withholding) times for a number of drugs used in food-producing animals and established maximum residues limits (MRLs) in food stuffs of animal origin including MRL for OTC and TC in milk (0.1μg/mL).

It has been reported that in 92% of cases, the cause

for the incidence of the antibiotic residues in milk was due to their administration in mastitis therapy (Schmidt et al., 2003). The occurrence of antibiotic residues in milk is strongly associated with certain variables such as milk production rate at the time of treatment, the type and amount of antibiotic used, the type of vehicle used in antibiotic formulations, and the disease state of the animal (Mercer et al., 1970).

Antimicrobials, anti-inflammatory, and hormones are the pharmacologically active substances most used for these purposes; however, an illegal or unsuitable use increases the risk of introducing harmful residues into human food chain. Adverse effects in consumers are connected with the intrinsic toxicity of a drug and/or its metabolites. Hence, the use of antimicrobial agents in food animals has made a lot of concerns regarding their impacts on human health.

The main applications of tetracycline in animal husbandry are for prophylaxis of bacterial infections and increasing the growth rates. Although the public health risks are difficult to define, it is accepted that antimicrobial drug residues may induce allergic reactions in sensitized individuals and may have negative effects on the composition of the human intestinal flora. In general, the excessive use of antimicrobials has led to the development and prevalence of multi-drug resistance in animal and human pathogens (Sarmah et al., 2006). Furthermore, milk contaminated with even low concentrations of antimicrobial residues may also create problems in the production process of fermented milk by-products, because such compounds may inhibit the growth of the starter cultures.

The first study on antibiotic residues in milk in Iran was carried out by Khavari (1961) in which 20 dairy cattle with clinical mastitis received an intramammary product containing antibiotics. Using microbiological tests, Khavari showed that 13 out of the 20 milk samples had antibiotic residues However, in another study, using microbiological tests, Abedi et al. (1984) did not find antibiotic residues in 325 milk samples collected from pasteurized dairy companies in Fars province. Another study assessed 200 raw milk samples in Shiraz (Fars province) for antibiotic contamination using the microbiological four-plate test (Liaghat et al., 1998). They reported that 10% of the raw milk samples from dairy companies and 13% of those from local markets were positive for antibiotic residues. However, they found no antibiotic residues in 100 pasteurized milk samples.

Desalegne (2008) collected 400 bulk milk samples randomly from dairy farms in Ethiopia. All samples were qualitatively screened for antibiotic residues by Delvotest SP assay. Out of 400 samples analyzed for antibiotic residue, 34 (8.5%) milk samples were positive for antibiotic residues. Then residue levels of the common antibiotics in positive samples were determined by HPLC. The antibiotic-residue positive samples which showed OTC residues higher than 100 ng/mL were 24 out of 34 (70.58%). Regarding penicillin G residual above MRL of 4 ng/mL, they were 7 (20.58%).

Rassouli et al. (2010), in a cross-sectional study, collected ninety milk samples during five sequential days from the products of six major dairy companies in Tehran in 2007. OTC and TC residues were extracted and quantified by an HPLC method with an ultraviolet detector. TCs residual were detected in seven (7.8%) milk samples. The OTC and TC in almost all samples were lower than 100 ng/mL. However, just in one milk sample out of 90 milk samples tested, the total residue levels of OTC and TC was more than MRL, 138.8 ng/mL.

Khosro khavar et al. (2011) studied OTC residues in infant formula in Tehran. They reported that the samples had no residues of OTC in infant formula from different companies.

Mesgari Abbasi collected 114 pasteurized, sterilized, and raw milk samples from markets of Ardabil (Mesgari Abbasi et al., 2011). Tetracycline, oxytetracycline, and chlortetracycline (TCs) residues extraction was carried out using solid phase extraction (SPE) method. The mean of total TCs residues in all samples (114 samples) was 97.6 ±16.9ng/mL and the means of pasteurized, sterilized, and raw milk samples were 87.1 ± 17.7, 112.0 ± 57.3 and 154.0±66.3ng/mL, respectively. 24.4%, 30%, and 28.6% of the pasteurized, sterilized, and raw milk samples, respectively, had higher TCs residues than the recommended MRL (100 ng/mL).

The method that was used in the present study for determination of TCs residues in milk was easy to validate, simple to perform, and more economical compared to the methods that used SPE cartridges. According to the results of this study, there were detectable TCs residues in 14 out of 432 (3.2%) of pasteurized milk samples; however, in seven cases (1.62%), the TCs levels were greater than the MRL. It was also noted that all milk samples containing detectable TCs residuals were collected in fall and winter in which it seems mastitis occur more frequently due to climatic changes, and as a result antibiotic therapy is carried out more often. It should be reminded that the milk samples analyzed in the present study represent the milk of a large number of dairy cows that were mixed together in milk tanks in dairy farms and further in dairy companies, and these processes greatly dilute the initial drug residues in milk.

In summary, with regard to the presence of TC residues above MRL in a limited number of milk samples, it is concluded that more studies on drug residues in food animal and the establishment of suitable regulations and inspection systems are needed to reduce the risks of antibiotic and other drug residues for public health.

Acknowledgments

The authors would like to acknowledge the Deputy of Research, Faculty of Vet. Med., University of Tehran, for financial support of this work.

References

1. Chopra, I., Howe, T.G.B., Linton, A.H. Linton, K.B., Richmond, M.H., Speller, D.C.E. (1981) The tetracyclines: Prospect at the beginning of the 1980s. J Anti Chem. 8: 5-21.
2. Ding, X., Mou, S. (2000) Ion chromatographic analysis of tetracyclines using polymeric column and acidic eluent. J Chromatogr A. 897: 205-214.
3. Fritz, J.W., Zuo, Y.G. (2007) Simultaneous determination of tetracycline, oxytetracycline, and 4-epitetracycline in milk by high-performance liquid chromatography. Food Chemistry. 105: 1297-1301.
4. Furusawa, N. (1999) Rapid and simple determination of oxytetracycline in milk products. J AOAC Int. 82: 770-772.
5. Ivona, K., Mate, D. (2002) Evaluation of the sensitivity of individual test organisms to residual concentrations of selected types of drugs. Slov Vet Res. 9: 78-82.
6. Iwaki, K., Okumura, N., Yamazaki, M. (1992) Determination of tetracycline antibiotics by reversed-phase high performance liquid chromatography with fluorescence detection. J Chromatogr. 623: 153-158.
7. Jacques, F.M.N., Loeffen, G., Schouten, J., Egmond, H.V., Keukens, H., Stegeman, H. (1998) Testing of raw milk for tetracyline residues. J Dairy Sci. 81: 2341-2345.
8. Kaplan, M.M., Abdussalam, M., Bijlenga, U. (1992) Specific and non-specific sensitizing agents FAO/WHO milk hygeine. WHO monograph series. 48: 56-58.
9. Khosrokhavar, R., Hosseini, M., Shoeibi, S., Jannat, B. (2011) Detection of oxytetracycline residue in infant formula by high performance liquid chromatography (HPLC). Iran J Pharm Res. 10: 221-224.
10. Mercer, H.D., Geleta, J.N., Wright, W.W. (1970) Milk out rates for antibiotics in intramammary infusion products used in the treatment of bovine mastitis: Relationship of somatic cell counts of milk production levels and drug vehicle. Am J Vet Res. 31: 1549-1560.
11. Mesgari Abbasi, M., Babaei, H., Ansarin, M., Nourdadgar, A., Nemati, M. (2011) Simultaneous determination of tetracyclines residues in bovine milk samples by solid phase extraction and HPLC-FL method. Adv Pharm Bull. 1: 34-39.
12. Rassouli, A., Abdolmaleki, Z., Bokaee, S., Kamkar, A., Shams, G.R. (2010) A cross-sectional study on oxytetracycline and tetracycline residues in pasteurized milk supplied in Tehran by an HPLC method. Int J Vet Res. 4: 1-3.
13. Sarmah, A.K., Meyer, M.T., Boxall, A.B. (2006) A global perspective on the use, sales, exposure pathways, occurrence, fate and effects of veterinary antibiotics in the environment. Chemosphere. 65: 725-759.
14. Schmidt, R.H., Rodrick, G.E. (2003) Food Safety Handbook. John Wiley & Sons, New Jersey, USA.
15. WHO technical report series No. 799. Report of the joint FAO/WHO expert committee on food Additives, WHO, Switzerland 1990.

Ticks fauna of sheep and goats in some suburbs of Mazandaran province, Iran

Ebrahimzadeh, E.*, Pazhoom, F., Nabian, S., Shayan, P., Bakhshani, A.

Department of Parasitology and Tick and Tick Born Diseases Center, Faculty of Veterinary Medicine, University of Tehran, Tehran, Iran

Key words:
ixodidae, sheep, ticks fauna

Correspondence
Ebrahimzadeh, E.
Department of Parasitology and Tick and Tick Born Diseases Center,
Faculty of Veterinary Medicine,
University of Tehran, Tehran, Iran

Email: eebrahimzade@ut.ac.ir

Abstract:

BACKGROUND: Ticks are obligatory blood sucking arthropods that can transmit important pathogens. **OBJECTIVES:** The distribution and diversity of ticks fauna were last studied in the north of Iran in 2007. Mazandaran province has a humid climate, which is favourable to animal husbandry such as sheep breeding. Due to humid climate, the likelihood of exposure to tick infestation is increasing. The aim of this study was to determine the ticks founa of sheep and goats that grazed on the outskirts of mazandaran in 2012. **METHODS:** During the first 7 months of 2012, a total of 1190 tick specimens were collected from the whole body of sheep and goats from 23 different points of Mazandaran province. Adult male ticks were identified under a stereomicroscope, according to the identification keys. **RESULTS:** The identified tick specimens belonged to six Genus and 11 species, including *Rhipicephalus turanicus* (47%), *Rhipicephalus bursa* (24.6%), *Haemaphysalis punctata* (17.16%), *Rhipicephalus sanguineus* (4%), *Haemaphysalis concina* (3%), *Haemaphysalis parva* (1%), *Hyalomma marginatum* (1%), *Hyalomma anatolicum* (0.6%), *Dermacentor marginatus* (0.6%), *Ixodes ricinus* (0.5%), and *Boophilus (Rhipicephalus) annulatus* (0.3%). *Rh. turanicus* was the most abundant tick. **CONCLUSIONS:** Due to climate change, regular monitoring of distribution patterns of ticks is an important concern to control the ticks and tick-borne diseases.

Introduction

Ticks are serious threat to the health of animals and human beings. They are haematophagus arthropods that can cause paralysis, anemia, skin irritation, and pathogen transmission. Important pathogens such as CCHF virus, *Anaplasma* spp, *Ehrlechia* spp, *Babesia* spp, and *Theileria* spp could be transmitted by various species of ticks.

The distribution of ticks in Iran were studied by Delpy (1936, 1938), Abbasian (1961), Mazlum (1968, 1971), Filippova (1976), Rahbari (1995, 2007 a, b), Razmi (2007, 2011), Nabian (2007, 2008a,b), and Telmadarraiy (2004).

Mazandaran province has a humid climate, which is favourable to animal husbandry such as sheep breeding. Due to humid climate, the likelihood of exposure to tick infestation is increasing.

The influence of moisture and temperature on the diversity of ticks is well known. Since weather condition changes for years in Iran, regular monitoring of distribution patterns of ticks is an important concern to control the ticks and tick-borne diseases (Rahbari et al., 2007a,b). The aim of this study was to determine ticks founa of sheep and goats that grazed on the outskirts of Mazandaran.

Materials and Methods

The area of study was Mazandaran province, which is located in the north of Iran. The province had an average temperature of 25°C in summer and about

9°C in winter, and the annual rainfall averages 615 mm in the eastern part of Mazandaran province and more than 886 mm in the western part in last year (2012). According to Iran Veterinary Organization, 2,023,260 sheep and 217,260 goats have been reported in 2011.

During the first 7 months of 2012, a total of 1351 animals (sheep and goats) from 23 different points of Mazandaran province were inspected. The tick samples were collected from the whole body of infested sheep and goats in some suburbs of Mazandaran province including 8 points from Ghaemshahr, 6 points from Sari, 2 points from Babol, 2 points from Mahmoodabad, 5 points from Savadkooh. In this study, Kou estakhr is the most mountainous area that is located in savadkooh with 1770 m above the sea level and Gol neshin is the low-laying area that is located near Sari. The height of other location is placed between 2 these points. Tick samples were counted and separately preserved in 70% ethanol. Adult male ticks were identified under a stereomicroscope, according to the identification keys (Mazlum, 1968, 1971; Walker et al., 2003; Estrada-Pena et al., 2004).

Results

In the present study, 321 (23.76%) out of the total 1351 inspected sheep and goats were infested with ticks. A total of 1190 ticks (590 female and 600 male) were collected from 321 animals (273 sheep and 48 goats). The occurrence of ticks on sheep and goats were 26% and 15.7%, respectively. Many inspected sheep and goats were free of ticks due to indiscriminate use of Ivermectin. Six genera including *Rhipicephalus*, Haemaphysalis, Hyalomma, Dermacentor, and Ixodes were determined in this study. The identified tick specimens belonged to six Genus and 11 species, including *Rhipicephalus turanicus* (47%), *Rhipicephalus bursa* (24.6%), *Haemaphysalis punctata* (17.16%), *Rhipicephalus sanguineus* (4%), *Haemaphysalis concina* (3%), *Haemaphysalis parva* (1%), *Hyalomma marginatum* (1%), *Hyalomma anatolicum* (0.6%), *Dermacentor marginatus* (0.6%), *Ixodes ricinus* (0.5%), and *Boophilus (Rhipicephalus) annulatus* (0.3%). *Rh. turanicus* was the most abundant of the studied ticks (Table1).

Table 1. Frequency of Tick species on the studied region.

Tick Species	No	%	Region
Rh. turanicus	282	47%	Ghaemshahr, Sari, Babol, Mahmoodabad, Savadkooh
Rh. bursa	148	24.6%	Ghaemshahr, Sari, Savadkooh
Haem. punctata	103	17.16%	Savadkooh
Rh. sanguineus	24	4%	Ghaemshahr, Sari, Savadkooh
Haem. concina	18	3%	Savadkooh
Haem. parva	6	1%	Savadkooh
Hy. marginatum	6	1%	Savadkooh
Hy. anatolicum	4	0.6%	Sari
D. marginatus	4	0.6%	Savadkooh
I. ricinus	3	0.5%	Savadkooh
B. annulatus	2	0.3%	Savadkooh
Total	600	100%	

Discussion

The north of Iran is in a favorable climate condition to sustain tick in the nature. The influence of weather condition on the distribution and abundance of tick species is well known. Therefore, climate change can cause diversity in tick species in a geographical area (Rahbari et al., 2007a).

Global warming will affect climate condition in Iran, and new ticks species and tick-borne diseases will be spread to Iran.

Rh. turanicus (47%) was the most abundant of the total ticks in the present study. Razmi et al. (2011) reported that *Rh. turanicus* had the highest frequency in northern and southern parts of Khorasan Razavi province. Nabian and Rahbari (2008) identified *Rh. turanicus* as a rare species in Zagros mountainous area. In Africa, *Rh. turanicus* is present at altitudes ranging from just above sea level to over 2000 m and in regions with annual rainfalls ranging from 100 mm to 1000 mm (Walker et al., 2000). In this study, *Rh. turanicus* was identified in low-laying area from the sea level (like Gol Neshin in Sari) and land with 1770 m above the sea level (kou estakhr). *Rh. turanicus* has been identified as a vector of *Babesia ovis* to the susceptible hosts (Shayan et al., 2007).

Nabian et al. (2007) found *Rh. Sanguineous* (42.37%) as the most prevalent species in Mazandaran province. Hosseini et al. (2010) reported *Rh. Sanguineous* (82.4%) as the most abundant species in Ghaemshahr suburbs. Shayeghi et al. (2005) recorded that *Rh. Sanguineous* (1.8%) had a low number in Mazandaran province (1.18%) in 2002-2003.

The frequency of *Rh.sanguineus* (4%) was low in the present study. This finding is in contrast with the results of Nabian et al. (2007) and Hosseini et al. (2010) and is in line with the finding of Shayeghi et al.(2005). The preferred host for *Rh.sanguineus* is the domesticated dog (Walker et al., 2000). The agent of canine tick fever, *Babesia* spp. in dogs and *Ehrlichia canis* can be transmitted by this tick.

In contrast with the study of Nabian et al. (2007) and Shayeghi et al. (2005) who did not find *Rh.bursa*, this species was observed as the second numerous species (24.66%) in the present study. Hosseini et al. (2010) found this species in a very small number in Ghaemshahr. Mazlum believed that *Rh.bursa* is a dominant tick in most sheep area (Mazlum,1968, 1971).

Rh.bursa prefers low to medium altitude mountain slopes and is present in steppe and semi-desert environments. However, in the present study *Rh. bursa* was found in land with 1770 m above the sea level (kou estakhr). *R.bursa* can transmit *B.bigemina*, *B.bovis*, *Anaplasma marginalae* to cattle, *B.equi*, *B.caballi* to horses, *B.motasi*, *B.ovis*, *A.ovis* to sheep. CCHF virus was isolated from this tick (Walker et al., 2000).

Haem. punctata (17.16%) was found as the third prevalent species in Mazandaran's countryside. Nabian et al. (2007) recorded this species in a large number (37.28%) in Mazandaran province. Hosseini et al. (2010) found this species in a very small number in Ghaemshahr. Shayeghi et al. (2005) did not find this species in Mazandaran province in 2002-2003. This species was reported by Mazlum (1968, 1971) in the mountainous areas in the north of Iran. In this study, *Haem. Punctate* was just identified in the mountainous area (kou estakhr). *Haem. punctata* is the vector of *B.motasi* and *B.major* and carries Rickettsia siberica and causes tick paralysis (Yin et al, 1996).

Haem. concina (3%) and *Haem. parva* (1%) were recorded in our study to have a small number. Nabian et al. (2007), Hosseini et al. (2010) and Shayeghi et al. (2005) did not report these two species in Mazandaran province. Filipova et al. (1976) mentioned *Haem.parva* and *Haem.concinna* are rare species encountered in Iran; they can be found in Caspian sea, mountainous, and semi-dessert zones of the country. Delpy (1938) found *Haem. concina* on sheep, cattle and horses in mountainous areas of Caspian zone. *Haem.parva* transmit *Theileria sergenti* and Crimen-Congo hemorrhagic fever virus (Shchelkanov et al., 2005). *Haem. concina* is observed in the east of Caspian sea zone and the southern mountainous areas (Rahbari et al. 2007b). This tick was found infected with *A.bovis*, *Rickettsia hulinii*, *Borrelia* and *Francisella tularensis* (Rahbari et al., 2007b). Haemaphysalis spp. were dominant species in kou estakhr in September.

Hy. marginatum (1%), *Hy.a. anatolicum* (0.6%), *D. marginatus* (0.6%), *I. ricinus* (0.5%) and *B.annulatus* (0.3%) were observed in a very small number during inspecting infested sheep and goats. Nabian et al. (2007) did not find *Hy. marginatum*, *D. marginatus* and found *Hy.a. anatolicum* (3.38%) and *I.ricinus* (3.38%) in a small number in Mazandaran. The frequency of *B.annulatus* was reported as 10.16% by them. Hosseini et al. (2010) observed *I.ricinus* (15.2%) and *B.annulatus* (1.2%); however, he did not find the other abovementioned species.

Shayeghi et al. (2005) reported the frequency of *Hy. marginatum* (1.66%), *Hy.anatolicum* (1.33%), *D.marginatus* (1.72%), *I.ricinus* (27.45%), *B. annulatus* (8.34%).

According to the finding of Vahedi-Noori et al. (2012) activity of *I.ricinus* in Mazandaran is dependent to the cold and humid month of the year, therefore probably this is the cause that we didn't find this tick in the summer in Mazandaran. *I. ricinus* was found in May and September in Savad Kooh. This tick is mostly found in Northern Turkey that has a high rain fall and tense forest (Aydin and Bakirci, 2007).

Walker et al. (2000) emphasized that *Borrelia burgdirferi* and *A. phagocytophilia* were transmitted by *I.ricinus*. Morisod et al. (1972) described that *B.bovis* was transmitted by this tick.

In the present study, *D.marginatus* was identified just in the mountainous area of Mazandaran province. This finding is in accordance with Nabian et al. (2008) who emphasized this tick could hardly adapt in low-lying areas from the sea.

Black sea climate and tick fauna in Turkey are similar to those of northern Iran (Aydin and Bakirci, 2007). *Amblyomma variegatum* have been found in the border of Turkey to the Syria, with warm and semidesert climate condition. This tick has not been reported from Iran until now.

Acknowledgments

This research was supported by grants from the university of Tehran. We are grateful to the Research Council of the University of Tehran and the Research Council of the faculty of Veterinary Medicine of the University of Tehran for financial support under project no. 27927/1/1.

References

1. Abbasian, L. (1961) Records of tick (Acarina: Ixodidae) occurring in Iran and their distributional data. Acarologia. 3: 546-59.
2. Aydin, L., Bakirci, S. (2007) Geographical distribution of ticks in Turkey. Parasitol Res. 101:163-166.
3. Delpy, L. (1936) Note sur les Ixodides dugenre Hyalomma (Koch). Annels deParasitologie. 14: 206-45.
4. Delpy, L. (1938) Les especes iranienes dugenre Haemaphysalis Koch 1844. Annalles de Parasitologie Humaine et Comparee. 16: 1-10.
5. Estrada-pena, A., Bouattour, A., Camicas, J.L., Walker, A.R. (2004) Ticks of Domestic animals in the mediterranean. A guide to the identification of species. Bioscience reports, London, UK.
6. Filopova, N.A., Neronov, V.M., Farhang-Azad, A. (1976) Data on ixodid tick fauna (Acarina, Ixodidae) of small mammals in Iran (in Russian). Ent Obozr. 55: 467-479.
7. Hosseini vasoukolaei, N., Telmadarraiy, Z., Vatandoost, H., Yaghoobi Ershadi, M.R., Hosseini vasoukolaei, M., Oshaghi, M.A. (2010) Survey of tick species parasiting domestic ruminants in Ghaemshahr County, Mazandaran province, Iran. Asian pac J Trop Med. 3: 804-806.
8. Mazlum, Z. (1968) Hyalomma asiaticum asiaticum (Schulze and Schlottke) 1929. Its distribution, hosts, seasonal activity, life cycle and role in transmission of bovine theileriosis in Iran. Acarologia. 10: 437-42.
9. Mazlum, Z. (1971) Ticks of domestic animals in Iran: Geographic distribution, host relation, and seasonal activity. J Vet Res, Univ Tehran, Iran. 27: 1-32.
10. Morisod, A., Brossard, M., Lambert, C., Suter, H., Aeschlimann, A. (1972) *Babesia bovis*: transmission by *Ixodes ricinus* (Ixodoidea) on the Rhone plain Schweiz Arch Tierheilkd. 114: 387-91.
11. Nabian, S., Rahbari, S. (2008) Occurrence of soft and hard ticks on ruminants in zagros mountainous areas of Iran. Iranian J Arthropod Borne Dis. 2: 16-20.
12. Nabian, S., Rahbari, S., Shayan, P., Haddadzadeh, H.R. (2007) Current status of tick fauna in North of Iran. Iran J Parasitol. 2:12-17.
13. Nabian, S., Rahbari, S., Shayan, P., Haddadzadeh, H.R. (2008). Identification of tick species of *Dermacentor* in some localities of Iran. 63: 123-126.
14. Rahbari, S. (1995) Studies on some ecological aspects of tick fauna of West Azarbayejan, Iran. J Appl Anim Res. 7: 189-94.
15. Rahbari, S., Nabian, S., Shayan, P. (2007a) Primary report on distribution of tick fauna in Iran. Parasitol Res. 101:175-S177.
16. Rahbari, S., Nabian, S., Shayan, P., Haddadzadeh, H.R. (2007b) Status of Haemaphysalis tick infestation in domestic ruminants in Iran. Korean J Parasitol. 45: 129-132.
17. Razmi, G.R., Glinsharifodini, M., Sarvi, S.H. (2007) Prevalence of ixodid ticks on cattle in Mazandaran province, Iran. Korean J Parasitol. 45: 307-310.
18. Razmi, G.R., Najarnejad, V., Rashtibaf, M. (2011) Determination the frequency of Ixodid ticks on the sheep in Khorasan Razavi province, Iran. Arch Razi Inst. 66: 129-132.
19. Shayan, P., Hooshmand, E., Rahbari, S., Nabian, S. (2007) Determination of *Rhipicephalus* spp. as vectors for *Babesia ovis* in Iran. Parasitol Res. 101: 1029-33.
20. Shayeghi, M., Piazak, N., Yazdi, F., Abolhasani, M. (2005) Geographical distribution of soft and hard ticks in Mazandaran province. Journal of School of Public Health and Institute of Public Health Research (In Persian). 3: 49-56
21. Shchelkanov, MIu., Kolobukhina, LV., Moskvina, TM., Aushev, ID., Kartoev, AA., Kelli, EI., Merkulova, LN., Grenkova, EP., Samokhvalov, EI., Petriaev, VG., Serobian, AG., Klimova, EA., Galkina, IV., Malyshev, NA., Aristova, VA., Slavskii, AA., Luk'ianova, NA., Deriabin, PG., Gromashevskii, VL., Efremenko, VI., Onishchenko, GG., L'vov, DK. (2005) Detection of the circulation of Crimean-Congo hemorrhagic fever virus in the piedmont steppes of the North Caucasus. Vopr Virusol. 50: 9-15.

22. Telmadarraiy, Z., Bahrami, A., Vatandoost, H. (2004) A survey on fauna of ticks in west azerbaijan province, Iran. Iran J Public Health. 33: 65-69.
23. Vahedi-Noori, N., Rahbari, S., Bokaei, S. (2012) The seasonal activity of *Ixodes ricinus* tick in Amol, Mazandaran province, Northern Iran. J Arthropod Borne Dis. 6: 129-135.
24. Walker, J.B., Keirans, J.E., Horak, I.G. (2000) The Genus *Rhipicephalus* (Acari, IXodidae) A guide to the brown ticks of the world. Cambridge University Press. Cambridge. New York, USA.
25. Walker, A.R., Bouattour, A., Camicas, J.L., Estrada-Pena, A, Horak, I.G., Latif,A, Pegram, R.G., Preston, P.M.(2003) Ticks of domestic animals in Africa, A guide to identification of species. Biosience Reports. Scotland, UK.
26. Yin, H., Lu, W., Luo, J., Zhang, Q., Lu, W., Dou, H. (1996) Experiments on the transmission of *Babesia major* and *Babesia bigemina* by *Haemaphysalis punctata*. Vet Parasitol. 67: 89-98.

Metabolic profile of pregnant, non-pregnant and male two-humped camels (*Camelus bactrianus*) of Iran

Omidi, A.[1*], Sajedi, Zh.[2], Montazer Torbati, M.B.[2], Mostafai, M.[3]

[1] *Department of Animal Health Management, School of Veterinary Medicine, Shiraz University, Shiraz, Iran*

[2] *Department of Animal Sciences, Agriculture Faculty, Birjand University, Birjand, Iran*

[3] *Research Centre for Agriculture and Natural Resources, Ardabil, Iran*

Key words:
Camelus bactrianus, pregnancy, camel

Correspondence
Omidi, A.
Department of Animal Health Management, School of Veterinary Medicine, Shiraz University, Shiraz, Iran

Email: aomidi@shirazu.ac.ir

Abstract:

BACKGROUND: The knowledge in blood constituents is important for assessing the physiological status and the health of animals. Only a limited number of two-humped camels (*Camelus bactrianus*) were reared in Ardabil province, northwest of Iran. **OBJECTIVES:** The present study was carried out to find out whether the sex and pregnancy affect thyroid hormones, lipid and lipoprotein profile, and selected biochemical factors in healthy Iranian Bactrian camels. **METHODS:** The evaluated herd contained twenty clinical healthy Bactrian camels, aged between four and thirteen years. Six of them were non-pregnant, five in the late period of pregnancy, and nine were male camels. Blood samples (10 mL) were collected from the jugular vein of camels in spring 2013 during two consecutive days. All samples were centrifuged at 3000× rpm for 15 min and sera were refrigerated at -21°C until analysis. Thyroid function tests were carried out by measuring serum levels of thyroid stimulating hormone (TSH), free and total thyroxin (fT4), (T4), and free and total triiodothyronine (fT3), (T3) by commercially available radio immunoassay kits. The biochemical parameters were measured using a standard autoanalyser (Hitachi717, Boehringer. Mannheim, Germany). **RESULTS:** The levels of fT4, HDL-Cholesterol, ALP, and glucose in the sera of pregnant camels were significantly lower than the male and non-pregnant camels. The serum levels of other parameters were not significantly different among the groups. **CONCLUSIONS:** The present study revealed that heavy pregnancy has a profound effect on certain serum biochemical parameters in Bactrian camels.

Introduction

In the central parts of Asia, there are two- humped camels, known as the bactrian. Bactrian camels endure temperature extremes, from -40 degrees in winter to +40 in the summer and can survive up to three days without food or water and up to one week in very cold weather. Camels are sexually mature when they are four or five. Mating takes place from December to February. After gestation for 12 to15 months, females give birth to a single calf weighing up to 45 kg. Calves can stand soon after birth, are weaned at one to two years, and stay with the mother until they reach maturity. The life span of the domestic bactrian camel is approximately 40 years. Bactrian camels are shorter and heavier than the one-humped dromedary. The domesticated bactrian camel is widely used in central Asia and western China because of its adaptation to harsh climates (Zongping, 2003). Only a limited number of two-humped camels (*Camelus bactrianus*) were reared in Iran, and most of them were kept at Jahanabad breeding center of Meshkinshahr in Ardabil province, northwest of Iran (Niasari-Naslaji et al., 2008). Our present knowledge about nutrition, physiology, and genetics of bactrian camel is limited because little research has been done. Compared to other domestic animals such as dairy cattle, sheep, and goats, our understanding about the physiological and hormonal changes that the camel undergoes during pregnancy is inadequate. Because of the long pregnancy period of camels, it was assumed that energy requirements of pregnant camels increase rapidly during the heavy pregnancy. This may affect the concentration of some biochemical parameters. Also, during pregnancy some metabolic changes occur that may alter blood constituents (El-Sherif and Assad, 2001; Khan and Ludri, 2002). Pregnancy is a dynamic process characterized by dramatic physiological changes that may influence hormonal functions and biochemical values in the animal. Thyroid function regulates a wide range of metabolic activities (Aziz khan et al., 2014). Appropriate thyroid gland function and its hormonal activity are crucial to sustain the reproductive performance, healthy pregnancy outcomes, and successful brain development in the fetus of animals (LaFranchi et al., 2005). Thyroid function significantly affects lipoprotein metabolism (Duntas, 2002; Eshratkhah and Sadaghian, 2010). The liver metabolizes lipids. Lipids play an important role in the pregnancy. They serve as hormones or hormone precursors, provide energy, and act as structural components in the cell membranes. Many researchers evaluated the normal concentrations of serum lipids and lipoproteins of the sheep (Eshratkhah and Sadaghian, 2010; Nazifi et al., 2002a), goats (Nazifi et al., 2002b), ewes (Piccione et al., 2009), cows (Mohebbi-Fani et al., 2012a; Mohebbi-Fani et al., 2012b), horses (Nazifi et al., 2005), pony mares (Watson et al., 1993), camel (Nazifi et al., 2000; Asadi et al., 2009), and women (An-Na et al., 1995). During pregnancy, blood serum constituents may be influenced by several factors such as breed, age, malnutrition, or season. Also, maternal tissues are involved in providing energy for reproduction processes, and growth of the fetus (Swansonk et al., 2004; Yokus et al., 2006). In sheep, during the late pregnancy, the blood serum lipid profile is characterized by increased concentration of total cholesterol, triglycerides, and lipoproteins (Schlumbohm et al., 1997). Variation in blood cholesterol content has been observed during pregnancy. Cholesterol is the precursor of the steroid hormones (Iriadam, 2007). Lipid profiles have been used to predict peripartum diseases (Nazifi et al., 2002b). The liver also plays an essential role in carbohydrates and amino acid metabolism (Ouajd and Kamel, 2009). Measurement of some blood constituents and enzymes (aspartate amino transferase concentrations, alanine amino transferase, alkalinephosphatase, and gammaglutamyl-trans-feraseare) need for evaluation of the health of the liver. Under normal circumstances, these enzymes exist within the hepatocytes; however, when the liver is injured, these enzymes enter the blood stream (Yap and Choon, 2010). Total protein and albumin are the proteins made by the liver. Serum creatinine, a marker for the assessment of renal function is the most common indicator of glomerular filtration rate (GFR). A decreasement in blood protein concentration during later stages of gestation was observed in sheep (Antunovic et al., 2002). It was also reported that plasma urea levels increased during week 10 of pregnancy, reaching a peak at parturition (El-Sherif and Assad, 2001), which in domestic ruminants was ascribed to the cortisolstimulated catabolism of proteins in the body (Silanikove, 2000). The Creatinine clearance test could be used as a practical method for GFR assessment in the dromedary camel in field conditions (Kamili et al., 2013). The present study was initiated with the aim to investigate and compare some biochemical blood parameters in healthy male, female, and pregnant Bactrian camels.

Materials and Methods

This study was conducted on female and male Iranian two-humped camels (*Camelus bactrianus*) in April 2013. The camels were reared at the Bactrian camels research center, Jahadabad, (90 km far from the city of Meshkinshahr; 47° 43′ 39.71″ North latitude, 38° 26′ 22.2″ East longitude, and 1320 m above sea level) in Ardabil province, Northwest Iran. The camel herd composition includes a dominant male and 26 females at different ages. The camels were kept in an enclosed area with about 1000 m2 of open space and pasture about 20 km2. Twenty adult camels, aged between four and thirteen years old were chosen for this study (Table 1). The pregnant camels were selected in consultation with cameleer who had recorded their mating history. Six non-pregnant camels, five in the last three months of pregnancy and nine male camels were selected for this experiment. All the animals were clinically healthy and free from internal and external parasites. The blood sample was collected into 10-ml vacuum tube and was chilled immediately after sampling and transported to the laboratory within 1 h after collection. Serum was harvested after centrifugation at 3000 rpm for 15 minutes, frozen, and stored at -21°C until analysis. Thyroid stimulating hormone (TSH), total tri-iodothyronine (tT3), and total thyroxine (tT4) concentrations were determined by radioim-munoassay method using commercial kits (Immuno-tech Company, Radiove, Prague, Chech Republic). The biochemical parameters were measured using a standard autoanalyser (Hitachi717, Boehringer. Mannheim, Germany). The level of total serum protein by Biuret reaction (Gornall et al., 1949), albumin by Bromocresol green dye binding method (McGinlay and Payne, 1988), and serum globulin was estimated by subtracting albumin from the total protein. Glucose and urea levels were measured with a clinical chemistry analyzer (Gilford Impact 400E, Gilford Systems, OH). The concentrations of calcium (Baginski et al., 1973) and inorganic phosphorus (Daly and Ertingshausen, 1972) were determined by an automated biochemical analyzer (Biotecnica, Targa 3000, Rome, Italy) using commercial kits (Parsazmoon, Tehran, Iran). The activity of aspartate aminotransferase (AST) and alanine aminotrans-ferase (ALT) were measured by the colorimetric method of Reitman and Frankel (Mansour et al., 1982), and gamma glutamyl-transferase (GGT) was measured by SZASZ method (Szasz, 1976). Serum enzyme activities were measured according to the specific reaction of each enzyme by using basic standard techniques. The serum was analyzed for cholesterol, HDL-cholesterol, and LDL-cholesterol by a modified Abell-Kendall/Levey-Brodie (AK) method (Burtis and Ashward, 1999), triglyceride by enzymatic method (Hinscha et al., 1980), and uric acid by phosphotungstic acid method (Elin et al., 1982). VLDL cholesterol was estimated as one-fifth of the concentration of triglycerides (Friedewald et al., 1972). Total lipid (TL) was measured using Raylander et al.'s approach (2006), the overall regression equation (TL = 0.9+1.3* [Cholesterol +Triglycerides]).

All results were expressed in SI unit (Burtis and Ashward, 1999). The data were analyzed by descriptive statistics and one way ANOVA followed by post hoc multiple comparisons of means using LSD tests with SPSS 16/PC software (Norusis, 1993). All values were expressed as mean and standard error (SEM) and ($p<0.05$ and $p<0.01$) were seen as statistically significant.

Results

The level of serum thyroid hormones (T3, T4, fT3 and fT4) and TSH are shown in Table 2. Table 3 shows the overall means±standard error (S.E.M) of the serum lipid profiles (Total cholesterol, triglyceride) and lipoproteins (HDL-cholesterol, LDL-cholesterol and VLDL-cholesterol). Some of serum biochemical parameters and liver enzymes (AST, ALP, ALT and GGT) in pregnant, non-pregnant, and male Bactrian camels are listed in Table 4. The levels of T4, HDL-Cholesterol, ALP, and glucose in the sera of pregnant camels were significantly lower than those of the male and non-pregnant camels ($p<0.01$ and 0.05 respectively). The serum levels of other parameters were not significantly different among the groups. In pregnant camels, the median serum thyroid hormones (T3, T4, fT3 and TSH) were lower than those of non-pregnant and male camels; nevertheless, the difference was not statistically significant. The average serum fT4 was significantly lower in pregnant camels than that of non-pregnant and males. There was no significant difference in serum lipid profiles and lipoproteins between non-pregnant, pregnant, and male camels; however, the value was lower in pregnant ones than that of non-pregnant and male ones. Serum creatinine and GGT were compared between these three groups, and results showed the values were higher in pregnant camels in comparison with non-pregnant and male camels; nonetheless, the differences were not statistically significant. We observed a decrease in serum AST level in pregnant camles compared to non-pregnant and male Bactrian camels.

Table 1. A summary of the age distribution of evaluating Bacterian camels.

Camel/year	Number	Range	Minimum	Maximum	Median	Mean ± Std. Error
Pregnant	5	3.00	10.00	13.00	13	11.80±0.73
Non- pregnant	6	1.00	4.00	5.00	5	4.66±0.21
Male	9	10.00	2.00	12.00	4	4.22±1.01

Discussions

The levels of fT4 in the sera of pregnant camels were significantly lower than those of the male and non-pregnant camels ($p<0.01$) as well as for T3, T4, fT3, and TSH, although not significant (Table 2). Reduction in total circulating thyroid hormones during pregnancy could be due to the increase in turnover rate or the decrease in hormone secretion from the thyroid gland. During pregnancy, hepatocytes increase their production of thyroidbinding globulin (TBG). High TBG and high estradiol concentration during pregnancy induced a reduction in free circulating hormones such as fT4 (Utiger, 1987). Thyroid failure is more common in females and epidemiological rate of prevalence rises with age. The serum TSH assay is an accurate test for detecting out-of-range circulating levels of thyroid hormones for either of hypothyroidism and hyperthyroidism (Nouh et al., 2008). Estrogens can alter the secretion rate and dynamics of thyroid hormones. It seems that fluctuations in thyroid activity may be due to varying concentrations of estrogens and progesterone during pregnancy. Progesterone can decrease TBG, which increases free thyroid hormones. Estrogen increases TBG levels, which can inactivate thyroid hormone. These processes slow the body metabolism and allow the storage of fat and energy for the fetus (Agarwal et al., 1989). However, our findings are in agreement with some other investigators who found that free hormone levels remain unchanged or decrease in pregnancy (Rahman et al., 2007). Nazifi et al. (2003) and Manalu et al. (1997) found that the concentrations of serum T4 and T3 and the dosage were higher in non-pregnant goats than those of the pregnant ones. Also, they showed that the concentration of T4 was higher in female goats compared with males. Comparison of the HDL-cholesterol concentrations revealed significant lower values in the females than the males. Significant lower HDL-cholesterol concentration was observed in the pregnant camels ($p<0.01$). The liver is the major site of cholesterol synthesis and acetate was used as a precursor in this process. Cholesterol biosynthesis begins with the conversion of 3 Acetyl CoA units into Mevalonate. During pregnancy, the synthesis of cholesterol fell markedly (Leoni, 1984). There was no significant difference in other serum lipid profiles and lipoproteins between non-pregnant, pregnant, and male camels. The findings of the current study about lipid profiles in Bactrian camels do not support our previous researches in dromedary camel species (Omidi et al., 2014). However, the findings of the current study are in agreement with the findings of Nath et al. (2005) and Krajnicakova et al. (2003) in cows, goats, buffaloes, and camels. The lower lipoproteins and lipid profiles level of these species near the parturition could be attributed to the increased utilization for steroid synthesis around parturition (Stocki, 1975). The quantity of creatinine depends on dietary intake, rate of synthesis of creatinine, and muscle mass. Serum creatinine and urea were compared between these three groups and results showed the values were higher in pregnant camels in comparison with non-pregnant and male ones; however, the differences were not statistically significant. Increase of creatinine concentration in pregnant animals could have been a consequence of the higher protein demands in late pregnancy which could have led to a reduction in the ability of kidneys to eliminate excess serotonin from plasma. Accordingly, Poljicak et al. (2009) found that the measured transaminase activity was higher in pregnant red and fallow deer females than non-pregnant ones. The higher activity of transaminases might indicate impairment in muscle and liver cells due to rapid gluconeogenesis associated with pregnancy. Beitz (2004) stated that the effect of adrenal corticoids on mobilization of amino acids from body proteins during pregnancy is associated with an increased rate of hepatic deamination. In the present research, there was no significant difference in serum total protein, albumin, and urea between non-pregnant, pregnant, and male camels; however, the values were lower in

Table 2. Mean ±standard error of mean of serum thyroid hormones and TSH in pregnant, non-pregnant and male camels (n=20). T3 - triiodothyronine, T4 - thyroxin, fT3- free triiodothyronin, fT4- free thyroxin, TSH- thyroid stimulation hormone. (**) Significant difference in p≤ 0.01. NS Non significant difference. (a) In each row, indicates significant differences with two others.

Variable	Unit	Bactrian camel			Significant
		Pregnant (n=5)	Non-pregnant (n=6)	Male (n=9)	
T3	(nmol/L)	114.56±17.87	149.56±14.94	121.46±15.69	NS
T4	(nmol/L)	4.43±0.99	6.58±0.79	6.79±0.51	NS
TSH	(mIU/L)	0.01±0.001	0.005±0.001	0.01±0.001	NS
fT3	(pmol/L)	1.86±0.18	2.55±0.31	2.58±0.29	NS
fT4	(pmol/L)	0.64±0.11a	0.97±0.06	1.06±0.06	**

Table 3. Mean ±standard error of mean of serum lipid profiles and lipoproteins in pregnant, non-pregnant and male camels (n=20). LDL- low-density lipoprotein, HDL- high-density lipoprotein, VLDL- very low-density lipoprotein, TL- total lipid. (**) Significant difference in p≤0.01. (NS) Non significant difference. (a) In each row, indicates significant differences with two others.

Variable	Unit	Bactrian camel			Significant
		Pregnant (n=5)	Non-pregnant (n=6)	Male (n=9)	
Total Cholesterol	(mmol/L)	27.60±3.70	32.16±2.95	36.11±2.80	NS
Triglycerid	(mmol/L)	23.80±2.65	36.66±6.60	34.00±2.71	NS
HDL- Cholesterol	(mmol/L)	7.00±0.89a	15.33±1.80	18.11±1.08	**
LDL- Cholesterol	(mmol/L)	15.8±4.31	9.83±1.45	11.22±1.10	NS
VLDL- Cholesterol	(mmol/L)	7.33±0.96	7.33±0.88	6.80±0.72	NS
Total Lipid	(g/L)	67.8±10.09	90.38±9.21	91.93±7.52	NS

Table 4. Mean ±standard error of mean of some of serum biochemical parameters and liver enzymes in pregnant, non-pregnant and male camels (n=20). AST, aspartate aminotransferase; ALT, alanine aminotransferase; ALP, alkaline phosphatase; GGT, Gama glutamine transferase. (*) Significant difference in p≤0.05. (**) Significant difference in p≤0.01. (NS) Non significant difference. (a) In each row, indicates significant differences with two others.

Variable	Unit	Bactrian camel			Significant
		Pregnant (n=5)	Non-pregnant (n=6)	Male (n=9)	
Glucose	mmol/L	68.60±16.01a	106.83±3.02	104.77±5.39	*
Calcium	mmol/L	10.78±0.35	9.55±0.199	10.1±0.35	NS
Phosphorus	mmol/L	4.58±0.61	7.08±0.66	7.18±0.78	NS
Albumin	g/L	2.86±0.25	2.98±0.22	3.03±0.15	NS
Total protein	g/L	5.74±0.31	5.76±0.37	5.84±0.24	NS
Urea	mmol/L	60.80±7.52	65.17±7.09	63.78±5.88	NS
Uric acid	mmol/L	0.2±0.04	0.22±0.06	0.18±0.5	NS
Creatinine	mmol/L	1.62±0.17	1.38±.07	1.41±0.09	NS
AST	IU/L	89.4±9.41	151.83±24.53	184.11±35.16	NS
ALT	IU/L	12.8±1.49	14.5±1.98	15.11±1.15	NS
ALP	IU/L	109.40±10.01a	345.66±68.36	381.77±51.92	**
GGT	IU/L	21.8±1.49	21.5±1.12	20.33±0.88	NS

pregnant camels than those of non-pregnant and male ones. With insufficient water supplies, there is an evidence of an increase in blood total protein, albumin, and urea concentration along with the pregnancy progress (El-Sherif and Assad, 2001; Poljicak, 2009). Rodriguez et al. (1996) found that glomerular filtration and urea clearance were significantly reduced during late pregnancy. In our study, the levels of glucose in the sera of pregnant camels were significantly lower than those of the male and non-pregnant camels. Our findings were in agreement with the findings of some researchers, e.g. Khan and Ludri (2002) and Saeed et al. (2009): They found significantly lower concentrations of glucose in pregnant goats than in non-pregnant ones with a tendency to decline in the group of the pregnant animals towards the end of gestation. The low level of glucose in pregnant camels may be due to developing fetus and mobilization of glucose from mother for providing the adequate energy of the fetus. Normal blood contains alkaline phosphatase (ALP) enzyme which catalyses the liberation of inorganic phosphates from phosphate esters (Bodansky, 1932). In this study, the level of ALP in male and non-pregnant camels was significantly higher than that of the pregnant camels. The level in the healthy animal is influenced markedly by age and to some extent by diet activity. The plasma ALP levels may increase during the diseases related to bone and liver (Shinowara, 1942). In cattle, sheep, and camels the effect of age on ALP was noticed by Vertor and Swaton (1969), where the serum ALP activity was considerably higher in young animals. A high level of ALP was reported by Elias and Yagil (1984) in the newborn calves. In Indian camels, ALP activities in the serum of male animals were significantly higher than those of the female animals (Kataria and Bhatia, 1991). Animals younger than three years of age had higher ALP activity than adult males. Progressive decline in ALP activity with the advancement of age in camels was also observed (NRCC, 1990). In this study, pregnant female camels were significantly older than the group of non-pregnant and male camels (Table 1). The ALP activity obtained from pregnant and non-pregnant camel was higher than the values reported by other researchers (Saeed et al., 2009; Khadjeh, 2002). There is not any relationship between the serum calcium or phosphorus levels and the variations observed in the ALP in pregnant and other camels (Table 4). It should be noted that all determinations were made with apparently healthy camels. No explanation other than an insufficient number of samples is readily available for the high and wide variation in serum ALP levels. The Major limitation of this study is that the number of Bactrian camels was relatively small in Iran (less than 200). Bactrian camel's research center in Jahadabad of Meshkinshahr is the only center of rearing two-humped camels. Our results may be influenced by this limitation. Future studies on the current topic are recommended.

Acknowledgements

We appreciate the support provided for this research by Shiraz University. We are also grateful to the bactrian camels research center (Jahadabad) staff for their help in conducting this project.

References

1. Agarwal, S.P., Khanna, N.D., Agarwal, V.K. (1989) Circulating concentrations of thyroid hormones in pregnant camels (*Camelus dromedarius*). Theriogenology. 31: 1239-1247.
2. An-Na, C., Man-Li, Y., Jeng-Hsiu, H. (1995) Alterations of serum lipid levels and their biological relevance during and after pregnancy. Life Sci. 56: 2367-2375.
3. Antunovic, Z., Sencic, D., Sperada, M. (2002) Influence of the season and the reproductive status of ewes on blood parameters. Small Rum Res. 45: 39-44.
4. Asadi, F., Shahroari, A., Pourkabir, M. (2009) Serum lipid, glucose, free fatty acid, and liver triglyceride in subadult and adult camels (*Camelus dromedarius*). Rev Med Vet. 12: 552-556.
5. Aziz Khan, F., Patil, S.K.B., Thakur, A.S. (2014) Lipid Profile in Thyroid Dysfunction: A Study on Patients of Bastar. J Clin Analic Med. 5: 12-14.
6. Baginski, E.S., Marie, S.S., Clark, W.L. (1973) Direct micro determination of serum calcium. Clin Chem Acta. 46: 46-54.
7. Beitz, D.C. (2004) Protein and amino acid metabolism. In: Duke's Physiology of Domestic Animals. Reece W.O. (ed.). Cornell University Press, Ithaca, USA. p. 535-553.
8. Bodansky, A. (1932) Hawk's Physiological Chemistry. Tata McGraw Hill Publishing Company Ltd. New Delhi, India.
9. Burtis, C.A., Ashward, E.R. (1999) Tietz Text Book of Clinical Chemistry. (3rd ed.). W.B. Saunders Company. Philadelphia, USA.
10. Daly, J.A., Ertingshausen, G. (1972) Direct method for determining inorganic phosphorus in serum with the centrifichem. Clin Chem. 18: 263-265.
11. Duntas, L.H. (2002) Thyroid disease and lipids. Thyroid. 12: 287-93.
12. Elias, E., Yagil, R. (1984) Hematological and serum biochemical values in lactating camels and their newborns. Refu Vet. 41: 7-13.
13. Elin, R.J., Johnson, E., Chesler, R. (1982) Four methods for determining uric acid compared with a candidate reference method. Clin Chem. 28: 2098-2100.

14. El-Sherif, M.M.A., Assad, F. (2001) Changes in some blood constituents of Barki ewes during pregnancy and lactation under semi-arid conditions. Small Rum Res. 40: 269-277.
15. Eshratkhah, B., Sadaghian, M. (2010) Relationship between the blood thyroid hormones and lipid profile in Moghani sheep; influence of age and sex. Comp Clinic Pathol. 19: 15-20.
16. Friedewald, W.T., Levy, R.I., Fredrickson, D.S. (1972) Estimation of the concentration of low-density lipoprotein cholesterol without the use of the preparative ultracentrifuge. Clin Chem. 18: 499.
17. Gornall, A., Bardawill, C.J., David, M.M. (1949) Determination of serum proteins by means of biuret reagent. J Biol Chem. 177: 751-759.
18. Hinscha, W., Ebersbach, W.D., Sundarama, P.V. (1980) Fully enzymic method of plasma triglyceride determination using an immobilized glycerol dehydrogenase nylon-tube reactor. Clin Chem Acta. 104: 95-100.
19. Iriadam, M. (2007) Variation in certain hematological and biochemical parameters during the peripartum period in Kilis does. Small Rum Res. 73: 54-57.
20. Kamili, A., Bengoumi, M., Oukessou, M. (2013) Assessment of glomerular filtration rate in normally hydrated and dehydrated dromedary camel by plasma exogenous creatinine clearance test. Emir J Food Agri. 25: 314-319.
21. Kataria, N., Bhatia, J.S. (1991) Activity of some enzymes in the serum of dromedary camels. Res Vet Sci. 51: 174-176.
22. Khadjeh, G.H. (2002) Concentration of serum enzymes in pregnant and non- pregnant Iranian one-humped camels. Indian J Anim Sci. 72: 391-392.
23. Khan, J.R., Ludri, R.S. (2002) Changes in blood glucose, plasma non-esterified fatty acids and insulin in pregnant and non-pregnant goats. Trop Anim Health Prod. 34: 81-90.
24. Krajnicakova, M., Kovac, G., Kostecky, M. (2003) Selected clinical biochemical parameters in the puerperal period of goats. Bull Vet Inst Pulawy. 47: 177-182.
25. LaFranchi, S.H., Haddow, J.E., Hollowell, J.G. (2005) Is thyroid inadequacy during gestation a risk factor for adverse pregnancy and developmental outcomes? Thyroid. 15: 60-71.
26. Leoni, S., Spagnuolo, S., ContiDevirgiliis, L. (1984) Cholesterol synthesis and related enzymes in rat liver during pregnancy. Experientia. 15: 703-4.
27. Manalu, W., Sumaryadi, M.Y., Kusumorini, N. (1997) Maternal serum concentration of total tri-iodothyronine, tetraiodothyronine and cortisol in different status of pregnancy during late pregnancy in ettawah-cross does. Asian Austral J Anim Sci. 10: 385-390.
28. Mansour, M.M., Farid, Z., Bassily, S. (1982) Serum enzyme tests in hepatosplenic schistosomiasis.Trans R Soc Trop Med Hyg. 76: 109-111.
29. McGinlay, J.M., Payne, R.B. (1988) Serum albumin by dye-binding: bromocresol green or bromocresol purple? The casefor conservatism. Ann Clin Biochem. 25: 417-21.
30. Mohebbi-Fani, M., Nazifi ,S., Bahrami, S. (2012a) Circulating thyroid hormones and indices of energy and lipid metabolism in normal and hormonally induced oestrus cows. J Basic Appl Sci. 8: 270-274.
31. Mohebbi-Fani, M., Nazifi, S., Rowghani, E. (2012b) Thyroid hormones and their correlations with serum glucose, beta hydroxybutyrate, nonesterified fatty acids, cholesterol, and lipoproteins of high-yielding dairy cows at different stages of lactation cycle. Comp Clin Pathol. 18: 211-216.
32. Nath, H.C., Baruah, K.K., Baruah, A. (2005) Serum cholesterol and protein in pre, peri and postpartum cows. Ind Vet J. 82: 519-521.
33. Naziffi-Habibabadi, S., Gheisari, H.R., Shakerlomani, F. (2003) Determination of serum thyroidal hormones of Iranian goats as influenced by age, sex, pregnancy and lactation. J Vet Med. (Tehran University). 4: 101-104.
34. Nazifi, S., Gheisari, H.R., Poorkabir, M.A. (2000) Serum lipids and lipoproteins in clinically healthy male camels (*Camelus dromedaries*). Vet Res Commun. 24: 527-531.
35. Nazifi, S., Gheisari, H.R., Shaker, F. (2002a) Serum lipids and lipoproteins and their correlations with thyroid hormones in clinically healthy goats. Vet Arhiv. 72: 249-257.
36. Nazifi, S., Saeb, M., Ghavami, S.M. (2002b) Serum lipid profile in Iranian fat-tailed sheep in late pregnancy, at parturition and during the post-parturition period. J Am Vet Med Assoc. 49: 9-12.
37. Nazifi, S., Saeb, M., Rategh, S. (2005) Serum lipids and lipoproteins in clinically healthy Caspian miniature horses. Vet Arhiv. 75: 175-182.

38. Niasari-Naslaji, A., Gharahdaghi, A.A., Mosaferi, S., Bahmani, N., Abarghani, A., Ghanbari, A., Gerami, A. (2008) Effect of sucrose extender with different levels of osmolality on the viability of spermatozoa in bactrian camel (*Camelus bactrianus*). Pajouhesh and Sazandegi (In Persian). 20: 112-117.
39. Norusis, M.J. (1993) SPSS for windows base system user's guide release 6.0. SPSS Inc, Michigan. 281-290.
40. Nouh, A.M., Ibrahim, A.M., Basher, M.A. (2008) Prevalence of thyroid dysfunction and its effect on serum lipid profiles in a Murzok, Libya Population. Thyroid Sci. 3: 1-6.
41. NRCC. (1990) Annual Report, National Research Centre on Camel. Bikaner, India.
42. Omidi, A., Montazertorbati, M.B., Sajedi, Z.H. (2014) Lipid profile and thyroid hormone status in the last trimester of pregnancy in single humped camels (*Camelus dromedarius*). Trop Anim Health Prod. 46: 609-14.
43. Ouajd, S., Kamel, B. (2009) Physiological Particularities of Dromedary (*Camelus dromedarius*) and Experimental Implications. Scant J Lab Anim Sci. 36: 19-29.
44. Piccione, G., Caola, G., Giannetto, C. (2009) Selected biochemical serum parameters in ewes during pregnancy, post-parturition, lactation and dry period. Anim Sci Papers Rep. 27: 321-330.
45. Poljicak, M., Terezija, S., Marenja, k. (2009) Comparative hematological and biochemical values in pregnant and non-pregnant red, Cervuselaphus, and fallow deer, Damadama, females. Folia Zool. 58: 36-44.
46. Rahman, H., AraChowdhury, M., TowhidulAlam, M. (2007) Serum thyroxine &triiodothyronine levels in normal pregnancy and pre-eclampsia. J Teach Assoc. 20: 6-10.
47. Raylander, L., Nilsson-Ehle, P., Hagmar, L. (2006) Simplified precisen method for adjusting serum levels of persistent organohalogen pollutants to total serum lipids. Chemosphere. 62: 333-336.
48. Rodriguez, M.N., Tebot, I., Le Bas, A. (1996) Renal functions and urea handling in pregnant and lactating Corriedale ewes. Can J Anim Sci. 76: 469-472.
49. Saeed, A., Khan, I.A., Hussein, M.M. (2009) Change in biochemical profile of pregnant camels (*Camelus dromedaries*) at term. Comp Clin Pathol. 18: 139-143.
50. Schlumbohm, C., Sporleder, H.P., Gurtler, H. (1997) The influence of insulin on metabolism of glucose, free fatty acids and glycerol in normo- and hypocalcaemia ewes during different reproductive states. Deut Tierärztl Woch. 104: 359-365.
51. Shinowara, G.Y., Jones, L.M., Reinhart, H.L. (1942) The estimation of serum inorganic phosphatase and acid and alkaline phosphatase activity. J Biol Chem. 142: 921- 933.
52. Silanikove, N. (2000) Effects of heat stress on the welfare of extensively managed domestic ruminants. Livest Prod Sci. 67: 1-18.
53. Stocki, V.M., Schuh, M., Schmid, S. (1975) The behavior of glucose, thyroxin, vitamin A, beta-carotene, methionine and vitamin B12 in blood of primiparous cattle during puerperium. Z Tierphysiol Tierenahr Futtermittelkd. 35: 282-288.
54. Swansonk, S., Kuzmuk, N., Schook, L.B. (2004) Diet affects nutrient digestibility, hematology, and serum chemistry of senior and weanling dogs. J Anim Sci. 82: 1713-1724.
55. Szasz, G. (1976) Reaction-rate method for gamma-glutamyltransferase activity in serum. Clin Chem. 22: 2051-5.
56. Utiger, R.D. (1987) The thyroid: physiology, hyperthyroidism, hypothyroidism and the painful thyroid. In: Endocrinology and Metabolism. Felig P, Baxter, J.D., Broadus, A.E., Frohman, L.A. (eds.). (2nd ed.) McGraw-Hill Inc, New York, USA. p. 409-412.
57. Vertor, W., Swaton, R. (1969) Alkaline phosphatase and acid phosphatase in cattle, sheep and camel serum with special reference to lymphatic leucosis in cattle. Mh Vet Med. 19: 384- 390. (Vet Bull 35: 390).
58. Watson, T.D.G., Burns, L., Packard, C.J. (1993) Effects of pregnancy and lactation on plasma lipid and lipoproteins concentrations, lipoprotein composition and post-heparin lipase activities in Shetland pony mares. J Reprod Fertil. 97: 563-568.
59. Yokus, B., Cakir, D.U., Kany, Z. (2006) Effects of seasonal and physiological variations on the serum chemistry, vitamins and thyroid hormone concentr-0ations in sheep. J Vet Med. 53: 271-276.
60. Zongping, L. (2003) Studies on the haematology and trace element status of adult Bactrian camels (*Camelus bactrianus*) in China. Vet Res Commun. 27: 397-405.

The evaluation of udder health status in Holstein dairy farms located in Qom province

Mahmoodi Afsah, T.[1]**, Vojgani, M.**[1]**, Gharagozlou, F.**[1]**, Akbarinejad, V.**[2*]

[1] *Department of Theriogenology, Faculty of Veterinary Medicine, University of Tehran, Tehran, Iran*

[2] *Young Researchers and Elites Club, North Tehran Branch, Islamic Azad University, Tehran, Iran*

Key words:
bulk tank milk, dairy cow, mastitis

Correspondence
Akbarinejad, V.
Young Researchers and Elites Club, North Tehran Branch, Islamic Azad University, Tehran, Iran

Email: v_akbarinejad@ut.ac.ir

Abstract:

BACKGROUND: Mastitis is the most economically important disease in dairy industry worldwide. Bulk tank milk (BTM) analysis has been suggested for monitoring the udder health status at herd level. **OBJECTIVES:** A cross-sectional study was conducted to evaluate udder health status in 15 Holstein dairy farms located in Qom province. **METHODS:** Bulk tank somatic cell count (BTMSCC) was analyzed using opto-fluoro-electronic counter. Standard plate count, preliminary incubation count, laboratory pasteurized count, and the number of environmental streptococci, *S. agalactiae*, *S. dysgalactiae*, *S. uberis*, *E. coli*, *K. pneumoniae*, coagulase negative streptococci, *S. aureus* and *C. bovis* were determined using specific culture media. Moreover, clinical and subclinical mastitis were diagnosed using physical examination and California mastitis test, respectively. **RESULTS:** Most herds had moderate to high BTMSCC and high bacterial counts. The prevalence of clinical and subclinical mastitis was 1.3% and 24.7%, respectively. **CONCLUSIONS:** The present study indicated inefficient stall management, udder hygiene, and milking practices in the herds investigated.

Introduction

Mastitis is the most economically important disease in dairy industry worldwide (Blosser, 1979, Harmon, 1994, Sargeant et al., 1998), which not only decreases milk production but also diminishes milk quality (Philpot and Stephen, 2000, Radostits et al., 2007). Mastitis might not be eradicated but can be controlled (Philpot and Stephen, 2000, Radostits et al., 2007). Control of mastitis necessitates the evaluation of udder health status leading to knowledge of the prevalence of mastitis and mastitis-associated pathogens. In this context, bulk tank milk (BTM) analysis has been applied to monitor udder health status at herd level, to troubleshoot herds with mastitis and to determine milk quality (Jayarao and Wolfgang, 2003, Radostits et al., 2007).

Qom province is located in the centre of Iran and has dry climate, with low humidity and scanty rainfall. In total, approximately 10,000 Holstein dairy cattle are raised in Qom province with daily milk production of 200,000 kg. Dairy farms located in Qom province provide milk for dairy industries not only in Qom province but also in adjacent provinces. A cross-sectional study was conducted to evaluate udder health status in 15 farms located in Qom province.

Materials and Methods

Dairy herds: The study was implemented from June to November 2012 in 15 dairy farms with 1,740 Holstein dairy cows. All herds were milked three times a day, had open shed housing, and utilized dried manure solids as bedding. All herds implemented some of the principles of mastitis control program

(Radostits et al., 2007) such as proper milking hygiene, use of functionally adequate milking machine, and post-milking teat dipping; however, none of the herds practiced pre-milking teat dipping.

BTM sample collection and analysis: BTM sample collection was performed as described by National Mastitis Council (Jayarao and Wolfgang, 2003). All BTM samples were transported on ice within 24 hours to the laboratory. BTM somatic cell count (SCC) was determined using an opto-fluoro-electronic counter (Fossomatic 90®; Foss Electric, Denmark). Standard plate count (SPC), preliminary incubation count (PIC), and laboratory pasteurized count (LPC) were determined using plate count agar (Merck, Germany). The number of environmental streptococci (ES) and *Streptococcus agalactiae* (*S. agalactiae*), *Streptococcus dysgalactiae* (*S. dysgalactiae*) and *Streptococcus uberis* (*S. uberis*) were determined using Modified Edward's agar (HiMedia, India). EMB and MacConkey agar (Merck, Germany) were used to count *E. coli* and *Klebsiella pneumoniae* (*K. pneumoniae*), respectively. Baird Parker's agar (Merck, Germany) was used to enumerate coagulase negative streptococci (CNS) and *Staphylococcus aureus* (*S. aureus*). Corynebacterium selective agar (Merck, Germany) was used to determine the number of *Corynebacterium bovis* (*C. bovis*). Plates for enumeration of SPC, PIC, and LPC were incubated at 32°C for 48 h. Plates for enumeration of CNS, ES, *S. aureus*, *Streptococci* spp., *E. coli*, *K. pneumonia*, and *C. bovis* were incubated at 37°C for 48h.

Clinical examination and california mastitis test (CMT): Initially, the quarters (n=6,960) were physically examined for the presence of the signs of clinical mastitis including warm, hard, and swollen quarter and/or abnormal milk appearance. Quarters that were not blind and were apparently healthy were then subjected to CMT to determine quarters with subclinical mastitis. In brief, 2 mL of milk were mixed with 2 mL of CMT reagent (DeLaval, Poland). Reactions were graded as 0, trace, 1+, 2+, and 3+ (Kasravi et al., 2010).

Statistical analysis: Initially, data were tested for normality using Kolmogorov-Smirnov test. Given that the assumptions of parametric tests were not achieved, spearman's rank correlation was used to analyze the relationship between data resulted from BTM analysis. All analyses were conducted in SAS Version 9.2 (SAS Institute Inc., USA). Correlations were considered significant at the $p<0.01$ level.

Results

BTM sample collection and analysis: Values for SCC and bacterial counts in BTM are summarised in Table 1 and 2. In terms of BTMSCC, SPC, PIC, LPC, CNS, and ES, 13%, 0%, 0%, 13%, 13%, and 0% of herds had low values, 47%, 0%, 0%, 67%, 0%, and 0% had moderate values, and 40%, 100% 100%, 20%, 87%, and 100% had high values, respectively (Table 3). *S. aureus*, *S. agalactiae*, and *K. pneumoniae*, which ideally must not be observed in BTM, were detected in 100% (15.15), 33% (5/15) and 87% (13/15) of herds, respectively. With regard to the count of *S. dysgalactiae*, *S. uberis* and *C. bovis*, 100% (15/15), 93% (14/15), and 60% (9/15) of herds had >500 CFU (the goal was BTM bacterial count of the mentioned bacteria). The goal for *E. coli* count in BTM was considered <50 CFU; however, all herds (100%; 15/15) had >50 CFU *E.coli* in BTM.

BTMSCC was correlated with SPC, PIC, *S. aureus*, *S. agalactiae* and *C. bovis* ($p< 0.01$; $r = 0.79$, 0.79, 0.76, 0.74 and 0.84, respectively; Table 4). SPC was correlated with PIC, ES, *S. aureus*, *S. dysgalactiae* and *C. bovis* ($p<0.01$; $r = 0.97$, 0.68, 0.78, 0.67 and 0.86, respectively). PIC was correlated with ES, *S. aureus*, *S. dysgalactiae* and *C. bovis* ($p<0.01$; $r = 0.68$, 0.79, 0.70 and 0.84, respectively). There was correlation between LPC and ES ($p<0.01$; $r=0.66$). CNS was correlated with ES, *S. dysgalactiae*, and *E. coli* ($p<0.01$; $r = 0.68$, 0.67 and 0.80, respectively). ES was correlated with *S. dysgalactiae* and *E. coli* ($p<0.01$; $r = 0.95$ and 0.75, respectively). *S. aureus* was correlated with *S. dysgalactiae* and *C. bovis* ($p< 0.01$; $r = 0.70$ and 0.73, respectively). *E. coli* was correlated with *S. dysgalactiae* and *K. pneumoniae* ($p< 0.01$; $r = 0.68$ and 0.71, respectively; Table 4).

Prevalence of clinical and subclinical mastitis: Values for prevalence of clinical and subclinical mastitis in each individual farm are presented in Table 5. In total, the proportion of blind quarters was 1.3% (89/6960). The prevalence of clinical and subclinical mastitis was 1.3% (90/6960) and 24.7% (1,721/6960), respectively. The proportion of trace, 1+, 2+,

Table 1. Somatic cell count (SCC), standard plate count (SPC), preliminary incubation count (PIC), laboratory pasteurized count (LPC), coagulase negative staphylococci (CNS), environmental streptococci (ES), *E. coli*, *S. aureus*, *S. agalactiae*, *S. dysgalactiae*, *S. uberis*, *C. bovis* and *K. pneumoniae* in bulk tank milk (BTM) in each individual farm.

Parameter	Farm 01	Farm 02	Farm 03	Farm 04	Farm 05	Farm 06	Farm 07	Farm 08	Farm 09	Farm 10	Farm 11	Farm 12	Farm 13	Farm 14	Farm 15
Number of cows	166	140	34	57	102	50	295	157	24	250	66	163	30	71	135
SCC (Cells/ml)	423000	481000	338000	963000	1273000	216000	211000	289000	142000	336000	218000	787000	173000	333000	437000
SPC (CFU/ml)	82000	84000	93000	116000	419000	41000	74000	49000	40000	74000	49000	115000	78000	122000	88000
PIC (CFU/ml)	176000	169000	216000	227000	963000	77000	128000	81000	5000	122000	72000	548000	149000	359000	159000
LPC (CFU/ml)	110	130	285	90	1250	100	125	100	75	105	125	350	130	100	145
CNS (CFU/ml)	1100	1000	2400	400	2200	1900	1000	1100	450	1000	2700	6000	1100	3400	3900
ES (CFU/ml)	15900	14500	19300	1400	21300	8100	11900	10900	4000	10900	8700	21000	11400	26500	24500
S. aureus (CFU/ml)	40	20	100	70	75	20	15	40	10	50	15	210	10	75	70
S. agalactiae (CFU/ml)	6200	5200	0	28000	17500	0	0	0	0	0	0	0	0	0	6200
S. dysgalactiae (CFU/ml)	7600	7200	8100	700	11200	2100	6800	2100	600	1800	1200	8100	1600	11600	10900
S. uberis (CFU/ml)	2100	1700	4900	150	4900	4500	1300	4600	2500	4500	4500	2500	5900	7400	5200
C. bovis (CFU/ml)	375	900	750	875	1500	350	200	400	100	500	300	1000	500	800	850
E. coli (CFU/ml)	481	322	482	121	349	325	209	316	60	428	371	1120	387	1388	491
K. pneumoniae (CFU/ml)	50	15	50	0	60	30	0	30	40	85	20	125	30	50	60

Table 2. Descriptive statistics of somatic cell count (SCC), standard plate count (SPC), preliminary incubation count (PIC), laboratory pasteurized count (LPC), coagulase negative staphylococci (CNS), environmental streptococci (ES), *E. coli*, *S. aureus*, *S. agalactiae*, *S. dysgalactiae*, *S. uberis*, *C. bovis* and *K. pneumoniae* in bulk tank milk (BTM).

Parameter	Minimum	Median	Maximum
Number of cows	24	102	295
SCC (Cells/ml)	142,000	336,000	1,273,000
SPC (CFU/ml)	40,000	82,000	419,000
PIC (CFU/ml)	50,000	159,000	963,000
LPC (CFU/ml)	75	125	1,250
CNS (CFU/ml)	400	1,100	6,000
ES (CFU/ml)	1,400	11,900	26,500
S. aureus (CFU/ml)	10	40	210
S. agalactiae (CFU/ml)	0	0	28,000
S. dysgalactiae (CFU/ml)	600	6,800	11,600
S. uberis (CFU/ml)	150	4,500	7,400
C. bovis (CFU/ml)	100	500	1,500
E. coli (CFU/ml)	60	371	1,388
K. pneumoniae (CFU/ml)	0	40	125

and 3+ grades of CMT was 38.0% (654/1721), 20.0% (344/1721), 21.2% (365/1721), and 20.8% (358/1721), respectively.

Discussion

Bulk tank milk analysis revealed moderate to high values of BTMSCC in the majority of the herds (87%), which shows the presence of intramammary infection within the herds (Philpot and Stephen, 2000, Bradley and Green, 2005). Major contagious pathogens of mastitis including *S. aureus* and *S.*

Table 3. Number and proportion of farms in different categories of bulk tank milk SCC and bacterial counts. [(a)]Categories and values were suggested by Jayarao et al. (10).

Parameter	Category (count)[a]	Number of farms (%)
BTMSCC	Low (<200,000)	2/15 (13)
	Moderate (200,000-400,000)	7/15 (47)
	High (>400,000)	6/15 (40)
SPC	Low (<5,000)	0/15 (0)
	Moderate (5,000-10,000)	0/15 (0)
	High (>10,000)	15/15 (100)
PIC	Low (<10,000)	0/15 (0)
	Moderate (10,000-20,000)	0/15 (0)
	High (>20,000)	15/15 (100)
LPC	Low (<100)	2/15 (13)
	Moderate (100-200)	10/15 (67)
	High (>200)	3/15 (20)
CNS	Low (<500)	2/15 (13)
	Moderate (500-1,000)	0/15 (0)
	High (>1,000)	13/15 (87)
ES	Low (<500)	0/15 (0)
	Moderate (500-1,000)	0/15 (0)
	High (>1,000)	15/15 (100)

Table 4. Spearman correlation coefficients. $^{(*)}p<0.01$. $^{(**)}p<0.001$. $^{(***)}p<0.0001$.

	BTM SCC	SPC	PIC	LPC	CNS	ES	*S. aureus*	*S. agalactiae*	*S. dysgalactiae*	*S. uberis*	*C. bovis*	*E. coli*	*K. pneumoniae*
BTMSCC	1	0.79**	0.79**	0.45	0.21	0.43	0.76*	0.74*	0.50	-0.14	0.87***	0.28	0.34
SPC		1	0.97***	0.48	0.35	0.68*	0.78**	0.54	0.67*	0.20	0.86***	0.48	0.33
PIC			1	0.51	0.34	0.68*	0.79**	0.50	0.70*	0.11	0.84***	0.48	0.37
LPC				1	0.56	0.66*	0.40	0.16	0.59	0.27	0.55	0.49	0.40
CNS					1	0.68*	0.53	-0.16	0.67*	0.61	0.32	0.80**	0.55
ES						1	0.61	0.16	0.95***	0.49	0.55	0.75*	0.58
S. aureus							1	0.27	0.70*	0.23	0.73*	0.60	0.61
S. agalactiae								1	0.21	-0.25	0.53	-0.11	-0.02
S. dysgalactiae									1	0.42	0.56	0.68*	0.54
S. uberis										1	0.17	0.57	0.46
C. bovis											1	0.38	0.38
E. coli												1	0.71*
K. pneumoniae													1

Table 5. Prevalence of clinical and subclinical mastitis. Numbers in parentheses are actual numbers.

Parameter	Farm 01	Farm 02	Farm 03	Farm 04	Farm 05	Farm 06	Farm 07	Farm 08
Number of quarters	664	560	136	228	408	200	1180	628
Proportion of blind quarters (%)	2.0 (13/664)	1.6 (9/560)	1.5 (2/136)	0.9 (2/228)	1.0 (4/408)	0.5 (1/200)	0.3 (4/1180)	2.4 (15/628)
Prevalence of clinical mastitis (%)	0.6 (4/664)	0.0 (0/560)	0.0 (0/136)	4.4 (10/228)	3.4 (14/408)	0.0 (0/200)	0.3 (4/1180)	0.2 (1/628)
Prevalence of subclinical mastitis (%)	19.4 (129/664)	16.4 (92/560)	33.1 (45/136)	34.6 (79/228)	38.5 (157/408)	18.0 (36/200)	13.6 (161/1180)	32.6 (205/628)
Proportion of grade trace quarters (%)	10.0 (13/129)	20.7 (19/92)	35.6 (16/45)	24.1 (19/79)	26.1 (41/157)	50.0 (18/36)	42.9 (69/161)	57.6 (118/205)
Proportion of grade 1+ quarters (%)	20.2 (26/129)	10.9 (10/92)	8.9 (4/45)	15.2 (12/79)	15.9 (25/157)	11.1 (4/36)	19.9 (32/161)	11.2 (23/205)
Proportion of grade 2+ quarters (%)	31.0 (40/129)	29.3 (27/92)	24.4 (11/45)	32.9 (26/79)	27.4 (43/157)	22.2 (8/36)	25.4 (41/161)	13.6 (28/205)
Proportion of grade 3+ quarters (%)	38.8 (50/129)	39.1 (36/92)	31.1 (14/45)	27.8 (22/79)	30.6 (48/157)	16.7 (6/36)	11.8 (19/161)	17.6 (36/205)

Parameter	Farm 09	Farm 10	Farm 11	Farm 12	Farm 13	Farm 14	Farm 15
Number of quarters	96	1000	264	652	120	284	540
Proportion of blind quarters (%)	1.0 (1/96)	2.1 (21/1000)	0.8 (2/264)	0.8 (5/652)	0.8 (1/120)	0.4 (1/284)	1.5 (8/540)
Prevalence of clinical mastitis (%)	0.0 (0/96)	2.7 (27/1000)	1.1 (3/264)	3.5 (23/652)	0.0 (0/120)	1.4 (4/284)	0.0 (0/540)
Prevalence of subclinical mastitis (%)	14.6 (14/96)	35.6 (356/1000)	35.6 (94/264)	27.0 (176/652)	13.3 (16/120)	22.9 (65/284)	17.8 (96/540)
Proportion of grade trace quarters (%)	50.0 (7/14)	50.0 (178/356)	45.7 (43/94)	31.8 (56/176)	31.3 (5/16)	40.0 (26/65)	27.1 (26/96)
Proportion of grade 1+ quarters (%)	28.6 (4/14)	27.5 (98/356)	30.9 (29/94)	24.4 (43/176)	25.0 (4/16)	24.6 (16/65)	14.6 (14/96)
Proportion of grade 2+ quarters (%)	14.3 (2/14)	12.9 (46/356)	16.0 (15/94)	20.5 (36/176)	31.2 (5/16)	21.5 (14/65)	23.9 (23/96)
Proportion of grade 3+ quarters (%)	7.1 (1/14)	9.6 (34/356)	7.4 (7/94)	23.3 (41/176)	12.5 (2/16)	13.9 (9/65)	34.4 (33/96)

agalactiae have the most contribution to the elevation of BTMSCC (Wilson et al., 1997, Olde Riekerink et al., 2006), which is probably the reason for correlation of BTMSCC with *S. aureus* and *S.*

agalactiae in the present study.

Moreover, the majority of BTM bacterial counts in the herds were substantially higher than goals. High SPC values could originate from milking cows with mastitis or contaminated teats, defective sanitation of milking equipment, or the delayed cooling of BTM (Jayarao and Wolfgang, 2003, Radostits et al., 2007). High PIC, affecting the keeping quality of milk, reflects substandard hygiene practices (Jayarao and Wolfgang, 2003). Correlation of *S. aureus* and environmental streptococci, particularly *S. dysgalactiae*, with SPC and PIC implies the contribution of these organisms to the rise of SPC and PIC. Intramammary infection with *S. aureus* increases bacterial count of individual cows, which could subsequently lead to elevation of SPC in BTM (Radostits et al., 2007). Jayarao et al., (2004) have also reported correlation of ES with SPC, and PIC. CNS, ES, *E. coli* and *K. pneumoniae* originates from not only intramammary infections, but also nonspecific contamination of cow skin, bedding, and water (Jayarao and Wolfgang, 2003). Elevation of the number of these organisms in BTM suggests defective stall management, udder hygiene, and milking practices (Godkin and leslie, 1993, Hayes et al., 2001, Jayarao et al., 2003, 2004). *C. bovis* is highly susceptible to teat disinfection and is, in turn, suggested as an indicator of teat dipping efficiency (Radostits et al., 2007). In this context, high number of *C. bovis* (which was strongly correlated with BTMSCC, SPC and PIC) in majority of herds indeed indicates inefficient teat-dipping. The considerably high count of environmental streptococci, particularly *S. dysgalactiae*, in all herds and its correlation with SPC and PIC implicates the need for improvement of stall management as well as proper implementation of pre-milking teat dipping in herds investigated (Radostits et al., 2007).

As it was previously indicated, the prevalence of subclinical mastitis (24.7%) was considerably higher than that of clinical mastitis (1.3%) in the present study (Philpot and Stephen, 2000, Radostits et al., 2007). The prevalence of clinical and subclinical mastitis in the present study is approximately comparable with that previously reported in Fars province (0.7% and 21.6%, respectively) (Hashemi et al., 2011).

In conclusion, the high BTM bacterial counts in the present study suggest defective stall management, udder hygiene, and milking practices. Although all herds practiced post-milking teat dipping, high values of *C. bovis* in the majority of the herds indicates substandard execution of teat disinfection.

Acknowledgements

The authors thank Dr. F. Moosakhani for his kind assistance in BTM sample analysis.

References

1. Blosser, T.H. (1979) Economic losses from and the national research program on mastitis in the United States. J Dairy Sci. 62: 119-127.
2. Bradley, A., Green, M. (2005) Use and interpretation of somatic cell count data in dairy cows. In Practice. 27: 310-315.
3. Godkin, M.A., Leslie, K.E. (1993) Culture of bulk tank as a screening test: A brief review. Can Vet J. 34: 601-605.
4. Harmon, R.J. (1994) Physiology of mastitis and factors affecting somatic cell counts in milk. J Dairy Sci. 77: 2103-2112.
5. Hashemi, M., Kafi, M., Safdarian, M. (2011) The prevalence of clinical and subclinical mastitis in dairy cows in the central region of Fars province, south of Iran. Iran J Vet Res. 12: 236-241.
6. Hayes, M.C., Ralyea, R.D., Murphy, S.C., Carey, N.R., Scarlett, J.M., Boor, K.J. (2001) Identification and characterization of elevated microbial counts in bulk tank milk. J Dairy Sci. 84: 292-298.
7. Jayarao, B.M., Pillai, S.R., Sawant, A.A., Wolfgang, D.R., Hegde, N.V. (2004) Guidelines for monitoring bulk tank milk somatic cell and bacterial counts. J Dairy Sci. 87: 3561-3573.
8. Jayarao, B.M., Wolfgang, D.R. (2003) Bulk-tank milk analysis. A useful tool for improving milk quality and herd udder health. Vet Clin North Am Food Anim Pract. 19: 75-92.
9. Kasravi, R., Bolourchi, M., Farzaneh, N., Seifi, H.A., Barin, A., Hovareshti, P., Gharagozlou, F. (2010) Relationship between in vitro antimicrobial sensitivity of bovine subclinical mastitis isolates and treatment outcome in lactating dairy cows. Iran J Vet Res. 11: 249-254.
10. Olde Riekerink, R.G.M., Barkema, H.W., Veenstra, S., Poole, D.E., Dingwell, R.T., Keefe, G.P. (2006)

Prevalence of contagious mastitis pathogens in bulk tank milk in Prince Edward Island. Can Vet J. 47: 567-572.

11. Philpot, W.N, Stephen, C.N. (2000) Winning The Fight Against Mastitis. (1st ed.) Westfalia Surge Inc. Bönen, Germany.
12. Radostits, O.M., Gay, CC. Hinchcliff, K.W., Constable, P.D. (2007) Diseases of the mammary gland. In: Veterinary Medicine. Radostits, O.M., Gay, CC. Hinchcliff, K.W., Constable, P.D. (eds.). (10th ed.) Saunders Ltd. Philadelphia, USA. p. 673-762.
13. Sargeant, J.M., Scott, M., Leslie, K.E., Ireland, M.J., Bashiri, A. (1998) Clinical mastitis in dairy cattle in Ontario: frequency of occurrence and bacteriological isolates. Can Vet J. 39: 33-38.
14. Wilson, D.J., Das, H.H., Gonzalez, R.N., Sears, P.M. (1997) Association between management practices, dairy herd characteristics, and somatic cell count of bulk tank milk. J Am Vet Med Assoc. 210: 1499-1502.

The effect of rumen protected methionine (RPMet) on milk composition of lactating Cashmere Rayeni goat

Nazem, M.N.[1], Sami, M.[2], Askari, N.[3*]

[1] *Department of Basic Sciences, Faculty of Veterinary Medicine, Shahid Bahonar University of Kerman, Kerman, Iran*

[2] *Department of Food Hygiene and Public Health, Faculty of Veterinary Medicine, Shahid Bahonar University of Kerman, Kerman, Iran*

[3] *School of Veterinary Medicine, Shahid Bahonar University of Kerman, Kerman, Iran*

Key words:
milk compositions, Rayeni Cashmere goat, RP Met

Correspondence
Askari, N.
School of Veterinary Medicine, Shahid Bahonar University of Kerman, Kerman, Iran

Email: nasrinaskari@yahoo.com

Abstract:

BACKGROUND: Methionine has been suggested as the first-limiting amino acid for milk production in ruminants. It is important how to increase milk protein yield and milk fat in dairy ruminants. **OBJECTIVES:** This study was set to investigate the effect of rumen protected methionine (RPMet) on milk composition of lactating Cashmere Rayeni goats. **METHODS:** 40 healthy singleton Cashmere Rayeni goats about 3 to 4 years of age, at the first day of lactation, were randomly divided into 2 equal control and experimental groups. The experimental group was supplemented with 5 gr/day RPMet for 60 days. Milk samples of 2 groups were taken on 30th and 60th days of the study. Milk protein, milk fat, milk lactose, and milk Solids-not-Fat (SNF) were determined using automatic analyzer. The results were statistically evaluated with SPSS. **RESULTS:** The supplementation with RPMet did not effect all of the above mentioned parameters during the 60 days of the experiment ($p>0.05$), except for the milk fat percentage of the experimental group which showed significant increase after 60 days ($p<0.05$). **CONCLUSIONS:** Our results about milk protein, milk lactose, and SNF were in agreement with previous studies that had not shown significant differences. Results about milk fat on the 30th day were in agreement with the results of several authors who reported that RPMet did not affect milk fat percentage or yield; however, in the present study milk fat increased significantly on the 60th day ($p<0.05$). To the best of the authors' knowledge, no study about the effects of RPMet on milk composition of Cashmere Rayeni goat has been done.

Introduction

The immense amount of nutrition-based research on dairy cows has been done with the primary goal to increase milk production and eventually to manipulate milk protein and milk fat yield.

Protein available for absorption in the ruminant intestine is derived from ruminal microbes and dietary protein that escapes degradation during passage through the rumen. Protein is one of the major limiting nutrients in the diets of lactating dairy cows (Yang et al., 2010). In the pasture fed dairy cow and goat, more than 50% of the protein ingested is degraded in the rumen into ammonia, and this extensive protein degradation may limit the amount of protein passing to the small intestine (Pacheco-Rios et al., 1999).

Methionine has been most often suggested as the first-limiting amino acid for milk production in ruminants; however, other amino acids have been proposed as first limiting or co limiting with methionine (Andereas et al., 2013; Izumi et al., 200; Leonardi et al., 2003; Yang et al., 2003). This is largely because of their low concentrations in feed protein as compared to their concentrations in milk and ruminally synthesized bacterial protein (Benefield et al., 2009; Bequette et al., 1998; Doepel et al., 2004; Lapierre et al., 2006). Supplementation of methionine postruminally has had positive effects on milk production and milk protein concentration (Armentano et al., 1997; Dinn et al., 1996; Noftsger et al., 2003). The implement of the protected amino acids in dairy cows' diet showed improvements of the production of milk and milk proteins (Overton et al., 1996; Pisulewski and Kowalski, 1999; Poljicak-Milas and Marenjak, 2007).

It is important how to increase milk protein yield and the efficiency of protein utilization and to avoid protein deficiency in early lactation (Yang et al., 2010). Several studies have been conducted to determine the effects of supplementation with Met on milk protein yield and composition, with varied responses. In some cases, an increase in milk protein and protein yield has been observed (Izumi et al., 2000; Koch et al., 1996; Robert et al., 1996), whilst in others there has been no response in milk protein yield (Overton et al., 1996; Papas et al., 1984). In this regard, some studies have suggested that supplementary dietary Met was associated with an increase in milk fat production (Robinson et al., 1998; Socha et al., 2008); whereas, some researchers have emphasized that Met had no effect on milk fat (Brodrick et al., 2008; Leonardi et al., 2003; Noftsger et al., 2003; Preynat et al., 2009). However, most of the studies have been undertaken with mixed rations, using different types of preserved forage and different ratios of forage to concentrate (Pacheco-Rios et al., 1999).

Although the data are rather variable regarding the amino acid supplements and their influence on the milk protein and milk fat synthesis in dairy cows, it could be suspected they have a similar effect on dairy goat performance (Kijora et al., 2002; Oliviera et al., 2001: Overton et al., 1996; Wang et al., 2003).

The objective of this study was to evaluate the effect of rumen protected methionine on the protein, fat, lactose, and SNF contents in milk of Cashmere Rayeni goat at two months of lactation.

Materials and Methods

40 healthy singleton Cashmere Rayeni goats about 3 to 4 years of age, at the first day of lactation, were randomly divided into 2 equal control and experimental groups. The experiment started at the beginning of the lactation period. Both groups were fed on the pasture. The experimental group was supplemented with 5 gr/day rumen protected methionine (RPMet) (3 gr/day pure RPMet; Mepron® M85, Degussa Corporation, Germany) manually for 60 days. The RPMet consisted of a DL-methionine core coated with pH sensitive copolymer to protect them from ruminal breakdown (Andereas et al., 2013).

Milk samples of the 2 groups were taken on the 30th and 60th days of the experience. Milk protein, milk fat, milk lactose, and milk SNF were determined using automatic analyser "Milcoscan 605" (A.S.N. Foss Eletronic). The results were statistically evaluated with SPSS (SPSS 16 Chi. USA, 2004).

Results

The results of the effect of RPMet on milk compositions measurements are reported in Tables 1 and 2.

The supplementation with RPMet did not influence milk protein, lactose, and SNF percentage during the 60 days of the study in Cashmere Rayeni goats ($p>0.05$). Also, no treatment effects were observed on the yields of milk fat on the first 30 days; however, 60 days from the beginning of the experience, there was a significant increase in milk fat percentage of the experimental group ($p<0.05$).

Discussion

Although AA utilization by dairy cows has received considerable attention from different research groups all over the world, there is relatively little published data on the effect of AA supplementation on milk production in pasture-fed animals.

Protein is one of the most valuable milk components, both in an economic and nutritional sense. The largest fraction of the milk proteins,

Table 1. Milk components in control and experimental group on 30th day. (*) p<0.05.

Milk components	Control group	Experimental group (RPMet)
	Mean±SE	Mean±SE
Protein (%)	3.41±.07	3.41±.07
Fat (%)	3.57±.45	2.82±.29
Lactose (%)	4.90±.10	4.96±.11
SNF (%)	9.28±.19	9.32±.18

Table 2. Milk components in control and experimental group on 60th day. (*) p<0.05.

Milk components	Control group	Experimental group (RPMet)
	(mean±SEM)	(mean±SEM)
Protein (%)	4.14±.06	4.23±.13
Fat (%)	2.46±.10*	2.92±.14*
Lactose (%)	5.80±.10	5.99±.18
SNF (%)	10.79±.16	11.15±.33

casein, determines the yield and quality of numerous products (Pacheco-Rios et al., 1999). Percentage of milk protein may be more sensitive index than milk yield to estimate the effect of RPMet on cows (Samuelson et al., 2001). Several studies have been carried out to determine the effect of RPMet on milk protein. The results of these studies differ and the values of RPMet are not yet clear (Izumi et al., 2001).

Casper et al. (1988) conducted a study on cows and found that supplementation of ruminally protected Met increased milk protein percentages. They concluded that methionine increased in mammary synthesis; nonetheless, it was not the first factor limiting milk production. RPMet tended to increase protein percentage in milk, which agreed with the data from other experiments (Casper et al., 1987; Misciatteilli et al., 2003; Rogers et al., 1987; Schingoethe et al., 1988; Wu et al., 1997).

Supplemental RPMet enhanced the production of milk protein (Armentano et al., 1997; Casper et al., 1988; Dinn et al., 1998; Misciatteilli et al., 2003), milk yield, and milk protein content (Illg et al., 1987). Kijora et al. (2002) in their research found a strong relationship between feed intake and protein content in the ration of dairy goats. On the other hand, supplementation with RPMet has also been reported to have no effect (Papas et al., 1984; Yang et al., 2010).

Our results about milk protein in this study were in agreement with previous studies that had not shown significant effect on milk protein. No significant effect of PRMet on protein percentage in milk may be due to low bioavailability of methionine from PRMet for protein synthesis (Yang et al., 2010).

Some researchers have shown that Met deficiencies have most often been suggested to affect milk fat synthesis because Met is a methyl donor in the transmethylation reactions of lipid biosynthesis (Robinson et al., 1998; Yang et al., 2010). Addition of methionine hydroxy analog to diets of dairy cows frequently has resulted in increased fat content of milk (Lundquist et al., 1983). Socha et al. (2008) reported that duodenal infusion of Met increased milk fat percentage and yield in cows during early lactation. Also, Misciatteilli et al. (2003) determined that early lactation cows fed RPMet had increased milk fat percentage compared with control cows. Specific mechanisms by which Met supplementation may affect milk fat, including ruminal effects (Soltan et al., 2012) or post absorption effects on lipid metabolism, remain largely speculative (Soltan et al., 2012).

Increased percentage of milk fat when RPMet was fed to cows or abomasal infusion of methionine was obtained in some experiments (Oldham et al., 1984; Overton et al., 1996; Robinson et al., 1998; Rogers et al., 1987; Yang et al., 2010). Clark and Oldham had suggested that supplementary dietary Met was associated with an increase in milk fat production (Clark et al., 1975; Oldham et al., 1984).

Our results about milk fat on the 30th day were in agreement with those obtained by several authors (Brodrick et al., 2008; Leonardi et al., 2003; Noftsger et al., 2003; Overton et al., 1996; Preynat et al., 2009) who reported that RPMet supplementation did not affect milk fat percentage or yield.

According to our results, after 60 days, only milk fat increased significantly (p<0.05).The specific reason for the increased percentage of milk fat in our experiment was unknown; however, several possibilities had been suggested in the literature. McCarthy et al. (1968) reported that Met might be important for synthesis of serum lipoprotein and as a methyl donor for synthesis of phospholipids, suggesting that a post-absorptive effect of Met on lipid metabolism is possible. Sharma and Erdman (1988) speculated that choline synthesized from Met was likely to have been at least partially responsible.

In this study, the percentages of lactose and SNF

in milk were not significantly affected when RPMet was fed, which was in agreement with the results found by other researches (Overton et al., 1996; Yang et al., 2010).

Differences in results from these experiments might have been caused by differences in the status of Met or other AA of the cows, the amount of methionine supplied in the protected product, and the efficacy of the protection scheme in delivering methionine to the small intestine (Yang et al., 2010).

The presented results indicate that the supplementation of the protected methionine (Mepron®, Degussa) cannot lead to an increase in milk components, total milk protein, and milk fat during the 30 days; however, after the 60th day, milk fat increased significantly ($p<0.05$). The results at the end of the 30th and 60th days (except milk fat on the 60th day) are in agreement with those of previous experiments conducted on Alpine goats (Bacar-Huskic et al., 1998; Poljicak-Milas and Marenjak, 2007) and the results obtained by some other researches in this field (Poljicak-Milas and Marenjak, 2007).

It is worth mentioning that parity and live weight of animals could have had an impact on the production results.

Acknowledgments

This research was financially supported by the research council of Shahid Bahonar University of Kerman.

References

1. Andereas, M.P., Vicini, J.L., Clark, J.H., Peirce-Sander, S. (2013) Effects of rumen-protected methionine on plasma free amino acids and production by dairy cows. J Nutr. 114: 2221-2227.
2. Armentano, L.E., Bertics, S.J., Ducharme, G.A. (1997) Response of lactating cows to methionine or methionine plus lysine added to high protein diets based on alfalfa and heated soybeans. J Dairy Sci. 80: 1194-1199.
3. Bacar-Huskic, L., Ljubic, Z., Magdalenic, B., Sakoman, M. (1998) Results of applying protected methionine to the diet of dairy goats. Krmiva. 40: 317-327.
4. Benefield, B.C., Patton, R.A., Stevenson, M.J., Overton, T.R. (2009) Evaluation of rumen - protected methionine source and period length on performance of lactating dairy cows within Latin squares. J Dairy Sci. 92: 4448-4455.
5. Bequette, B.J., Backwell, F.R.C., Crompton, L.A. (1998) Current concepts of amino acid and protein metabolism in the mammary gland of the lactating ruminant. J Dairy Sci. 81: 2540-2559.
6. Brodrick, G.A., Stevenson, R.A., Patton, N.E., Lobos, J.J. Olmos Colmenero. (2008) Effect of supplwmwnting rumen-protected methionine on production and nitrogen excretion in lactation dairy cows. J Dairy Sci. 91: 1092-1102.
7. Casper, D.P., Schingoethe, D.J., Yang, C.M.J., Mueller, C.R. (1987) Protected methionine supplementation with an extruded blend of soybeans and soybean meal for dairy cows. J Dairy Sci. 70: 321-330.
8. Casper, D.P., Schingoethe, D.J. (1988) Protected methionine supplementation to a barley-based diet for cows during early lactation. J Dairy Sci. 71: 164-172.
9. Clark, J.H. (1975) Lactational responses to postruminal administration of proteins and amino acids. J Dairy Sci. 58: 1178-1197.
10. Dinn, N. E., Shelford, J. A., Fisher, L. J. (1998) Use of the cornell net carbohydrate and protein system and rumen-protected lysine and methionine to reduce nitrogen excretion from lactating dairy cows. J Dairy Sci. 81: 229-237.
11. Doepel, L.D., Pacheco, D., Kennelly, J.J., Hanigan, M.D., Lopez, I.F., Lapierre, H. (2004) Milk protein synthesis as a function of amino acid supply. J Dairy Sci. 87: 1279-1297.
12. Fisher, L.J. (1972) Response of lactating cows to the intravenous infusion of amino acids. Can J Anim Sci. 52: 377-384.
13. Illg, D.J., Sommerfeldt, J.L., Schingoethe, D.J. (1987) Lactational and systemic responses to the supplementation of protected methionine in soybean meal diets. J Dairy Sci. 70: 620-629.
14. Izumi, K., Kikuchi, C., Okamoto, M. (2000) Effect of rumen-protected methionine on lactation performance of dairy cows. Research farm, Rakuno Gakuen University, Ebet su. p. 1235-1238.
15. Kijora, C., Peters, K.J., Rexroth, H., Chowdhury, S. (2002) Einfluss des Energie- und Proteinniveaus

sowie der Proteinqualität auf die Milchleistung der Bunten. Deutschen Edelziege. Arch Tierz Dummerstorf. 45: 255-268.

16. Koch, K.L., Whitehouse, L., Garthwaite, B.D., Wasserstrom, V.M., Schwab, C.G. (1996) Production responses of lactating Holstein cows to rumen-stable forms of lysine and methionine. J Dairy Sci. 79: 239.
17. Koenig, K.M., Rode, L.M. (2001) Ruminal degradability, intestinal disappearance and plasma methionine response of rumen-protected methionine in dairy cows. J Dairy Sci. 84: 1480-1487.
18. Lapierre, H.D., Pacheco, R., Berthiaume, D.R., Ouellet, C.G., Schwab, P. Dubreuil, G., Holtrop, S., Lobley, G.E. (2006) What is the true supply of amino acids for a dairy cow? J Dairy Sci. 89: E1-E14.
19. Leonardi, C., Stevenson, M., Armentano, L.E. (2003) Effect of two levels of crude protein and methionine supplementation on performance of dairy cows. J Dairy Sci. 86: 4033-4042.
20. Lundquist, R.G., Linn, J.G., Otterby D.E. (1983) Influence of dietary energy and protein on yield and composition of milk from cows fed methionine hydroxy analog. J Dairy Sci. 66: 475-491.
21. McCarthy, R.D., Porter, G.A., L.C. Griel, J.R. (1968) Bovine ketosis and depressed fat test in milk: A problem of methionine metabolism and serum lipoprotein aberration. J Dairy Sci. 51: 459-462.
22. Misciatteilli, L., Kristensen, V. F., Vestergaard, M., Welsbjerg, M.R., Sejrsen, K., Hvelplund, T. (2003) Milk production nutrient utilization and endocrine responses to increased postruminal lysine and methionine suooly in dairy cows. (7th ed.) National Academic Press, Washington. DC, USA.
23. Noftsger, S., St-Pierre, N.R. (2003) Supplementation of methionine and selection of highly digestible rumen undegradable protein to improve nitrogen efficiency for milk production. J Dairy Sci. 86: 958-969.
24. Oldham, J.D. (1984) Protein-energy interrelationships in dairy cows. J Dairy Sci. 67: 1090-1114.
25. Oliviera, M.D.S., Oliviera, E., Nalim, M.D., Motta, L.O. (2001) Effect of methionine addition in the diet on milk production by dairy cows. Ars Veterinaria. 17: 130-136.
26. Overton, T.R., LaCount, D.W., Cicela, T.M., Clark, J.H. (1996) Evaluation of a ruminally protected methionine product for lactating dairy cows. J Dairy Sci. 79: 631-638.
27. Pacheco-Rios, D., McNabb, W.C., Hill, J.P., Mackenzie, D.D.S. (1999) The effects of methionine supplementation upon milk composition and production of forage-fed dairy cows. Can J Anim Sci. 79: 235-241.
28. Papas, A.M., Sniffen, C.J., Muscato, T.V. (1984) Effectiveness of rumen-protected methionine for delivering methionine postruminally in dairy cows. J Dairy Sci. 67: 545-552.
29. Pisulewski, P.M., Rulquin, H., Peyraud, J.L., Verite, R. (1996) Lactational and systemic responses of dairy cows to postruminal infusion of increasing amounts of methionine. J Dairy Sci. 79: 1781-1791.
30. Pisulewski, P.M., Kowalski, Z.M. (1999).The effect of protected lysine and methionine on milk yield and its composition in lactating cows fed grass silage-based rations. J Anim Feed Sci. 8: 341-353.
31. Poljicak-Milas, N., Marenjak, T.S. (2007) Dietary supplement of the rumen protected methionine and milk yield in dairy goats. Arch Tierz Dummerstorf. 50: 273-278.
32. Preynat, A.H., Lapierre, M.C., Thivierge, M.F., Palin, J.J., Mate, Desorchers, A., Girard, C.L. (2009) Effects of supplements of folic acid, Vitamin B12 and rumen-protected methionine on whole body metabolism of methionine and glucose in lactating dairy cows. J Dairy Sci. 92: 677-689.
33. Robert, J.C., Sloan, B.K., Denis, C. (1996) The effects of graded amounts of rumen protected methionine on lactational responses in dairy cows. J Dairy Sci. 79: 194.
34. Robinson, P.H., Chalupa, W., Sniffen, C.J., Julien, W.E., Sato, H. (1998) Ruminally protected lysine or lysine and methionine for lactating dairy cows fed a ration designed to meet requirements for microbial and postruminal protein. J Dairy Sci. 81: 1364-1373.
35. Rogers, J.A., Krishnamoorthy, U., Sniffen, C.J. (1987) Plasma amino and milk protein production by cows fed rumen-protected methionine and lysine. J Dairy Sci. 70: 789-798.
36. Samuelson, D.J., Denise, S.K., Roffler, R., Ax, R.L., Armstrong, D.V. (2001) Response of Holstein and brown swiss cows fed alfalfa at two stages of lactation. J Dairy Sci. 84: 917-928.
37. Schingoethe, D.J., Casper, D.P., Yang, C., Illg, D.G., Smonnerfeldt, J.L. (1988) Lactational response to soybean meal, heated soybean meal and extruded soybeans with ruminally protected methionine. J

Dairy Sci. 71: 173-180.
38. Sharma, B.K., Erdman, R.A. (1988) Abomasal infusion of choline and methionine with or without 2-amino-2-methyl-1-propanol for lactating dairy cows. J Dairy Sci. 71: 2406-2411.
39. Socha, M.T., Schwab, C.G., Putnam, D.E., Whit-house, N.L., Garthwaite, B.D., Ducharme, G.A. (2008) Extent of methionine limitation in peak, early and mid-lactation dairy cows. J Dairy Sci. 91: 1996-2010.
40. Soltan, M.A., Mujalli, A.M., Mandour, M.A., El-Shinway Abeer, M. (2012) Effect of dietary rumen protected methionine and/or choline supplement-ation on rumen performance characteristics and productive performance of early lactating cows. Pak J Nutr. 11: 221-230.
41. Wang, J.T., Wan, W.J., Xu, G.Q., Cui, G.Y. (2003) Effects of protected methionine on production performance of dairy cows. China Dairy Cattle. 1: 15-17.
42. Wu, Z., Fisher, R.J., Polan, C.E., Schwab,C.G. (1997) Lactational performance of cows fed low or high ruminally undegradable protein prepartum and supplemental methionine and lysine. J Dairy Sci. 80: 722-729.
43. Yang , W.R., Sun , H., Wang, Q.Y., Liu, F.X., Yang, Z.B. (2010) Effects of Rumen-Protected Methionine on Dairy Performance and Amino Acid Metabolism in Lactating Cows. Am J Anim Vet Sci. 5: 1-7.

Effect of dietary chitosan on immune response and disease resistance in *Cyprinus carpio*

Alishahi, M.[1*], Esmaeili Rad, A.[2], Zarei, M.[3], Ghorbanpour, M.[4]

[1] *Department of Clinical Sciences, Faculty of Veterinary Medicine, Shahid Chamran University of Ahvaz, Ahvaz, Iran*

[2] *Graduated Student from the Faculty of Veterinary Medicine, Shahid Chamran University of Ahvaz, Ahvaz, Iran*

[3] *Department of Pathobiology, Faculty of Veterinary Medicine, Shahid Chamran University, Ahvaz, Iran*

[4] *Department of Food Hygiene, Faculty of Veterinary Medicine, Shahid Chamran University of Ahvaz, Ahvaz, Iran*

Key words:
Aeromonas hydrophila, chitosan, *Cyprinus carpio*, immune response

Correspondence
Alishahi, M.
Department of Clinical Sciences, Faculty of Veterinary, Shahid Chamran University, Ahvaz, Iran

Email: alishahimoj@gmail.com

Abstract:

BACKGROUND: Occurrence of resistance against antibiotics and inadequate efficacy of some vaccines necessitates studies of natural immunostimulators in aquaculture. Shrimps shell derived from Chitosan can be used as immune stimulators in fish. **OBJECTIVES:** In this study, the effects of oral administration of chitosan, derived from shrimp shell, on some immune responses and disease resistance in *Cyprinus carpio* were studied. **METHODS:** Three hundred healthy fish weighing 42.4+8.1 g were divided into 4 equal groups: the first group (G10) was fed with food supplemented with 10 mg kg^{-1} chitosan, the second (G5) and third groups (G2.5) were fed with food supplemented with 5 mg kg^{-1} and 2.5 mg kg^{-1}, respectively. The control group was fed with basal feed (without chitosan). All groups were treated for 60 days. Blood samples were taken on 0, 20, 40, and 60 days post- experiment; In addition, some immunological indices, including serum lysozyme activity, serum bactericidal activity, Nitro Blue Tetrazolium (NBT) reduction activity, serum proteins, white blood cell count (WBC), and differentiated count were measured. At the end of the treatment, fish were challenged with live *Aeromonas hydrophila* and mortality rate was recorded for 14 days. **RESULTS:** Oral administration of chitosan (0.5 and 1%) significantly enhanced NBT reduction activity and resistance to *A. hydrophila* infection ($p=0.012$). Serum lysozyme and bactericidal activity, serum total protein and globulin, WBC and leukocytes ratio showed no significant change among the groups ($p>0.05$). **CONCLUSIONS:** This study indicates that oral administration of shrimp shell chitosan may have a positive effect on some immune parameters and resistance against bacterial infection in *Cyprinus carpio*.

Introduction

Fish culture is an important industry around the world. There is essential attention to improve this industry in closed and small areas. Due to intensive culture, over-crowding leads to poor physiologic conditions and increasing susceptibility to diseases (Sakai, 1999). Vaccination and antibiotics are used for treating and controlling fish diseases; however, there are limited vaccines for fish diseases, and utilization of antibiotics is not safe because of the development of antibiotic-resistant bacteria strain; in addition, these ways are very expensive (Siwicki et al., 1994; Sakai, 1999; Salisbury et al., 2002). Reducing mortality due to opportunistic pathogens, preventing viral diseases, enhancing efficacy of anti-microbial agents, and vaccines as well as increasing resistance to parasites are benefits of using immune-stimulants (Bricknell and Dalmo, 2005). Enhancing aquatic organism immune status by dietary administration of immune-stimulants is an acceptable practice (Sakai, 1999). Different immune-stimulants have been reported to enhance natural (innate) immunity in fish. These materials include: killed bacteria and bacterial products (Nayak et al., 2007; Aly et al., 2008; Geng et al., 2011), herbal extracts (Dugenci et al., 2003; Selvaraj et al., 2006; Alishahi et al., 2010), some vitamins (Nayak et al., 2007; Cerezuela et al., 2009), Levamisole (Findlay and Munday, 2000; Gopalakannan and Arul, 2006), nucleotides (Low et al., 2003), hormones (Yada et al., 2002), and some biopolymers such as Chitin (Esteban et al., 2000; Cuesta et al., 2003). Recently optimized usage of food industries wastes or by-products as food additives have been increased to better conservation of environment (Esteban et al., 2000). One of these by-products is chitosan.

Chitosan is an amino-oligosaccharide (a linear homo-polymer of ß-(1-4)-2-amino-deoxy-D-glucose) and is obtained with alkaline de-acetylation from Chitin (poly (ß -(1-4)-N-acetyl-D-glucose-amine), obtained from crustaceans exoskeleton, insects cuticle and cell wall of some microbes. Chitosan has biological activities such as immune-modulatory, adjuvant, anti-microbial, wound healing, analgesic, anti-oxidant, anti-tumor, etc. (Seferian and Martinez, 2001; No et al., 2002; Okamoto et al., 2002; Qin et al., 2002; Dutta et al., 2004; Boonyo et al., 2007; Harikrishnan et al., 2012; Ramesh and Maridass, 2010); meanwhile, chitosan has industrial activities such as stimulation of plant growth, preservative, thickener, and stabilizer for sauces and coating of fruit in food technology, seed coating, frost protection in agriculture technology and clarifying water, removal of metal ions and ecological polymers and reducing odor in water treatment (Muzzarelli et al., 1989; Ohta et al., 1999; Rinaudo, 2006). Nowadays, Chitosan is examined to enhance immune status and bacterial and viral diseases protection in aquaculture (Dautremepuits et al., 2004; Gopalakannan and Arul, 2006; Lin et al., 2011; Geng et al., 2011). Seferian and Martinez, (2001) reported immunostimulating and adjuvant effects of Chitosan in intraperitoneal route i. Meanwhile, Anderson and Siwicki (1994) showed immunostimulating effects of chitosan in injection or in immersion routs in rainbow trout.

Common carp cultivates as an important world-wide warm-water fish in earthen pond of cyprinid polyculture system in Iran. Annual production of this species is around 20000 tones. Annual production of farmed shrimp in Iran is about 10000 tons, and around 40 percent of this production is by-products like shell which is left in the environment as waste materials. Therefore, these large amounts of shrimp shell, which nowadays contaminate the environment, can be changed to chitosan and used as a food supplementary material in common carp. Therefore, in this study the effect of oral administration of different levels of chitosan, obtained from farmed shrimp shell, on immune responses of common carp were investigated. To the best of our knowledge, it is the first study which evaluates the effect of chitosan derived from Peneous vanameii as an immunostimulant in common carp.

Materials and Methods

Fish and experimental design: Three hundred healthy common carp, *Cyprinus carpio*, weighing 42.4+8.1 g, were obtained from a fish farm in Ahvaz, Khouzestan province, Iran. They were kept in a 300 l. tank for acclimation for two weeks. Water quality factors were recorded during the experiment: temperature, 25±1°C; Dissolved oxygen, 8-10 ppm; pH, 7.8±0.2; NO_2 <0.01ppm and NH_3 <0.1ppm. Water exchange rate was 20% of water volume daily.

Fish were divided into 4 groups in triplicates; groups 1 to 4 were fed with basal diet without chitosan supplementation (as control group), 2.5, 5 and 10 g kg^{-1} chitosan, respectively. Five fish were randomly collected from each group on days 0, 20th, 40th, and 60th of the experiment and anesthetized with 100 ppm MS-222 in de-chlorinated water. Blood samples were taken from caudal vein with a 2cc sterile syringe. Heparinized blood was used for hematological assays. Sera were separated from blood sample via centrifugation, for immunological assays. The sera were stored at -20 °C until they were used.

Diet preparation: Commercial common carp

food (Beyza feed mill, Shiraz, Iran) was used. Chitosan was grinded by a grinder machine, then was suspended in distilled water, and finally added to diet and mixed completely according to mentioned dosages. After air-drying, the feed were stored at 4 °C until used (Webster et al., 1997).

Extraction of chitin from shrimp shell: The shrimp shells were washed under running tap water to remove soluble organics, adherent proteins, and other impurities. The shells were then dried at room temperature and grounded. For demineralization of the shells, cold 0.25 M HCl (300 mL) was added to 50.0 g dried and grounded shrimp shells. This extraction was allowed to proceed for 15 min at 4°C. The suspension was then filtered and additional 300 ml of cold 0.25 M HCl was added to the pellet. After 30 min of cold extraction, the suspension was filtered again. The pellet was washed to neutrality with tap water, rinsed with distilled water, and then oven-dried at 70°C overnight. Deproteinization of the chitin was carried out using 1.0 M NaOH (15 mL/g) at 70°C for 20 h. Then, the extract was cooled to room temperature, filtered, and washed with tap water until neutrality was achieved. The pellet was finally washed with ethanol (96%) and dried at 70°C.

Preparation of chitosan: The conversion of chitin to chitosan involved deacetylation using strong alkaline treatment. The chitin (1 g) was put into 15-20 ml 50% NaOH at 70°C for 20 h. Then, the extract was cooled, filtered, and washed with tap water until neutrality. The pellet was finally washed with ethanol (96%) and dried at 70°C.

Obtaind: Obtained chitosan characterization: Molecular weight: 580±12 KD, deacetylation rate: % 83.5±%2.7, colure and solubility, white powder soluble in water and PBS (pH=5)

Immunological parameters (Serum lysozyme activity): Serum lysozyme activity was measured following Ellis (1990) and Nayak et al. (2008). Based on turbidometric method, lyophilized and its activity were measured. The lyophilized *Micrococcus lysodeikticus* (Sigma, USA) at a concentration of 0.2 mg mL^{-1} (in 0.02 M sodium citrate buffer) were added to sera ratio of 1:10 v/v in the same buffer. Immediately after adding *M. lysodeikticus*, the first OD was read at 450 nm. The second OD was read 60 minutes later. Lysozyme activity was expressed as units mL^{-1} where one unit is defined as the decrease in absorbance of 0.001 min^{-1}.

Serum bactericidal activity: Serum bactericidal activity was measured according to Kajita et al. 1990 with slight modification. Sera samples from each subgroup were diluted three times with 0.1% gelatin-veronal buffer (GVBC2) (pH 7.5, containing 0.5 mM mL^{-1} Mg2C and 0.15 mM mL^{-1} Ca2C). The bacteria *Yersinia ruckerii* (live, washed cells used earlier) was suspended in the same buffer to make a concentration of 1×10^5 cfu mL^{-1}. The diluted sera and bacteria were mixed at 1:1, incubated for 90 min at 25°C, and shaken. One control group containing bacterial suspension in same buffer was also incubated for 90 min at 25°C. The numbers of viable bacteria was then calculated by counting the colonies from the resultant incubated mixture on TSA plates in duplicate (two plates per sample) after 24 h incubation. The bactericidal activity of test serum was expressed as percentage of colony forming units in test group to that in control group.

Nitroblue-tetrazolium (NBT) reduction: A part of each blood sample was utilized for determining respiratory burst activity that was evaluated by the reduction of nitroblue-tetrazolium (NBT), following Anderson and Siwicki et al. (1994). 1 mL of heparinized blood from fish of each group was mixed with 100 ml of 0.2% NBT (Sigma, USA) solution for 30 min at 25°C after incubation; 50 ml from the mixture above was added with 1 mL of N-diethyl methyl formamide (Qualigens, India) and then centrifuged at 3000 × g for 5 min. The optical density of the supernatant was measured at 620 nm.

Total serum protein, Albumin and globulin: Total protein of each sample was analyzed following Lowry et al.'s (1951) method. Albumin content was measured using a standard albumin estimation kit (Zistchem Diagnostics, Iran) and the globulin content was estimated by subtracting albumin from total protein.

White blood cell count (WBC), Differential cell count: Leucocyte total count was made in a Neubauer counting chamber. Blood smears were stained with Giemsa, then 100 leucocytes were counted under the microscope (1000X) and the percentage of different types of leucocytes was calculated following Schaperclaus et al. (1991).

Challenge with bacterium: Virulent strain of *A. hydrophila* (isolated from common carp mortality in

Iran) was used for disease resistance assay. Thirty fish from each group were intraperitoneally injected with the bacterial suspension (2.1×10^7 CFU per fish $=LD_{50}$), and the mortality of challenged fish was recorded daily for 14 days. The cause of death was ascertained by re-isolating the infecting organism from kidney and liver of the dead fish. The cumulative daily mortality curve was drawn according to Misra et al.'s method (2006).

Statistical analysis: For statistical analysis of data SPSS software version 13 was used. Analysis of Variance (ANOVA) was used for comparison of means among the groups. Duncan complementary test was used for determining the significant differences among the groups. A p-value of <0.05 was accepted as significant.

Results

The serum lysozyme activity in all groups fed with different level of chitosan is shown in Figure 1. The results showed that lysozyme activity was not significantly affected by feeding chitosan supplemented food ($p=0.087$).

Serum bactericidal activity was not affected by oral administration of different levels of chitosan in common carp; however, slight improvement in bactericidal activity was seen in G1 and G2 (Figure 2).

As showed in Figure 3, although there was a significant enhancement of NBT reduction activity in G10 and G5 at days 20, 40 and 60 of experiment ($p=0.035$), no significant change was induced in G2.5 ($p=0.52$).

Total serum protein, albumin, and globulin of treatments were shown in Table 1. Total protein and immunoglobulin in G10 increased in all sampling period, but not significantly ($p=0.085$).

The results suggested that WBC value and blood Leukocytes ratio showed no significant differences in chitosan treated groups ($p>0.05$) (Table 2).

Mortality percentage of common carp fed on different level of chitosan-supplemented diet and the control diet after challenging with *A. hydrophila* is presented in Figure 4. Mortality in G10 and G5 decreased significantly ($p<0.05$). The mortality percentage was highest (76.7% ± 6.7) in the control group and lowest (60% ± 4.78) in G5 Chitosan group.

Discussion

Recently, chitin and chitosan have been used to increase the resistance of fish by enhancing the non-specific defense mechanisms (Harikrishnan et al., 2012). In this study, some immune responses of common carp were stimulated following oral administration of chitosan. Although slight increase in lysozyme activity was seen in G10 and G5 in some sampling periods, the changes among treatments were not significant ($p=0.087$).

Lysozyme is an important element of innate immunity of fish. It is a lytic enzyme that destroys peptidoglycan layer of gram-positive bacteria and activates complement system and phagocytes (Ellis, 1990). Similar report by Cha et al. (2008) showed that 1% chitosan-coated diet did not enhance lysozyme activity compared to control in Paralichthys olivaceus. Lin et al. (2011) also reported that dietary 0.2% chitosan (produced by microbial fermentation of the crustaceans shell) in diet did not affect lysozyme activity in *Cyprinus carpio* koi. Geng et al. (2011) showed that supplementation of food with 0.3% commercial chitosan did not affect lysozyme activity in Rachycentron canadum. In spite of these reports, there are some work in which chitosan has the stimulating effect on serum lysozyme activity. Gopalakannan and Arul (2006) reported that using of 1% chitosan in common carp has increasing effect on lysozyme activity. Lin et al. (2012) also found that oral administration of oligo-chitosan has a positive effect on lysozyme activity especially when it used along with probiotic. These contradictory results can be referred to the types of chitosan origin, purification procedure and quality of obtained chitosan or differences in fish species.

Although the serum bactericidal activity was enhanced by oral administration of 5 and 10 mg kg-1 chitosan in food, this enhancement was not significant. Similarly, Maqsood et al. (2010) found that serum bactericidal activity in carp fed on diet supplemented with 2 and 5 percent chitosan increased, but 1% chitosan did not affect serum bactericidal activity. Also, supplementation of food of Viscum album extract (Family Loranthaceae) in common carp enhanced serum bactericidal activity in the study of Alishahi et al. (2012). Divyagnaneswari

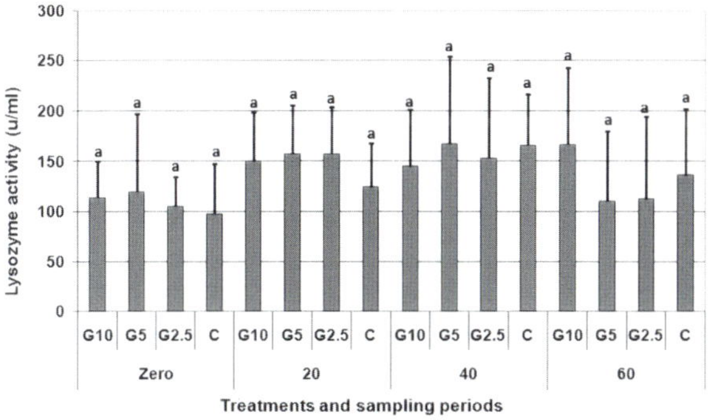

Figure1. The effects of dietary chitosan on serum lysozyme activity (units mL^{-1}) of common carp in each sampling period. Data showed as Mean±SD, n= 15. G10: carp fed with 10g/kg chitosan supplemented food, G5: carp fed with 5 g/kg chitosan supplemented food, G2.5: carp fed with 2.5 g/kg chitosan supplemented feed, C: carp fed with non-supplemented food (Mean±SD, n= 15). Significant differences (p<0.05) are marked by different letters.

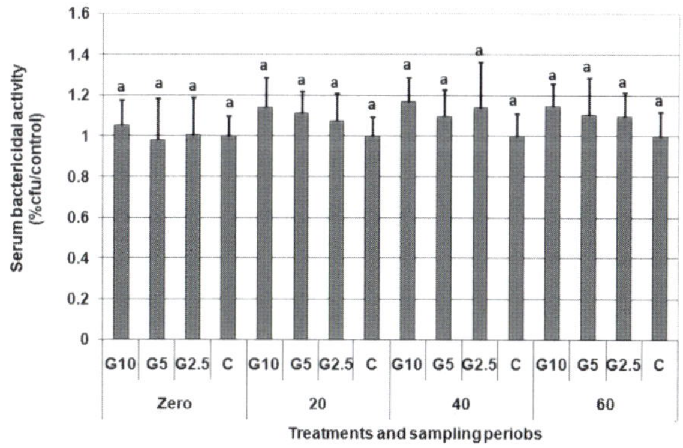

Figure 2. The effects of dietary chitosan on serum bactericidal ativity (as percentage of control group) of common carp in each sampling period. Data showed as Mean±SD, n=15. G10: carp fed with 10g/kg chitosan supplemented food, G5: carp fed with 5 g/kg chitosan supplemented food, G2.5: carp fed with 2.5 g/kg chitosan supplemented feed, C: carp fed with non-supplemented food (Mean±SD, n= 15). Significant differences (p<0.05) are marked by different letters.

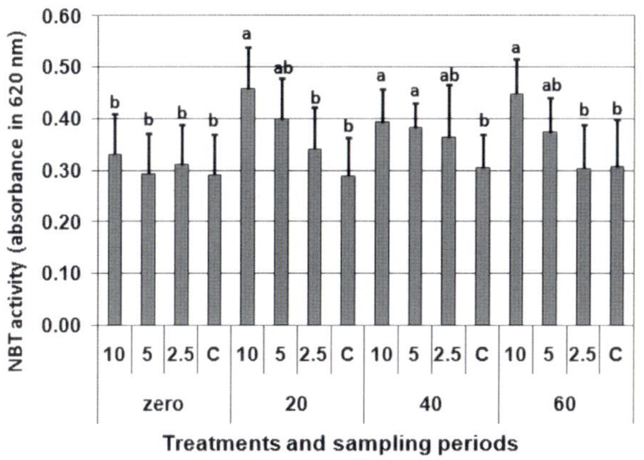

Figure 3. The effects of chitosan enriched diet on NBT activity in common carp in each sampling period. G10: carp fed with 10g/kg hitosan supplemented food, G5: carp fed with 5 g/kg chitosan supplemented food, G2.5: carp fed with 2.5 g/kg chitosan supplemented feed, C: carp fed with non-supplemented food (Mean±SD, n= 15).

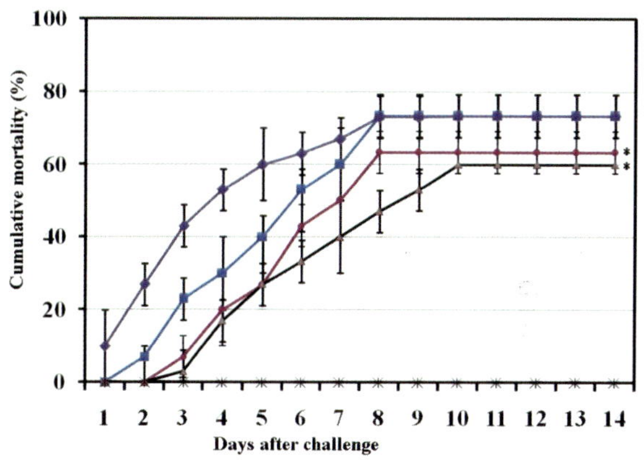

Figure 4. Cumulative mortality of common carp challenged with *A. hydrophila* following oral administration of chitosan-supplemented food. Data showed as Mean±SD, n= 15. G10: carp fed with 10g/kg hitosan supplemented food, G5: carp fed with 5 g/kg chitosan supplemented food, G2.5: carp fed with 2.5 g/kg chitosan supplemented feed, C: carp fed with non-supplemented food (*significant differences with control group, p< 0.05).

G 2.5 — G 5 — G 10 — Control ✻ PBS

et al. (2007) in tilapia and Katija et al. (1990) in rainbow trout reported increase of serum bactericidal activity after administration of biological immunostimulants. The increased serum bactericidal activity in chitosan treated groups indicates that various humoral factors are involved in innate and/or adaptive immunities which are elevated in the serum to protect the fish effectively from infection (Das et al. 2009). Thus, chitosan proved to be as an effective immunostimulant in preventing the establishment of bacterial infection in common carp.

The NBT activity as an indicator for respiratory burst activity in G10 and G5 groups enhanced significantly compared with the control groups (p=0.035). The present result is similar to Siwicki et al. (1994), Lin et al. (2011), Lin et al. (2012), and Gopalakannan and Arul's (2006) reports. Geng et al. (2011) also reported that using of dietary 0.3% and

Table 1. The effect of different level of dietary chitosan of total protein, albumin, and immunoglobulin in common carp in each sampling period. Data showed as Mean±SD, n= 15. G10: carp fed with 10g/kg hitosan supplemented food, G5: carp fed with 5 g/kg chitosan supplemented food, G2.5: carp fed with 2.5 g/kg chitosan supplemented feed, C: carp fed with non-supplemented food. Significant differences (p<0.05) are marked by different letters.

Parameters	Treatments	Day zero	days 20	days 40	days 60
Total protein	G10	2.75±0.32[a]	2.98±0.21[a]	2.93±0.22[a]	2.90±0.28[a]
	G5	2.75±0.32[a]	2.86±0.36[a]	2.72±0.48[a]	2 a.67±0.26[a]
	G2.5	2.75±0.32[a]	2.69±0.46[a]	2.67±0.47[a]	2 a.68±0.29[a]
	C	2.75±0.32[a]	2.70±0.21[a]	2.64±0.52[a]	2.70±0.24[a]
Albumin	G10	1.27±0.22[a]	1.28±0.28[a]	1.19±0.31[a]	1.29±0.34[a]
	G5	1.27±0.22[a]	1.27±0.16[a]	1.30±0.22[a]	1.30±0.43[a]
	G2.5	1.27±0.22[a]	1.20±0.20[a]	1.27±0.29[a]	1.30±0.24[a]
	C	1.27±0.22[a]	1.12±0.26[a]	1.22±0.33[a]	1.28±0.38[a]
Immunoglobulin	G10	1.45±0.20[a]	1.71±0.22[a]	1.68±0.38[a]	1.62±0.36[a]
	G5	1.45±0.20[a]	1.59±0.28[a]	1.51±0.25[a]	1.36±0.37[a]
	G2.5	1.45±0.20[a]	1.50±0.36[a]	1.41±0.29[a]	1.36±0.35[a]
	C	1.45±0.20[a]	1.57±0.35[a]	1.42±0.29[a]	1.41±0.27[a]

Table 2. Leukocyte count and differential count in common carp fed with different level of chitosan. Data showed as Mean±SD, n= 15. G10: carp fed with 10g/kg hitosan supplemented food, G5: carp fed with 5 g/kg chitosan supplemented food, G2.5: carp fed with 2.5 g/kg chitosan supplemented feed, C: carp fed with non-supplemented food. Significant differences (p<0.05) are marked by different letters.

Parameters	Treatments	Days zero	days 20	days 40	days 60
WBC	G10	5.29±2.38[a]	4.73±2.19	5.72±3.18[a]	4.34±1.20[a]
	G5	5.19±2.08[a]	5.67±2.59[a]	5.77±2.59[a]	4.62±1.29[a]
	G2.5	5.21±1.89[a]	4.37±1.26[a]	6.02±3.50[a]	4.72±1.37[a]
	Control	5.12±1.81[a]	4.5±1.84[a]	5.92±3.65[a]	4.47±1.43[a]
Lymphocyte	G10	57.75±6.63[a]	57.1±5.25[a]	62.83±6.61[a]	60.8±6.17[a]
	G5	56.55±6.12[a]	59.8±7.90[a]	62.16±7.49[a]	60.83±4.30[a]
	G2.5	59.5±6.13[a]	58±10.93[a]	55.83±6.79[a]	62.33±8.26[a]
	Control	55.75±7.13[a]	57.5±2.12[a]	54±5.2[a]	58.5±6.36[a]
Heterophile	G10	24.63±6.12[a]	27.3±4.68[a]	21.83±8.61[a]	26.16±3.37[a]
	G5	22.24±6.04[a]	27.67±4.1[a]	21.83±3.76[a]	25.83±4.57[a]
	G2.5	24.1±5.2[a]	28.5±9.86[a]	22.5±2.73[a]	28±4.38[a]
	Control	25.22±5.77[a]	26±6.5[a]	22.5±9.57[a]	28.2±5.65[a]
Monocyte	G10	14.66±4.64[a]	16.17±3.71[a]	13.5±4.18[a]	13.4±4.66[a]
	G5	13.45±4.22[a]	11.50±4.96[a]	16.16±4.49[a]	12.6±4.87[a]
	G2.5	14.23±4.11[a]	12.57±6.60[a]	19±7.21[a]	15±4.08[a]
	Control	15.06±3.9[a]	14.5±2.12[a]	16.66±2.88[a]	13.5±2.12[a]
Heterophile	G10	0.37±0.13[a]	0.44±0.13[a]	0.37±0.16[a]	0.44±0.13[a]
	G5	0.47±0.45[a]	0.56±0.37[a]	0.55±0.27[a]	0.55±0.28[a]
	G2.5	0.39±0.13[a]	0.37±0.11[a]	0.47±0.16[a]	0.44±0.13[a]
	Control	0.37±0.17[a]	0.57±0.18[a]	0.41±0.12[a]	0.37±0.13[a]
Monocyte	G10	0.71±0.17[a]	0.61±0.18[a]	0.67±0.13[a]	0.63±0.11[a]
	G5	0.67±0.19[a]	0.63±0.19[a]	0.63±0.15[a]	0.72±0.13[a]
	G2.5	0.73±0.18[a]	0.71±0.17[a]	0.67±0.16[a]	0.66±0.15[a]
	Control	0.63±0.23[a]	0.67±0.18[a]	0.67±0.15[a]	0.59±0.18[a]

0.6% chitosan enhanced the respiratory burst activity in Rachycentron canadum.

Total serum protein and globulin slightly increased in carp fed on diet supplemented with 5 and 10 mg kg-1 chitosan (p=0.085). Our result is similar to what Siwicki et al. (1994) reported. They observed no significant change in serum proteins following dietary administration of chitosan in rainbow trout. Besides Dugenci et al. (2003) also showed that 1% Zingiber officinale supplemented diet as an immunostimulant plant in rainbow trout did not increase total plasma protein. On the other hand, Harikrishnan et al. (2012) reported enhancement of total serum protein and globulin following feeding the fish with 1% and 2% chitosan supplemented food in Epinephelus bruneus.

The effect of dietary chitosan on Leukocyte numbers and differential count showed that neither leukocyte numbers nor leukocytes ratio affected significantly, in other work on chitosan similar results were reported: Gopalakannan and Arul (2006) reported that dietary 1% chitosan in common carp did not enhance Leucocyte numbers. Besides Chang et al. (2006) show total leucocyte numbers were unaffected by dietary 0.5%, 1% and 2% chitosan in Jappanese sea bass. Similarly, Supplementation of rainbow trout diet with chitosan had no effects on total leucocyte numbers (Siwicki et al., 1994). However, the present results contradict with the findings of other studies: Maqsood et al. (2010) reported that 1%, 2%, and 5% dietary chitosan in food can increase WBC in common carp. Lin et al. (2011) also showed that dietary 0.2% chitosan, produced by microbial fermentation of the crustaceans shell, in *Cyprinus carpio* koi had an enhancement effect on WBC count. Meshkini et al. (2012) reported that although 0.25% dietary chitosan enhanced significantly WBC and Leukocyte ratio, 0.50% and 1% chitosan did not enhance these parameters significantly. The contradictory results can be caused by different chitosan extraction procedure and fish species. It is possible that chitosan quality and origin cause these effective different results.

Mortality percentage of common carp fed on chitosan-supplemented diet (5 and 10 mg kg^{-1}) significantly decreased in comparison with the control group ($p<0.05$). This might be due to the enhancement of the non-specific immune system of the fish by chitosan. Maqsood et al. (2010) observed that supplemented diet with 1 and 2 percent chitosan cause decrease in mortality rate following bacterial challenge. Gopalakannan and Arul (2006) also reported that the RPS in the chitosan-supplemented group of common carp challenged with *Aeromonas hydrophila* was significantly higher than the control and chitin supplemented group. Rairakhwada et al. (2007) reported that the highest RPS (100%) was recorded in 0.5% levan fed and the lowest RPS was recorded in 1% levan fed fish. Alishahi et al. (2010) reported that enhancement of protection against *A. hydrophila* infection in common carp fed on 5% Aloe vera extract supplemented diets.

This study indicates that supplementation of food with 0.5 and 1% chitosan induced enhancement of some immune parameters and resistance against bacterial infection in *Cyprinus carpio*. Then, shrimp shell derived chitosan can be used for increasing resistance against bacterial infection and immunostimulation in common carp.

Acknowledgments

This work was financially supported by the research council of Shahid Chamran University, Ahvaz, Iran.

References

1. Alishahi, M., Ranjbar, M.M., Ghorbanpour, M., Peyghan, R., Mesbah, M., Razi jalali, M. (2010) Effects of dietary *Aloe vera* on specific and nonspecific immunity of common carp (*Cyprinus carpio*). J Vet Res. 4: 85-91.
2. Alishahi, M., Ghorbanpour, M., Peyghan, R. (2012) Effects of *Viscum album* linnaeus and *Nigella sativa* linnaeus extracts on some immune responses of common carp *Cyprinus carpio* Linnaeus. Asian Fisher Sci. 25: 15-28
3. Al Sagheer, F.A., Al-Sughayer, M.A., Muslim, S., Elsabee, M.Z. (2009) Extraction and characterization of chitin and chitosan from marine sources in Arabian Gulf. Carbohydr Polym. 77: 410-419.
4. Aly, S.M., Ahmed, Y.A.G., Ghareeb, A.A.A., Mohamed, M.F. (2008) Studies on *Bacillus subtilis* and *Lactobacillus acidophilus*, as potential probiotics, on the immune response and resistance of *Tilapia nilotica* (*Oreochromis niloticus*) to challenge infections. Fish Shellfish Immunol. 25: 128-36.
5. Anderson, D.P., Siwicki, A.K. (1994) Duration of protection against Aeromonas salmonicida in brook trout immunostimulated with glucan or chitosan by injection or immersion. Progress Fish Culturist. 56: 258-61.
6. Benhabiles, M.S., Salah, R., Lounici, H., Drouiche, N., Goosen, M.F.A., Mameri, N. (2012) Antibacterial activity of chitin, chitosan and its oligomers prepared from shrimp shell waste. Food Hydrocoll. 29: 48-56.
7. Boonyo, W., Junginger, H.E., Waranuch, N., Polnok, A., Pitaksuteepong, T. (2007) Chitosan and trimethyl chitosan chloride (TMC) as adjuvants for inducing immune responses to ovalbumin in mice following nasal administration. J Control Release. 121: 168-175.
8. Bricknell, I., Dalmo, R.A. (2005) The use of im-

munostimulants in fish larval aquaculture. Fish Shellfish Immunol. 19: 457- 472.

9. Cerezuela, R., Cuesta, A., Meseguer, J., Esteban, M.A. (2009) Effects of dietary vitamin D3 administration on innate immune parameters of sea bream (*Sparus aurata* L.). Fish Shellfish Immunol. 26: 243-248.
10. Cha, S., Lee, J., Song, C., Lee, K., Jeon, Y. (2008) Effects of chitosan-coated diet on improving water quality and innate immunity in the olive flounder, Paralichthys olivaceus. Aquaculture. 278: 110-118.
11. Chang, Q., Liang, M., Wang, J., Sun, J. (2006) Influence of chitosan on the growth and non-specific immunity of Japanese sea bass (*Lateolabrax japonicus*). Mar Fish Res. 27: 17-22.
12. Cuesta, A., Meseguer, J., Esteban, M.A. (2003) In vitro efiect of chitin particles on the innate cellular immune system of gilthead sea bream (*Sparus aurata* L.). Fish Shellfish Immunol. 15: 1-11.
13. Das, B.K., Pradhan, J., Sahu, S. (2009) The effect of Euglena viridis on immune response of rohu, *Labeo rohita* (Ham.). Fish Shellfish Immunol. 26: 871-876.
14. Dautremepuits, C., Betoulle, S., Paris-Palacios, S., Vernet, G. (2004) Humoral immune factors modulated by copper and chitosan in healthy or parasitised carp (*Cyprinus carpio* L.) by Ptychobothrium sp. (Cestoda). Aquat Toxicol. 68: 325-338.
15. Divyagnaneswari, M.D., Christybapita, A., Dinakaran, R. (2007) Enhancement of nonspecific immunity and disease resistance in *Oreochromis mossambicus* by *Solanum trilobatum* leaf fractions. Fish shellfish immunol. 23: 249-259.
16. Dugenci, S.K., Arda, N., Candan, A. (2003) Some medicinal plants as immunostimulant for fish. J Ethnopharmacol. 88: 99-106.
17. Dutta, P.K., Dutta, J., Tripathi, V.S. (2004) Chitin and chitosan: Chemistry, properties and applications. J Sci Ind Res. 63: 20-31.
18. Ellis, A.E. (1990) Lysozyme assay. In: Techniques in Fish Immunology.Stolen, J.S., Fletcher, D.P., Anderson, B.S., Robertson, B.S. (eds.). SOS Publication, Fair Haven, USA. p. 101-103.
19. Esteban, M.A., Mulero, V., Cuesta, A., Ortun, J., Meseguer, J. (2000) Effects of injecting chitin particles on the innate immune response of gilthead sea bream (*Sparus aurata* L.). Fish Shellfish Immunol. 10: 543-554.
20. Findlay, V.L., Munday, B.L. (2000) The immunomodulatory effects of levamisole on thenonspecific immune system of Atlantic salmon, *Salmo salar* L. J Fish Dis. 23: 369-378.
21. Geng, X., Dong, X., Tan, B., Yang, Q., Chi, S., Liu, H., Liu, X. (2011) Effects of dietary chitosan and *Bacillus* subtilis on the growth performance non-specific immunity and disease resistance of cobia, *Rachycentron canadum*. Fish Shellfish Immunol. 31: 400-406.
22. Gopalakannan, A., Arul, V. (2006) Immunomodulatory effects of dietary intake of chitin, chitosan and levamisole on the immune system of *Cyprinus carpio* and control of *Aeromonas hydrophila* infection in ponds. Aquaculture. 255: 179-187.
23. Harikrishnan, R., Kim, J., Balasundaram, C., Heo, M. (2012) Immunomodulatory effects of chitin and chitosan enriched diets in *Epinephelus bruneus* against *Vibrio alginolyticus* infection. Aquaculture. 326-329: 46-52.
24. Katija, Y., Sakai, M., Atsuta, S., Kobayash, M. (1990) The immunonodulatory effects of levamisole on rainbowtrout. Fish Pathol. 25: 93-98.
25. Lin, S., Mao, S., Guan, Y., Luo, L., Luo, L., Pan, Y. (2012) Effects of dietary chitosan oligosaccharides and *Bacillus* coagulans on the growth, innate immunity and resistance of koi (*Cyprinus carpio* koi). Aquaculture. 342-343: 36-41.
26. Lin, S., Pan, Y., Luo, L., Li, L. (2011) Effects of dietary b-1, 3-glucan, chitosan or raffinose on the growth, innate immunity and resistance of koi (*Cyprinus carpio* koi). Fish Shellfish Immunol. 31: 788-794.
27. Low, C., Wadsworth, S., Burrells, C., Secombes, C.J. (2003) Expression of immune genes in turbot (*Scophthalmus maximus*) fed a nucleotide-supplemented diet. Aquaculture. 221: 23-40.
28. Lowry, O.H., Rosebrough, N.J., Farr, A.L., Randall, R.J. (1951) Protein measurement with the folin phenol reagent. J Biol Chem. 193: 265-275.
29. Maqsood, S., Singh, P., Samoon, M.H., Balange, A.K. (2010) Effect of dietary chitosan on non-specific immune response and growth of *Cyprinus carpio* challenged with *Aeromonas hydrophila*. Int Aquat Res. 2: 77-85.
30. Meshkini, S., Tafy, A., Tukmechi, A., Farhang-Pajuh, F. (2012) Effects of chitosan on hematological parameters and stress resistance in rainbow trout (*Oncorhynchus mykiss*). Vet Res Forum. 3: 49- 54.

31. Misra, C.K., Das, B.K., Mukherjee, S.C., Meher, P.K. (2006) The immunomodulatory effects of tuftsin on the non-specific immune system of Indian Major carp, *Labeo rohita*. Fish Shellfish Immunol. 20: 728-738.

32. Muzzarelli, R.A.A., Weckx, M., Filippini, O. (1989) Removal of trace metal ions from industrial waters, nuclear effluents and drinking water, with the aid of cross-linked N- *Carboxymethyi Chitosan*. Carbohydr Polym. 11: 293-306.

33. Nayak, S.K., Swain, P., Mukherjee, S.C. (2007) Effect of dietary supplementation of probiotic and vitamin Con the immune response of Indian major carp, *Labeo rohita* (Ham.). Fish Shellfish Immunol. 23: 892- 896.

34. Nayak, S.K., Swain, P., Nanda, P.K., Dash, S., Shukla, S., Meher, P.K., Maiti, N.K. (2008) Effect of endotoxin on the immunity of Indian major carp, Labeo rohita. Fish Shellfish Immunol. 24: 394-399.

35. No, H., Park, N.Y., Lee, S.H., Meyers, S.P. (2002) Antibacterial activity of chitosan and chitosan oligomers with different molecular weights. Int J Food Microbiol. 74: 65-72.

36. Ohta, K., Taniguchi, A., Konishi, N., Hosoki, T. (1999) Chitosan treatment affects plant growth and flower quality in *Eustoma grandiflorum*. Hort Sci. 34: 233-234.

37. Okamoto, Y., Kawakami, K., Miyatake, K., Morimoto, M., Shigemasa, Y., Minami, S. (2002) Analgesic effects of chitin and chitosan. Carbohydr polym. 49: 249-252.

38. Qin, C., Du, Y., Xiao, L., Li, Z., Gao, X. (2002) Enzymic preparation of water-soluble chitosan and their antitumor activity. Int J Biol Macromol. 31: 111-117.

39. Rairakhwada, A.K., Pal, Z.P., Bhathena, N.P., Sahu , A.J., Mukherjee, S.C. (2007) Dietary microbial levan enhances cellular non-specific immunity and survival of common carp (*Cyprinus carpio*) juveniles. Fish Shellfish Immunol. 22: 477-486.

40. Ramesh, U., Maridass, M. (2010) Wound healing effect of chitosan in fresh water fish *Cyprinus carpio*L. Int J Biol Techol. 1: 99-102.

41. Rinaudo, M. (2006) Chitin and chitosan: Properties and applications. Prog Polym Sci. 31: 603-632.

42. Rødde, R.H., Einbu, A., Varum, K.M. (2008) A seasonal study of the chemical composition and chitin quality of shrimp shells obtained from northern shrimp (*Pandalus borealis*). Carbohydr Polym. 71: 388-393.

43. Sakai, M. (1999) Current research status of fish immunostimulants. Aquaculture. 172: 63-92.

44. Salisbury, J.G., Nicholls, T.J., Lammerding, A.M., Turnidge, J., Nunn, M.J. (2002) A risk analysis frame work for the long-term management of antibiotic resistance in food-producing animals. Int J Antimicrob Agents. 20: 153-164.

45. Schaperclaus, W., Kulow, H., Schreckenbach, K. (1991) Hematological and serological technique. In: Fish Disease. Kothekar, V. S. (ed.). Oxonian Press, New Delhi, India. p. 71-108.

46. Seferian, P.G., Martinez, M.L. (2001) Immune stimulating activity of two new chitosan containing adjuvant formulations. Vaccine. 19: 661-668.

47. Selvaraj, V., Sampath, K., Sekar, V. (2006) Adjuvant and immuno-stimulatory effects of b-glucan administration in combination with lipopolysaccharide enhances survival and some immune parameters in carp challenged with *Aeromonas hydrophila*. Vet Immunol Immunopathol. 114:15-24.

48. Siwicki, A.K., Anderson, D.P., Rumsey, G.L. (1994) Dietary intake of Immunostimulants by rainbow trout affects non-specific immunity and protection against furunculosis. Vet Immunol Immunopathol. 41: 125-139.

49. Webster, C.D., Tiu, L.G., Tidwell, J.H., Grizzle, J.M. (1997) Growth and body composition of channel catfish, *Ictalurus punctatus*, fed diets containing various percentages of canola meal. Aquaculture. 150: 103-112.

50. Yada, T., Uchida, K., Kajimura, S., Azuma, T., Hirano, T., Grau, E.G. (2002) Immunomodulatory effects of prolactin and growth hormone in the tilapia, *Oreochromis mossambicus*. J Endocrinol. 173: 483-492.

A histological study of the corneosclera layer (*Fibrous tunic*) of ostrich (*Struthio camelus*)

Mansoori, F.[*]**, Roshani, H.**

Department of Basic Sciences, School of Veterinary Medicine, Shahid Bahonar University of Kerman, Kerman, Iran

Key words:
cornea, histology, ostrich, sclera

Correspondence
Mansoori, F.
Department of Basic Sciences,
School of Veterinary Medicine,
Shahid Bahonar University of
Kerman, Kerman, Iran

Email: fmansori_2000@uk.ac.ir

Abstract:

BACKGROUND: The Ostrich is an interesting subject concerning animal evolution and morphology studies. It has been speculated that ostrich eyes would have distinct tissue structures and this has not been previously studied in detail. **OBJECTIVES:** The aim of the present study was to investigate the histology of the outer layer of the ostrich. **METHODS:** Ten mature ostriches were chosen from an ostrich breeding center in Jupar, Kerman, Iran. All of them were in a good shape and healthy condition. After slaughter, their heads were kept in 10% formalin solution for 7 days and then the eyes were removed. Routine histological techniques were done and 6-µm-thick sections were cut. Sections were stained with standard hematoxylin and eosin (H&E) and Masson's trichrome and PAS. The sections were studied under a light microscope. **RESULTS:** The cornea of ostrich had both dermal and sclera components and the two distinct parts were separated by a distinct zone; in addition, the sclera was divided into an episclera zone and a sclera proper zone. **CONCLUSIONS:** The outer layer of the episclera composed of connective fibers loosely attached to the sclera proper. The inner layer of the sclera consisted of dense connective tissues with two cartilaginous parts continuing over the oraserrata that composed dense connective fibers and ossicles.

Introduction

The eye of ostrich is very large in comparison with the size of the head and the brain, the weight ratio of the two eyes to the brain being almost 1 to 1 (kingsmith, 1971).

The wall of the eyeball is divided into three layers: the outer *fibrous tunic* (corneaosclera layer), the middle vascular tonic(uvea), and the inner or nervous layer. The sclera is the outer fibrous layer of eye which covers most of the eye posteriorly and the cornea anteriorly (Banks, 1993).

The sclera is usually made up of collagenous fibers and may contain ossified cartilage in some teleost species (Kunz, 2004). Scleral ossicles or scleral cartilages display a large degree of variation in presence or absence, number, and morphology with indoors the teleost eye .(Mansoori, Sattari and Franz-Odendaal, 2008; Franz-Odendaal and Hall, 2006). Two distinct scleral ossicle morphologies have recently been identified, and the number of these elements decreased from the ancestral arrangement of four scleral ossicles per eye to the present arrangement of two or less scleral ossicles per eye (Franz-Odendaal, 2008).

The cornea is a curved non-vascular and clear window which mainly consists of an epithelium superimposed a basement membrane (Kapoor and Hara, 2001).The cornea is a transparent window which mainly consists of an epithelium overlying a basement membrane (Kapoor and Hara, 2001), and an endothelium with a basement membrane known as Descemet's membrane separating it from the stroma (Kapoor and Hara, 2001). Although the histology of ostrich eyes from numerous species has been undertaken, no detailed study has been carried out.

Materials and Methods

For this study, the eyes from ten light-adapted ostriches that were killed for reasons other than ocular lesions were examined by using light microscopy. After the ostriches were slaughtered, their heads were kept in 10% formalin solution for 7 days and then the eyes were removed and kept in 10% formalin solution for two more days.

Routine histological techniques were undertaken, and 6-μm-thick sections were cut. Sections were stained with standard hematoxylin and eosin (H&E) and Masson's trichromeand. Histological study was performed using a light microscope, and photographs were taken for detailed illustration of the results (Fig. 1).

Results

The cornea: In this study, we found that the cornea of ostrich had both dermal and sclera components, and the two distinct parts were separated by a distinct zone. The outer dermal portion was composed of four layers: (1) an anterior non-keratinizing stratified squamous epithelium; (2) Bowman's membrance is composed of a compact , acellular, collangenous matrix (3) substantiapropria which is the greater part of the thickness of the cornea it is transparent but not completely homogeneous since it is composed of bundles of collagen fibres ;(4) This was the only component present here, and (5) a posterior single layer of cuboidal to flattened cuboidal cells Figs. 4-6.

The sclera: The sclera was divisible into an episclera zone and a sclera proper zone. The outer layer of the episclera was composed of connective fibers loosely attached to the sclera proper. The inner layer of the sclera consisted of dense connective tissues with two cartilaginous parts continuing over the oraserrata. These two parts were joined together by means of connective fibrils at the posterior of the globe and changed into the corneal connective tissue at the anterior end. The transition from sclera proper to scleral cornea which occurred at the corneoscleral junction or limbus included vessels extention. In this case we see the osteofication and diiffiuse into the cornea and because the age of these ostrich was low the ossicle had not been created (Figs. 2-3 & 7-8).

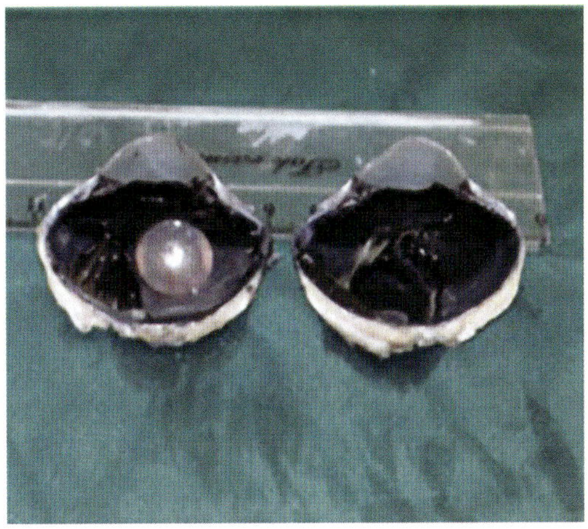

Figure 1. Sagittal section of Ostrich eye.

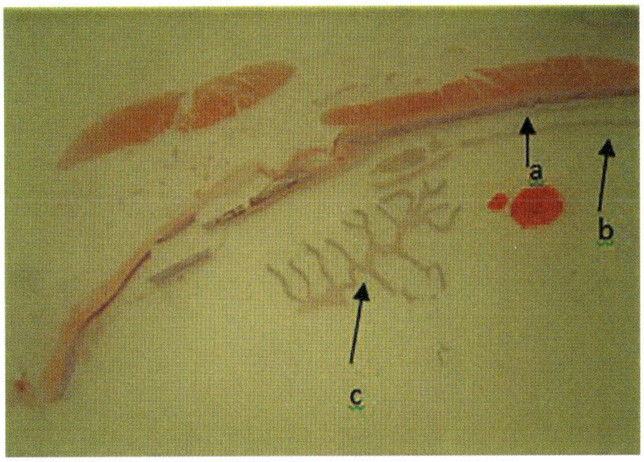

Figure 2. Sagittal section of Ostrich. a, scleral crtilage connective. tissue between two cartilages; c, ora serrata; d, limbus; e cornea. H&E, ×20.

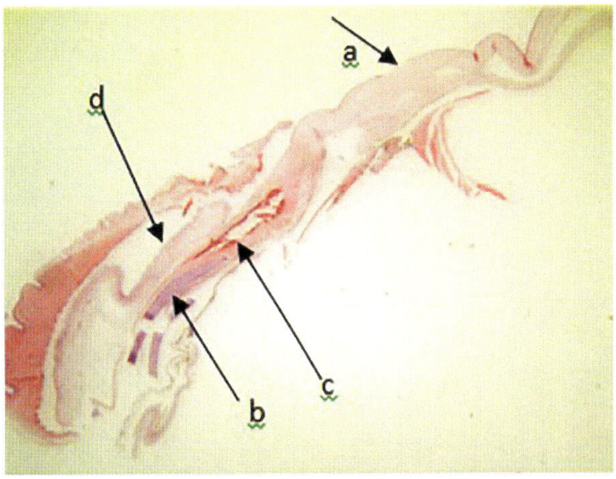

Figure 3. Sagital section of Ostrich . a, sclera ; b tissue between two. Cartilages; c, ora serata ; d , limbus; e cornea , H&E, ×40

Discussion

The sclera: Two cartilaginous segments with

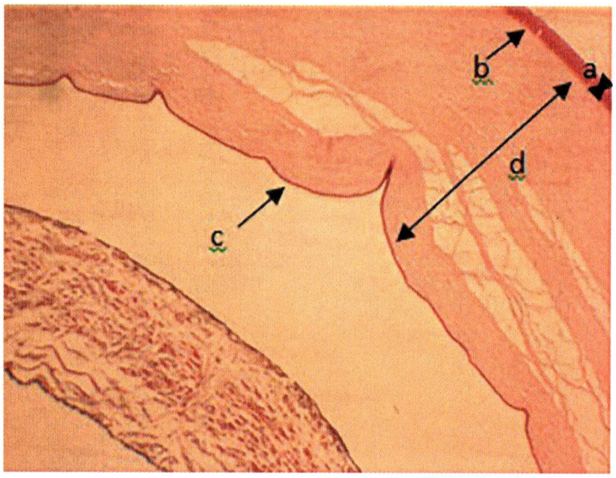

Figure 4. Sagittal section of the cornea. a, epithelium; b, Bowman's layer; c, dermal stroma; d ; scleral stroma. H&E, ×200.

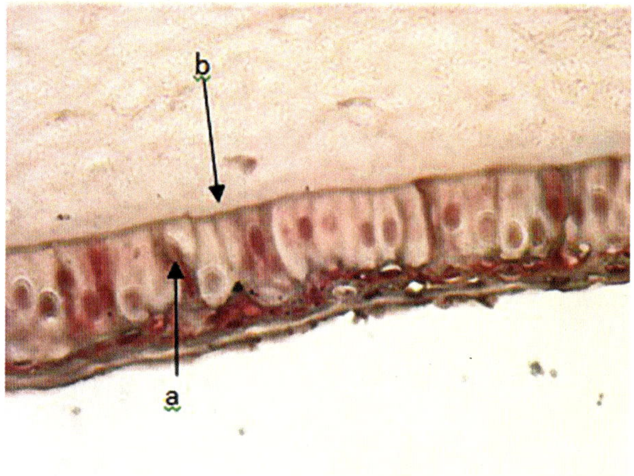

Figure 5. Sagittal section of the ostrich cornea . a, epithelium; b, Bowman's layer; stroma. Masson's trichrome, ×400.

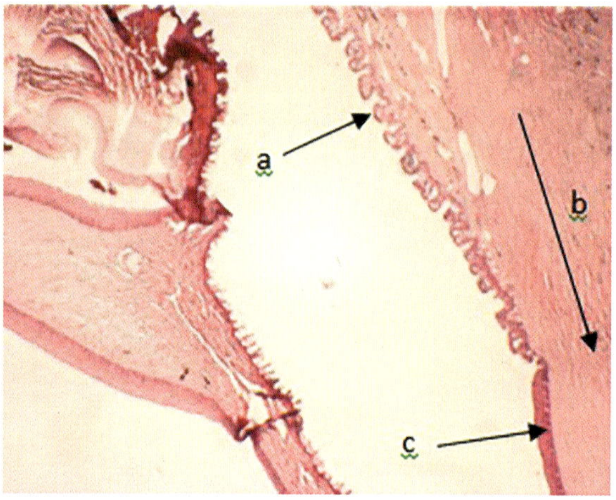

Figure 6. Sagittal section of ostrich eye. A.cunjuctiva. b;connective tissue between two cartilages; c.cornea. H&E, ×200.

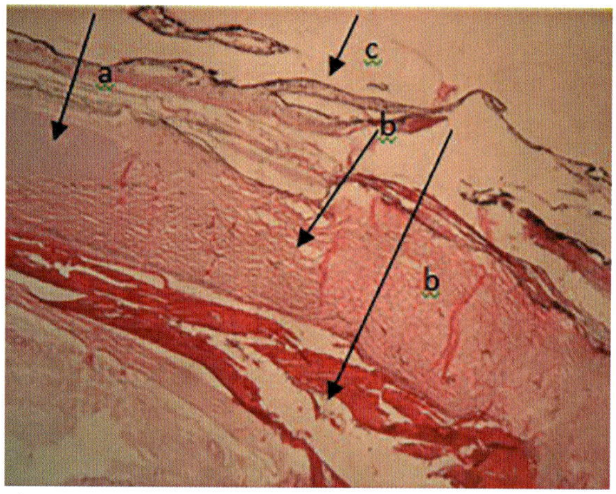

Figure 7. Sagittal section of ostrich eye a, scleral cartilage. b, connective tissue between two cartilages; c, ora serrata.

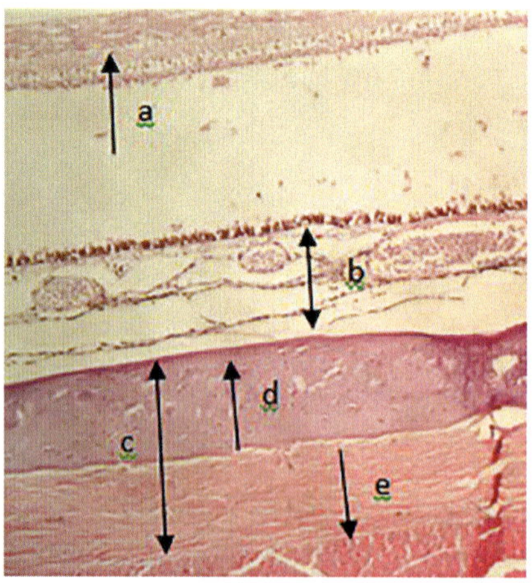

Figure 8. Sagittal section of ostrich eye a. Retina. b,choroid ; c.sclera d, scleral. cartilage;e.connective. tissues.

connective tissue correlation were seen in the sclera of the *Struthio camelus* eye. The first extensive investigation on the distribution of scleral ossicles in the living teleosts was done by (Franz-Odendaal, 2008) and suggested that having no ossicles is more common among teleosts. Chondrostei (bichirs, sturgeons, etc.) and Neopterygii (bow-fins, gars, etc.) do not have scleral ossicles (Franz-Odendaal and Hall, 2006). The oldest actinopterygian fossil has four ossicles; within Chondrostei, the same trend is seen, while modern Chondrostei have none (Franz-Odendaal, 2008). Fish without scleral ossicles have a continuous cartilage element within the sclera (Franz-Odendaal and Ryan, 2007). When two parts of the ossicles are present, these two elements are joined to one another by means of a cartilaginous bridge (Franz-Odendaal and Hall, 2006).

There is a strong correlation between fish habitats, activity level, and presence/absence of scleral ossicles.

Accordingly, fish that inhabit deep sea environments are most likely to lack scleral ossicles, and 100 % of those that are very active have two ossicles per eye (Franz-Odendaal, 2008). Tuna and swordfish, which are fast swimmers, have large bony rings in their eyes (Nakamura and Yamaguchi 1991).

The cornea: The stratified cuboidal epithelium of the dermal cornea in the Struthio camel us was continuous with the conjunctiva. A corneal epithelium continuous with the conjunctiva and the skin appears to be present in all aquatic vertebrates (Kapoor and Hara, 2001).

A Bowman layer has been identified in only a few species of some birds. In spite of the claim that the Bowman's layer is a normal component of the teleost cornea, it was not present in the species examined by Collin and Collin (Collin and Collin, 1998; 1995). It is an unorganized membrane in some trout species 1968), but it is seen in the cornea of s, at the anterior stroma adjacent to the epithelial cells. This layer is also easily recognizable in the lamprey *Petromyzon marinus* (Van Horn and Edelhauser, 1969; Pederson and Van Horn, 1971) and in cartilaginous fish. The two separated parts of the dermal stroma present in the rabbit fish cornea are in accordance with the investigation of Collin and Collin (Collin and Collin, 1995) on the pipefish *Corythoichthyes paxtoni* and the salamander fish Lepidoga-laxiassalamandroides. Aquatic vertebrate corneas possess one stroma, but up to three stromata are present in some deep sea species (Collin and Collin, 1998). The results of this study confirmed the presence of numerous cells in the dermal stroma as is demonstrated in the Florida garfish *Lepisosteus platyrhincus* (Collin and Northcutt, 1993). The region separating the two stromata of *Struthio camelus* eye occasionally had connective tissue fibrils. This region may be filled with a granular material as in the pipefish (Collin and Collin, 1995) or mucoid tissue as in the salamander fish L. salamandroides (Collin and Collin, 1994) and the eel *Anguilla anguilla* (Walls, 1963). In the deep-sea gadiforme, *Coryphaenoide sarmatus*, which has one layer of dermal stroma and two layers of scleral stroma, a mucoidlayer separates the two main parts: dermal and scleral In some species, an autochthonous layer which thickens towards the periphery and terminates at the scleral margin has been reported (Kapoor and Hara, 2001). Munk (1968) described the same layer in the cornea of Amiacalva in a light microscopic study. Electron microscopic studies demonstrated that the autochthonous layer may be an iridescent layer (Kapoor and Hara, 2001). Corneal iridescence has been observed in some species (Collin and Collin, 1998; 1995; 1994). Light microscopic investigation of the *S. javus* cornea confirmed the presence of a connective tissue layer between the separating layer and the scleral stroma. This finding, when compared with reported data, suggests that this layer may represent an iridescent layer. Among bony fish, Descemet's membrane as the basement membrane of the corneal endothelium is present in most species (Kapoor and Hara, 2001), but it was not seen in the eye of *S. javus*. It is also absent in the sea lamprey *P. marinus* (Van Horn, Edelhauser, 1969; Pederson, Van Horn, 1971). Although there is a single layer of endothelial cells in the posterior cornea in bony fish examined by Collin and Collin (Collin and Collin, 1998; 1995; 1994; 2000; Collin and Northcutt, 1993), there was no cellular layer in the posterior cornea of the eye of the rabbit fish, and also a complete absence of the endothelium is seen in some cartilaginous fish.

References

1. Banks W.J. (1993) Applied Veterinary Histology. Mosby Year Book (3rd ed.) St Louis, USA.
2. Kunz, Y.W. (2004) Developmental Biology of Teleost Fishes. Introduction, Springer. Dordrecht, The Netherlands.
3. Mansoori, F., Sattari, A., Kheirandish, R., Asli, M. (2012) A histological study of the outer layer of rabbit fish (*Siganus javus*) eye. Comp Clin Pathol. p. 1-4.
4. Franz-Odendaal, T.A. (2008) Scleral ossicles of Teleostei: Evolutionary and developmental trends. Anat Rec. 291: 161-8.
5. Franz-Odendaal, T.A., Hall, B.K. (2006) Skeletal elements within teleost eyes and a discussion of their homology. J Morphol. 267: 1326-37.
6. Kapoor, B.G., Hara, T.J. (2001) Sensory Biology of Jawed Fishes: New Insights. Science Publishers. Cincinnati, Ohio, USA.
7. Franz-Odendaal, T.A., Ryan, K., Hall, B.K. (2007) Developmental and morphological variation in the

teleost craniofacial skeleton reveals an unusual mode of ossification. J Exp Zool B Mol Dev Evol. 308: 709-21.

8. Collin, S.P., Collin, H.B. (1998) A comparative study of the corneal endothelium in vertebrates. Clin Exp Optom. 81: 245-54.
9. Collin, H.B., Collin, S.P. (1995) Ultrastructure and organization of the cornea, lens and iris in the pipefish, *Corythoichthyes paxtoni* (Syngnathidae, Teleostei). Histol Histopathol 10: 313-323.
10. Van Horn, D.L., Edelhauser, H.F., Schultz, R.O., (1969) Ultrastructure of the primary spectacle and cornea of the sea lamprey. J Ultrastruct Res. 26: 454-64.
11. Pederson, H.J., Van Horn, D.L., Edelhauser, H.F., (1971) Ultrastructural changes associated with loss of transparency in the primary spectacle and cornea of spawning sea lamprey. Exp Eye Res. 12: 147-50.
12. Collin, S.P., Northcutt, R.G. (1993) The visual system of the florida garfish, *Lepisosteus platyrhincus* (Ginglymodi). Brain Behav Evol. 42: 295-320.
13. Collin, S.P., Collin, H.B. (1994) The fine structure of the cornea of the salamanderfish, *Lepidogalaxias salamandroides* (Lepidogalaxiidae, Teleostei). Cornea. 15: 414-26.
14. Munk, O. (1968) The eyes of Amia and Lepisosteus (Pisces, Holostei) compared with the brachiopterygian and teleostean eyes. Vidensk Meddr dansk naturh Foren. 131: 109-27.
15. Collin, H.B., Collin, S.P. (2000) The corneal surface of aquatic vertebrates: microstructures with optical and nutritional function? Philos Trans R Soc Lond B Biol Sci. 355: 1171-6.

Occurrence of parasitic protozoa in wild waterfowl in southern coastal Caspian sea lagoons

Shemshadi, B.[1*], **Ranjbar-Bahadori, Sh.**[1], **Faghihzadeh-Gorji, S.**[2]

[1]*Department of Parasitology, Faculty of Veterinary Medicine, Garmsar Branch, Islamic Azad University, Garmsar, Iran*

[2]*Graduated from the Faculty of Veterinary Medicine, Garmsar Branch, Islamic Azad University, Garmsar, Iran*

Key words:
Caspian sea, parasitic protozoa, waterfowl

Correspondence
Shemshadi, B.
Department of Parasitology, Faculty of Veterinary Medicine, Garmsar Branch, Islamic Azad University, Garmsar, Iran

Email: bshemshadi@yahoo.com

Abstract:

BACKGROUND: Protozoa are common in poultry and other birds and can cause mild to severe disease. **OBJECTIVES:** This study was concerned with the prevalence of parasitic protozoa in wild waterfowl in Caspian sea lagoons in the North of Iran. **METHODS:** A total of 293 waterfowl belonging to various genera including *Tadorna tadorna* (common shelduck), *Aythya fuligula* (Tufted duck), *Aythya ferina* (Common puchard), *Spatula clypeata* (Shoveler), *Anser anser* (greylag goose), *Cygnus Cygnus* (Whooper Swan), *Anas strepera* (Gadwall), *Anas Penelope* (Eurasian Widgeon), *Anas crecca* (common teal), and *Anas platyrhynchos* (mallard) were sampled and tested for intestinal, tracheal, and blood protozoa between winter 2010 and spring 2011. **RESULTS:** The results showed that 184 birds of 293 (62.8%) harbored protozoan parasites. The highest prevalence of protozoan contamination belonged to *Giardia* spp (24.2%) and the lowest belonged to *Haemoproteus* spp. (6.1%). *Thricomunas gallinea*, *Plasmodium* spp., and *Cryptosporidium* spp. were found in 7.2%, 8.2%, and 17% of waterfowl, respectively. Moreover, statistical analyses showed that the highest rate of giardiosis was in female *Aythya fuligula* (43.75%). However, tricomuniasis belonged to *Anas crecca* (30.5%). On the other hand, female *Cygnus cygnus* had the highest rate of cryptosporidiosis (44.7%), and more infection to *Haemoproteus* and *Plasmodium* spp. were observed in *Anas platyrhynchos*, concurrently. **CONCLUSIONS:** Migration of various species of waterfowl toward the northern parts of Iran has an important impact on parasitic diseases in birds and human in these regions.

Introduction

Waterfowl are hosts to a wide variety of internal and external parasites, such as protozoa, that infect many of vertebrate hosts, including mammals and birds (Bennett et al., 1977). Most of these parasites are common pathogenic species in humans. Protozoa are common parasite in a wide variety of birds and can cause mild to severe disease. Some enteric protozoa, such as *Giardia* and *Cryptosporidium*, are pathogenic and have been associated with drinking water related outbreaks (Current et al., 1986; O'Donoghue, 1995; Hsu et al., 1999). They may be found in water following direct or indirect contamination by the feces of humans or other animals such as waterfowl. Coccidian are found in birds, also *Histomonas* species cause a disorder of the ceca and liver in many birds (Silvanose et al., 1998), Trichomonas species affect the upper gastrointestinal tract of turkeys and chickens (Cooper and Petty, 1988). *Haemoproteus* spp. is common among many bird species, and causing severe myositis in avian hosts (Atkinson, 2009; Zabransky et al., 2008).

There are nearly 520 species of birds in Iran and Passeriformes order includes a big population of birds in this fauna (Mansoori, 2008). These birds are all in close contact with human residential areas as well as native and industrial poultry and other domestic fowls; as a result, there is a potential risk to contaminant other birds and human (Halajian et al., 2011).

Some of waterfowl nest in Northern provinces, while the rest are migratory birds that spend the winter in Iran or flyover the country during migration. Mazandaran and Gilan are two of the 31 provinces of Iran, along the Caspian sea. Population estimates of waterfowl, waders, and water birds in these provinces have been reported about 1.6 million in Gilan and 1.2 in Mazandaran. However, within the last five years, some significant changes in population and diversity have taken place (Barati & Khalilipoor, 2006).

Because of a lack of confident information and very few publications concerning the protozoan infection of waterfowl such as duck, goose, and swan in lagoons of Mazandaran and Gilan Provinces, northern Iran, this study was conducted to evaluate parasitic protozoa in wild waterfowl in Caspian sea lagoons.

Materials and Methods

Sample collection: A total of 293 waterfowl including twenty *Tadorna tadorna*, sixteen Aythya fuligula, thirteen *Aythya ferina*, twenty-three *Spatula clypeata*, seventeen *Anser anser*, forty-four *Cygnus Cygnus*, thirty-four *Anas strepera*, twenty-seven *Anas Penelope*, thirty-six *Anas crecca*, and sixty-three *Anas platyrhynchos* were live trapped or killed with shotguns from 4 localities from 2 provinces in Southern coastal Caspian sea lagoons between winter 2010 and spring 2011.

Each bird was sexed by cloacal examination in the field, and it was confirmed by gonad examination. Then, intestinal, tracheal, and blood protozoa were diagnosed in the laboratory.

After taking blood samples, the intestines from below the pancreas to above the anus and sections of the upper respiratory tract were removed from the abdominal cavity of each bird. Each sample was placed in an individual container and labeled.

Intestinal content examination: Immediately after the arrival of a sample in the lab, 1cm was cut from each end of the intestine with a sterile scalpel to eliminate any cross-contamination during processing. The fecal material was then forced into a sterile 50mL centrifuge tube containing 10 mL of a 2.5% (wt/vol) $K2Cr2O7$ to maintain the (oo) cysts during storage. Fecal samples were then kept at 4°C less than 4 weeks before processing (Kuhn, 2002).

Fecal specimens were tested for *Giardia* spp. by examining trichrome-stained direct smears of fecal pellets (Spaulding et al., 1983). Slides were screened at × 400 magnifications, and cysts of *Giardia* spp. were confirmed at × 1,000 magnification. Internal characteristics that were used to identify the cysts were included two to four nuclei, median bodies, and axonemes.

The modified zeilnelson staining technique was used to identify *Cryptosporidium*, the oocysts appear as pink to red, spherical to ovoid, bodies on a green background. According to Henriksen and Pohlenz's (1981) instruction, fecal and tracheal smears were prepared on a microscope slide, air dried and fixed with methanol for 5 min. Fixed smears were stained with dilute carbol fuchsin (1:10) for 3 to 5 min and washed with tap water. Smears were decolorized using acid alcohol, then counterstained with 0.5% Malachite Green solution for 1 min. Smear slides were dried in air and examined under the microscope at 400 × magnification.

Intestinal contents of samples were tested by saline wet mount preparation to survey the presence of intestinal protozoa such as trichomonas (Silvanose et al., 1998).

Tracheal examination: Swabs were taken from tracheal mucosa, the buccal cavity and pharynx, were spread onto cover slips that were fixed in schadin and stained with trichorom for examination of tracheal Trichomonas contamination.

As described previously, tracheal smears were examined based on Henriksen and Pohlenz' (1981) instruction for *Cryptosporidium* spp.

Blood examination: Blood samples were collected from the brachial vein. Then, they were placed in EDTA for hematological investigations.

Blood smears were fixed with 90% methanol and stained with Giemsa. The blood smear was examined at least for 20 min, which included examination of the periphery of the smear for diagnose of large hematozoans such as *Plasmodium*, *Haemoproteus* and *Leucocytozoon*. Medium (400×); high (1000×) magnification were used to scan further until at least 50,000 red blood cells were viewed. Quantification of parasite intensity followed recommendations by Godfrey et al. (1987).

Statistical analysis: Data analysis of the relationship between prevalence rates and different areas were evaluated by the SPSS and Chi-square test. Statistical significance was defined as $p<0.05$.

Results

In this study, out of the 293 examined waterfowl, 184 birds (62.8%) harbored protozoan parasites. Result comparison showed that the highest prevalence of protozoan contamination belonged to *Giardia* lamblia (24.2%), also giardiosis was observed in all examined species; however, the infection rate was different between 43.75% in *Aythya fuligula* and 8.3% in *Anser anser* (Figure 1).

Thricomunas gallinea was found in 7.2% of samples, the highest rate of tricomuniasis belonged to *Anas crecca* (30.5%). Intestinal form of tricomuniasis was not found in samples, however, tracheal form was found only in *Anas strepera* and *Anas crecca* without significant difference between males and females.

The rate of contamination of the examined waterfowl to intestinal *Cryptosporidium* spp. oocyst was 17%, and tracheal form was not observed in this study. *Cygnus cygnus* had the highest rate of contamination and *Spatula clypeata* was in the second place, meanwhile *Cryptosporidium* was not found in *Tadorna tadorna*, *Aythya ferina* and *Anser anser* (Figure 2).

Plasmodium spp. and *Haemoproteus* spp were observed in blood samples of the studied waterfowl. The total rate of contamination to *Plasmodium* spp. (8.2%) was higher than *Haemoproteus* spp. (6.1%), but the prevalence rate was not different significantly ($p>0.05$). *Haemoproteus* spp. was not found In *Spatula clypeata* and *Tadorna tadorna* species (Figure 3), while *Aythya ferina* and *Spatula clypeata* samples were free from *Plasmodium* spp. contamination (Figure 4).

The highest rate of infection to *Haemoproteus* and *Plasmodium* spp. was observed in *Anas platyrhynchos* concurrently. The prevalence of *Haemoproteus* was differente in male (10.6%) and female (8.2%) ($p<0.05$), but there was not any significantly difference between male (13.6%) and female in *Plasmodium* infection (14.7%), ($p>0.05$).

Leucocytozoon spp. and microfilariae were not observed in examined blood samples.

Discussion

Waterfowl can act as a main source of different types of parasites; they can pick up infection from their habitat, carry and spread them in the environment, including drinking water supplies and also domestic animals (Graczyk et al., 1998). Moreover, it is estimated that 80 to 96% of surface waters in the United States are contaminated with *Cryptosporidium* and *Giardia* (Hansen, 1991).

The contributions of *Giardia* cysts and *Cryptosporidium* oocysts from avian species to the concentrations of cysts and oocysts in water samples are largely unknown, as are the extent of transmission of bird-vectored organisms to mammalian hosts and the importance of these parasites in avian species (Erlandsen, 1990).

Migration of various species of waterfowl toward the northern parts of Iran has important impact on parasitic diseases in birds and human in Northern part of Iran.

Giardia spp. commonly was reported from various birds including budgerigars (*Melopsittacus undulatus*), cockatiels (*Nymphicus hollandicus*), love birds (*Agapornis* spp.), grey-cheeked parakeets (*Brotogeris pyrrhopterus*) and other psittacines (Greiner & Ritchie, 1994). *Giardia* cysts are commonly found in sewage and surface waters and occasionally in drinking water. In Canada, a cross-sectional survey in 72 municipalities performed between 1991 and 1995, Wallis et al. (1996) found that 72.6%, 21% and 18.2% of raw sewage, raw water, and treated water samples, respectively, contained *Giardia* cysts. In a similar study, fecal samples were taken from wild ducks on the lower Rio Grande River around Las Cruces, from 2000 to 2001.

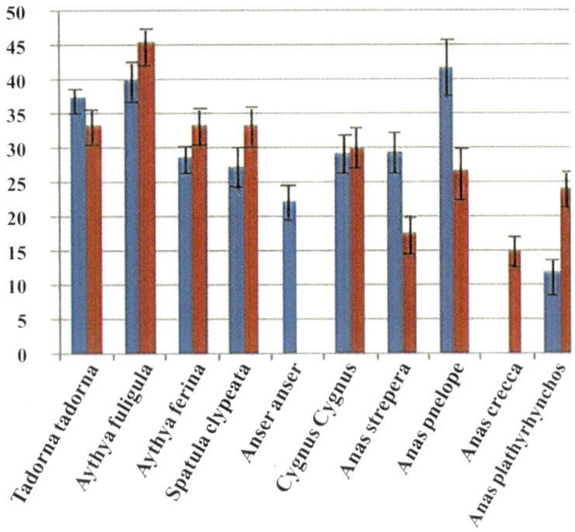

Figure 1. Prevalence rate of waterfowl with *Giardia* spp contamination. Male Female

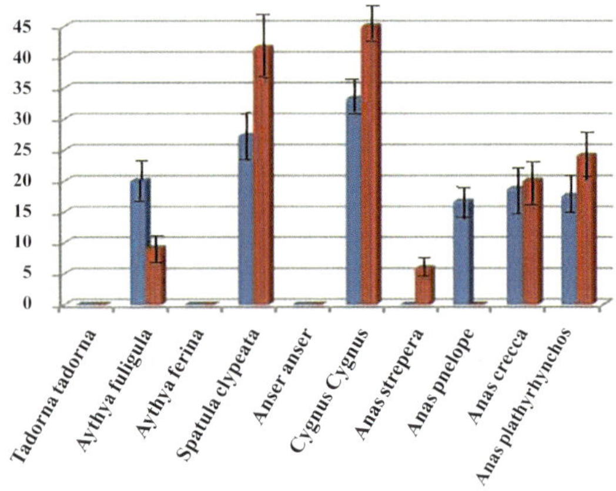

Figure 2. Prevalence rate of waterfowl with intestinal *Cryptosporidium* spp. contamination. Male Female

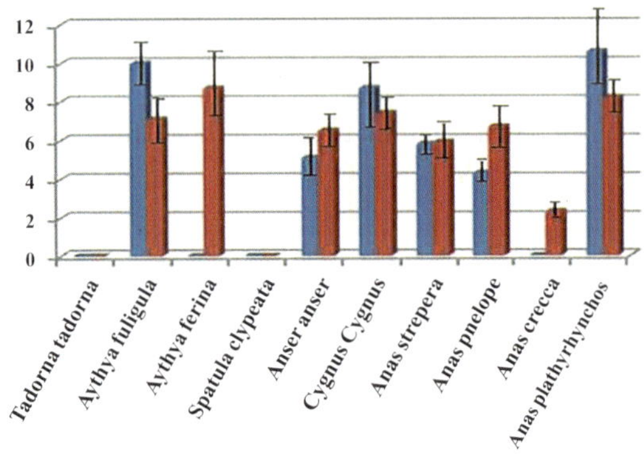

Figure 3. Prevalence rate of waterfowl with *Haemoproteus* spp. contamination. Male Female

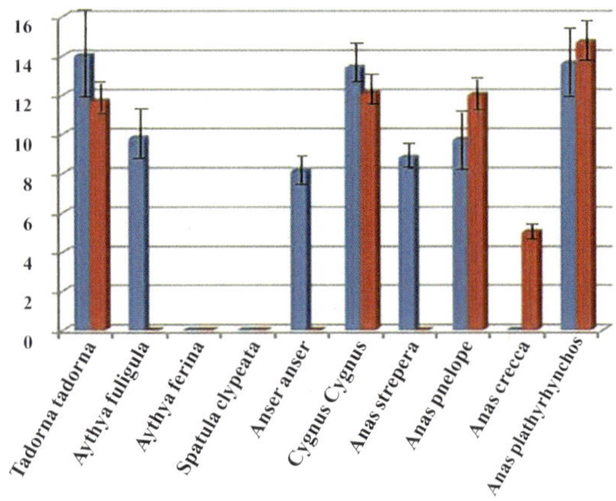

Figure 4. Prevalence rate of waterfowl with *Plasmodium* spp. contamination. Male Female

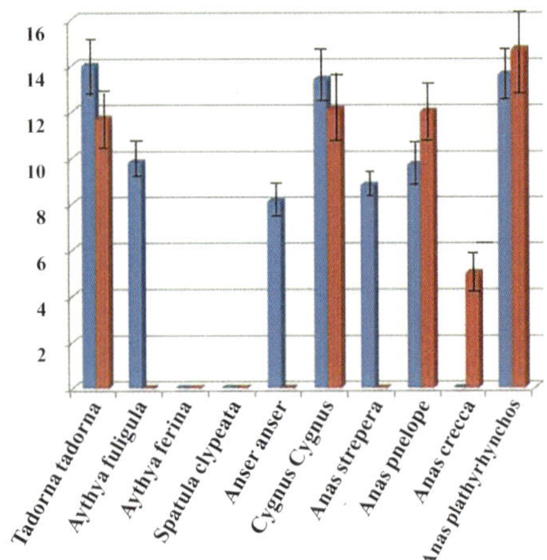

Figure 5. Prevalence rate of waterfowl with *Plasmodium* spp. Contamination. Male Female

The results of this study indicated that 49% of the ducks were carriers of *Cryptosporidium*, also 28% of the ducks were positive for *Giardia* (Kuhn et al., 2002). In our study, prevalence of giardiosis was 24.2%, which is very close to the result of Kuhn et al.'s (2002). In the present study, the infection rate of giardiosis in females was 25.3% and in male ducks was 23.1%. There was no significant difference between giardiosis rate in male and female ducks in most species ($p<0.05$), excluding *Anser anser* for which the infection rate in males was higher than in females, and *Anas crecca* for which the infection rate in females was higher than in males ($p>0.05$).

Trichomonas gallinarum has been documented from the lower digestive tract and caeca of chickens and other gallinaceous birds (McDougald, 1997). Silvanose (1998) studied captive houbara bustards, 49 (43%) were found positive to protozoa including 34 (29.8%) *Trichomonas gallinarum*; 12 (10.5%) *Chilomastix gallinarum*; one (0.9%) *Lophomonas* spp.; one (0.9%) *Giardia* spp., all the birds infected with *T. gallinarum* and *C. gallinarum* appeared clinically normal. In the current study, 21(7.2%) of the examined waterfowl were infected; the rate of infection was higher than houbara bustards study. In addition, *Anas strepera* and *Anas crecca* were the only species that *Trichomonas gallinarum* were found in them. The prevalence rate of *Thricomunas gallinea* in waterfowl trachea was 7.2%, which was considerably less than that reported by Silvanose (1998). However, intestinal trichomoniasis was not found in our study. The highest rate of infection was found in *Anas crecca* males which was significantly higher than in females ($p<0.05$).

Humans and animals are important reservoirs for *Cryptosporidium*. Human cryptosporidiosis has been reported in more than 90 countries (Fayer et al., 2000). Contaminated drinking water, recreational water, and food are very important and are a major pathway for transmission. *Cryptosporidium* oocysts are commonly found in sewage and surface waters and occasionally in treated water (Ranjbar-Bahadori et al., 2013). To date, only two valid species of *Cryptosporidium* (*Cryptosporidium baileyi* and *Cryptosporidium meleagridis*) have been proven to cause infections in birds (Current, 1986; Slavin, 1955), and *Cryptosporidium* has been detected in more than 30 species of birds including geese (*Anser anser*), tundra swans (*Cygnus* sp.), black-headed gulls (Larus ridibundus), chickens (Gallus gallus) (Shemshadi et al., 2011), turkeys (Meleagris gallopavo), mallards (*Anas platyrhynchos*), and (Cairina moschata) Muscovy ducks (O'Donoghue, 1995). In this study, intestinal *Cryptosporidium* infection rate were in *Cygnus Cygnus* 36.0%, *Spatula clypeata* 32.3%, *Anas platyrhynchos* 22.1%, *Anas crecca* 11.8%, *Anas penelope* 11.2% and *Anas strepera* 6.2%, which were similar in most species to the results of a study carried out in Canada on drinking water. However, in *Anas strepera* and *Anas crecca*,the difference was considerable, no infection was found in *Tadorna tadorna* and *Aythya ferina* species.

Thul et al. (1980) studied 213 wood ducks (Aix sponsa) in the Atlantic Flyway for blood parasites from 1976 to 1977. They found *Haemoproteus* nettionis was the most common parasite, occurring in 56% of the northern wood ducks; *Leucocytozoon* simondi (20%), *Plasmodium* circumflexum (6%), and also they found (18%) microfilariae. Fakhar et al. (2012) . Respectively It has shown the prevalence rate of infection by *Plasmodium* spp., and *Haemoproteus* spp. (2.3%), and (6.6%), in Iranian duck, goose, turkey, poultry, and pigeon and also they found only ducks and turkeys were infected with *Plasmodium* spp. In this study, it was determined that *Plasmodium* spp. exists in blood smear of 24 (8.2%) of the examined waterfowl. The results of *plasmodium* infection rate of the current study is more similar to Thul et al.'s (1980) than the rate has been reported by Fakhar et al. (2012). *Anas platyrhynchos* had the highest infection rate (14.2%) of *Plasmodium* spp. in this study, while *Aythya ferina* and *Spatula clypeata* blood examination were negative.

The prevalence rate of H. columbae in North of Iran has been reported 17.47%. Also, the prevalence of *Haemoproteus* in birds in Costa Rica, Alaska, and Japan revealed rates lower than 10%. In the United states, Colombia, Bulgaria and Queensland the prevalence rate ranged from 20-30% (Yousefi et al., 2010). Prevalence of *H. crumenium* from 42 nestling wood storks during 2003 that was reported by Cody et al. was (7.2%). Also, the rate of infection showed by Fedynich et al. (1998) in Georgia was (3 of 75; 4%) and in this study the prevalence of *Haemoproteus* spp. (6.1%) was completely lower than the rate of infection has reported by Yousefi et al. (2010) in the North of Iran, but slightly higher than that published by Fedynich et al. (1998) in Georgia (3 of 75; 4%) and published by Forrester and Spalding (2003) collected in Florida (4 of 98; 4%), but it was close to the results demonstrated by Zabransky et al. (2008).

In this study, *Leucocytozoon* spp., and microfilariae were not observed in the examined blood samples, also in Zabransky study in 2008, *Leucocytozoon* sp., *Plasmodium* sp. and micro-filariae were not found.

Therefore, with regard to our findings, migration of various species of waterfowl toward the northern parts of Iran can be an important source for transmission of parasitic diseases to other birds and even human.

Acknowledgments

The authors are particularly indebted to laboratory staffs of the Faculty of Veterinary Medicine, Garmsar branch, Islamic Azad University, specially Mr. Mohammad Gholibeigi for supporting this research.

References

1. Atkinson, C.T. (2009) *Haemoproteus*, in parasitic diseases of wild birds. Atkinson, C.T., Thomas, N.J., Hunter, D.B. (eds.). Wiley-Blackwell, Oxford, UK. p. 116-119.
2. Barati, A., Khalilipoor, O.G. (2006) Changes in abundance and diversity of wintering waterfowl on the southern coast of the Caspian sea. Water birds around the world. United Kingdom Department for Environment, Food and Rural Affairs, by DBA. Thompson. p. 368-369.
3. Bennett, G.F., Greiner, E.C., Whiteley, P.L., Norman, F.I. (1977) Blood parasites of some waterfowl from Victoria, Australia. J Wildlife Dis. 13: 242-247.
4. Cooper, J.E., Petty, S.J. (1988) Trichomoniasis in Free-Living Goshawks (*Accopiter gentilis*) from Great Britain. J Wildlife Dis. 24: 80-87.
5. Current, W.L., Upton, S.J., Haynes, T.B. (1986) The life cycle of *Cryptosporidium baileyi* sp. (Apicomplexa: Cryptosporidiiae) infecting chickens. J Protozool. 33: 289-296.
6. Erlandsen, S.L., Bemrick, W.L., Wells, C.L., Feely, L.K, Campbell, S.R., Van Keulen, H., Jarroll, E.L. (1990) Axenic culture and characterization of *Giardia* ardeae from the great blue heron (*Ardea herodias*). J Parasitol. 76: 717-724.
7. Fakhar, M., Kalani, H., Rahimi-Esboei, B., Armat, S. (2012) Hemoprotozoa in free-ranging birds from rural areas of Mazandaran province, northern Iran. Comp Clin Pathol. 22: 509-512.
8. Fayer, R., Morgan, U., Upton, S.J. (2000) Epidemiology of *Cryptosporidium*: transmission, detection, and identification. Int J Parasitol. 30: 1305-1322.
9. Fedynich, A.M., Bryan, A.L.J., Harris, M.J. (1998) Hematozoa in the endangered wood stork from Georgia. J Wildlife Dis. 34: 165-7.
10. Forrester, D.J., Spalding, M.G. (2003) Parasites and Diseases of Wild Birds in Florida. University Press of Florida, Gainesville, USA.
11. Godfrey, R.D.J., Fedynich, A.M., Pence, D.B. (1987) Quantification of hematozoa in blood smears. J Wildlife Dis. 23: 558-65.
12. Graczyk, T.M., Fayer, R., Trout, J.M., Lewis, E.J., Farley, C.A., Sulaiman, I., Lal, A.A. (1998) *Giardia* sp. cysts and infectious *Cryptosporidium parvum* oocysts in the feces of migratory Canada geese (*Branta canadensis*). Appl Environ Microbiol. 64: 2736-2738.
13. Greiner, E., Ritchie. B. (1994) Parasites. In: Avian Medicine: Principles and Application. Harrison, G., Harrison, L., Ritchie, B. (eds.). Lake Worth, FL: Wingers, USA. p. 1007-1029.
14. Hansen, J.S., Ongerth, J.E. (1991) Effects of time and watershed characteristics on the concentration of *Cryptosporidium* oocysts in river water. Appl Environ Microbiol. 57: 2790-2795.
15. Halajian, A., Eslami, A., Mobedi, I., Amin, O., Mariaux, J., Mansoori, J., Tavakol, S. (2011) Gastrointestinal Helminths of Magpies (*Pica pica*), Rooks (*Corvus frugilegus*) and Carrion crows (*Corvus corone*) in Mazandaran province, north of Iran. Iranian J Parasitol. 6: 38-44.
16. Hsu, B.M., Huang, C., Jiang, G.Y., Hsu, C.L.L. (1999) The prevalence of *Giardia* and *Cryptosporidium* in Taiwan water supplies. J Toxicol Environ Health. 57: 149-160.
17. Henriksen, S.A., Pohlenz, J.F.L. (1981) Staining of Cryptosporodia by modified Ziehl-Neelsen technique: a brief communication. Acta Vet Scand. 25: 322-326.
18. Kuhn, R.C., Rock, C.M., Oshima, K.H. (2002) Occurrence of *Cryptosporidium* and *Giardia* in wild ducks along the Rio grande river valley in southern New Mexico. Appl Environ Microbiol. 68: 161-165.
19. Mansoori, J.A. (2008) Guide to the Birds of Iran. (2nd ed.) Farzan Book Publishing. Tehran, Iran (In Persian).
20. McDougald, L.R., Fuller, L., Mattiello, R. (1997) A survey of Coccidia on 43 poultry farms in Argentina. Avian Dis. 41: 923-9.
21. O'Donoghue, P.J. (1995) *Cryptosporidium* and cryptosporidiosis in man and animals. Int J Parasitol. 25: 139-195.
22. Ranjbar-Bahadori, Sh., Mostoophi, A., Shemshadi, B. (2013) Study on *Cryptosporidium* contamination in vegetable farms around Tehran. Trop Biomed. 30: 1-6.
23. Shemshadi, B., Rangbar-Bahadori, Sh., Mozafari, A. (2011) Study on cryptosporidiosis incidence in broilers in Garmsar region, Iran. Comp Clin Pathol. 20: 143-149.
24. Silvanose, C.D., Bailey, T.A., Samour, J.H., Naldo, J.L. (1998) Intestinal protozoa and associated

bacteria in captive Houbara bustards (*Chlamydotis undulata*) in the United Arab Emirates. Avian Pathol. 28: 94-97.

25. Slavin, D. (1955). *Cryptosporidium meleagridis* (sp. nov.). J Comp Pathol. 65: 262-266.
26. Spaulding, J.J., Pacha, R.E., Clark, G.W. (1983) Quantitation of *Giardia* cysts by membrane filtration. J Clin Microbiol. 18: 713-715.
27. Tachezy, J., Tachezy, R., Hampl, V., Sedinová, M., Vanacova, S., Vrlik, M., VanRanst, M., Flegr, J., Kulda, J. (2002) Cattle pathogen *Tritrichomonas foetus* (Riedmuller, 1928) and pig commensal *Tritrichomonas suis* (Gruby & Delafond, 1843) belong to the same species. J Eukar Microbiol. 49: 154-163.
28. Thul, J.E., Forrester, D.J., Greiner, E.C. (1980) Hemato-zoa of wood ducks (*Aix spons*) in the Atlantic flyway. J Wildlife Dis. 16: 383-390.
29. Wallis, P.M., Erlandsen, S.L., Isaac-Renton, J.L., Olson, M.E., Robertson, W.J., Van Keulen, H. (1996) Prevalence of *Giardia* cysts and *Cryptosporidium* oocysts and characterization of *Giardia* spp. isolated from drinking water in Canada. Appl Environ Microbiol. 62: 2789-97.
30. Youssefi, M.R., Grami sadeghian, A., Esfandian, B. (2010) Prevalence of *Heamoproteus columbae* infection in Columba livia in North of Iran. World J Zool. 5: 275-277.
31. Zabransky, C.J., Webb, S.L., Fedynich, A.M., Bryan, A.L. (2008) Blood parasites in Wood Storks (*Mycteria americana*) from the Southeastern United States. J Parasitol. 94: 1178-1179.

Prevalence, intensity and associated risk factors for ovine tick infestation in two districts of Semnan area

Changizi, E.

Deparment of Pathobiology, Faculty of Veterinary Medicine, Semnan University, Semnan, Iran

Key words:
Dermacentor marginatus, *D. raskemensis*, *Hyalomma marginatum marginatum*, tick

Correspondence
Changizi, E.
Deparment of Pathobiology, Faculty of Veterinary Medicine, Semnan University, Semnan, Iran

Email: echangizi@semnan.ac.ir

Abstract:

BACKGROUND: Ticks are the most important vectors which transmit several arthropod-borne diseases such as theileriosis, babesiosis, and anaplasmosis. **OBJECTIVES:** An epidemiological study was conducted in Semnan area to determine the current situation of tick infestation in sheep and assess the efficacy of usage of CIS-cypermethrin against tick infestation under field condition. **METHODES:** Sampling was done monthly on 5% of a sheep herd in a population of 1000 sheep for one year. Ticks were collected, counted, and diagnosed. **RESULTS:** Ticks species affecting sheep were *Hyalomma marginatum marginatum* in winter quarters and in summer pasture; *Dermacentor marginatus* and *D. raskemensis* were the prominent ticks. In the middle of autumn and during the winter, no ticks were detected from the animals. The preferred sites of tick attachment to infested animals were perineal region and ears in winter quarters; however, in the summer pastures, the ticks were found only under the neck area and on the sternum. There was a significant difference between the numbers of male ticks on ewe and lamb; however, these phenomena were not recorded for female ticks. In this regard, CIS-cypermethrin deeping treatment reduced the rate of infestion (almost 100%) after one day of treatment. Nonetheless, in the next sampling after 4 weeks, the rate of infestation increased again and reached 50%. **CONCLUSIONS:** In order to control the tick infestation, it is recommended that spraying be done monthly on the infected areas.

Introduction

The ticks have great health importance due to the pathogenic factors they impose on the host during blood feeding. These arthropods have been on earth for at least 300 million years (Bowman & Nuttall, 2008). The mentioned arthropods are parasites located temporarily on vertebrata hosts and feed (Kettle, 1995). Ticks are economically the most important external parasite of sheep and other domestic species in tropical and subtropical countries (Jongejan & Uilenberg, 1994). More than 80% of the cattle population is infested with ticks (FAO, 2002), which cause harm to animals through blood loss, general stress and irritation, depression of immune function, and damages to skins (Jongejan & Uilenberg, 1994). The main losses that ticks impose to their hosts are the diseases which they transmit. Theileriosis is the most important disease in many areas of Iran, transmitted to sheep through tick (Heidarpour Bami et al., 2010). The economic loss resulting from nagging and irritation and depreciation of the value of skins and hides (up to 30%) are also significant (Bowman & Nuttall, 2008).

There are many ways to control the contamination of livestock to ticks; however, use of chemical acaricide is still one of the most important methods to control such parasites on animals. Incorrect use of such acaricide has led to resistance of animals to tick infestation in many countries. The mentioned acaricide are applied by dipping, spraying, or powdering; however, deeping has been proved to be the most common method of chemical fighting with Ticks (Abbas et al., 1995; FAO, 2002).

The purpose of this study was to assess the tick infection in sheep herd in winter quarters and summer pasture of "Sangsar" area (Province of Semnan), intensity and prevalence of ticks and the influence of deeping sheep with cypermethrin in field situation.

Materials and Methods

Sampling: In order to evaluate the infestation rate of different types of hard ticks in the herds of sheep in winter quarters and summer pasture of "Sangsar" area (North parts of Semnan), a herd of 1000 sheep was selected. The sampling was performed monthly on almost 5% of the population of the herd (in total 629), consisting of ewes (352) and lambs (277) in various regions located in winter quarters of Darjazin (an arid area in proximity of Semnan with the longitude of 53.357 and latitude of 35.639 and 1300 m above the sea level) and the mountainous area of Najafdar (in the north of Firoozkooh with the longitude of 52.383 and latitude of 35.783 and 2600 m above the sea level). Ticks were collected and kept in a labeled container consisting of alcohol 70% and Glycerin 5%, then they were sent to the lab. In the lab, the ticks of each animal were counted and recorded. The gender and species of the ticks were diagnosed using Estrada-Pena keys and by help of Parasitology department of faculty of Veterinary Medicine, University of Tehran (Estrada-Pena et al., 2004). Prevalence was calculated using the following formula (Thrusfield, 1995).

Prevalence = No, of infested cases during specified period/ population at risk during that specified time period × 100

The mentioned herd was in winter quarter until the early of June (The pastures around Darjazin town) and then went to the summer pasture in the north of Firoozkuh in Najafdar region. Due to the short path (about 150 km), the herd moved as usual and, after 2 to 3 weeks, reached the pastures of Najafdar village. In the movement from winter quarters to the summer pasture, at the end of June, acaricide was used on the herd against Arthropods.

To deep the sheep, Mac-Tomeil containing (10%) CIS-cypermethrin, made by Keshavarz National Chemistry Company, was used. First, the batch capacity along with the needed acaricide was calculated, then they were mixed in a bin of water (1:1000). Then the solution was added and mixed using a long wood stick. To ensure the uniformity of the solution in the bath, two sheep were passed through the bath as samples. The two sheep were batched again. Each sheep was bathed for one minute and attempt was made to keep the sheep head beneath the water. Upon deeping, every sheep was kept in bathing pan for at least 10 minutes (O'Brien et al., 1997). After the bath capacity was reduced by 10%, it was replenished at the dilution 1:800. To study the effect of acaricide on sheep, the day after use, two weeks after use, and 4 weeks after use, the external surface of sheep bodies were examined accurately, and hard ticks were taken off. The table of variables being studied consisting of type, age, gender, and the attachment location of the tick were provided in the two studied areas (Table 1). The probable relationships of the mentioned variables with the infestation of domestic livestock to hard ticks were analyzed with SPSS.

Results

On the whole, during a year and 12 samplings in each month on the sheep, 629 livestock, including 352 ewes and 277 lambs, were checked and a total of 1505 hard ticks (646 female ticks & 859 male ticks) were collected. Two species of Dermacentor: *D. marginatus* and *D. raskemensis* and one species of Hyalomma; *H.m.marginatum* were isolated from sheep in Najafdar (summer pasture) which were located in Firoozkuh and winter quarters in Mahdishahr, Darjazin village, respectively (Table 1).

In the examination of 5% of the herd, one day after deeping, on the first day of July, the ticks gathered were all dried up and killed, and no live tick was taken off. However, in the sampling performed 2 weeks later, among 53 animals examined, 12 (22.6%) were infected to ticks and 64 ticks were separated from them.

Due to the effects of the acaricide on reducing the incidence and severity of infection, the number of ticks isolated in these samples was not considered in the overall calculation.

Table 1. Frequency distribution of ticks on sheep during different months of year in Darjozain (valley) and Firuzkuh (Mountain).

Date 2010-2011	No: collected ticks	Prevalence	Male ticks	Female ticks	Average of ticks on infested animal	Average of female ticks on infested animal	Average of male ticks on infested animal	location	Site of attachment	Genus of the tick
15th May	179	70%	125	54	5.11	2	3.7	Valley	Ear, perineum	*Hyalomma*
11th June	170	74%	102	67	4.59	2.23	3.21	Mountain	Sternum	*Dermacentor*
1th July	0	0	0	0	0	0	0	Mountain	-	-
16th July	64	22.6%	37	27	5.3	2.25	3.08	Mountain	Sternum	*Dermacentor*
6th Aug	185	50%	112	73	7.4	3.31	5.33	Mountain	Sternum	*Dermacentor*
3rd Sep	519	82%	298	221	12.65	5.52	8.27	Mountain	Sternum	*Dermacentor*
7th Oct	358	72%	183	175	9.83	4.26	5.58	Valley	Sternum	*Dermacentor*
11th Nov	0	0	0	0	0	0	0	Valley	-	-
5th Dec	0	0	0	0	0	0	0	Valley	-	-
30th Dec	0	0	0	0	0	0	0	Valley	-	-
4th Feb	0	0	0	0	0	0	0	Valley	-	-
15th Mar	0	0	0	0	0	0	0	Valley	-	-
10th Apr	44	22	21	24	4	3	1.81	Valley	Ear, perineum	*Hyalomma*
17th May	50	28	29	21	3.57	2.1	3.2	Mountain	Sternum	*Dermacentor*

A total of 715 Hyalomma ticks and 790 Dermacentor ticks were isolated from the ewes and lambs, respectively. The number of ticks on lambs was significantly ($p \leq 0.01$) higher than the number of ticks on ewes. In this survey, 487 female and 372 male ticks were isolated from lambs and ewes, respectively. 343 female ticks were isolated from ewes and 303 female ticks from the lambs. Although there was a significant difference between the number of male ticks on ewe and lamb ($p \leq 0.01$), there was not a significant relationship between the number of female ticks on ewe and lamb. The results indicated that there was a significant relationship between the population of male and female ticks ($p < 0.01$). The more the number of male ticks, the more the number of female ticks and vice versa. In other words, the ticks attracted and affected each other.

In all months of the year except April, the number of male ticks on the host was more than the number of female ticks. The average prevalence of infestation was 56.85%, and the mean intensity of infestation was 7.56 (Table 1).

Discussion

Existence of both dry and desert and cold and mountains climates, with a distance of about 20 km from each other, has created a unique opportunity to study the animal's tick infestation in different regions. In this study, a flock of sheep was studied for a year for tick infection. Therefore, in contrast to other studies where numerous herds zone sampling are performed, ticks isolated were of less variety (Sohrabi et al., 2013; Yakhchali & Hajihasanzadehzarza, 2004).

In spring when the herd pastured in low areas (Darjazin village), the *H. m. marginatum* ticks were observed that attaching to the ear and perineal region of the animal. In the early summer when the herd moved to the higher levels of the mountainous area of Firoozkuh (Najafdar village), the ticks changed to *D. marginatus* and *D. raskemensis* that were living under the neck and on the sternum.

H. marginatum ticks were isolated from sheep in spring. The most common hard ticks of sheep and goats reported in Salehabad city Torbatejam were *H. marginatum* (Yakhchali & Ranjbargarmabolia, 2008). Also, in a study in DarrehShahr of Ilam Province, *H. marginatum* has been reported as the most abundant sheep tick (Sharifinia et al., 2014). In a study conducted in the city of Kermanshah on sheep, in the east which has less rainfall than the western areas, the most common spesies was *H. marginatum* ticks (in the western part of the city with the most rainfall *Rhipicephalus turanicus* was the most frequent tick isolated) (Sohrabi et al., 2013). Yakhchali and Hosseini (2006) identified *Rhipicephalus bursa* as the dominant species of hard ticks on sheep and goats around Urmia's villages. Differences in species diversity in different areas show the compatibility of different species with different climatic conditions.

In Iran, three species including *D. marginatus*, *D. raskemensis*, and *D. niveus* have been reported from 6 provinces. In this study, of the mountainous regions of Semnan Province, Nabian has reported that only *D. raskemensis* and the isolation of *D. marginatus* from the animals in this area were unsuccessful (Nabian et al., 2008). *D. marginatus* is a species that has been reported in Asia, Europe, and North Africa. These ticks are usually found at elevations of 800 to 1000 meters above sea level (Estrada-Pena & Eastrada-Pena, 1991). Nabian has reported this tick from the provinces of Kurdistan, Ardabil, East Azerbaijan, and Zanjan. *D. marginatus* was the dominant tick on most of the sheep in early summer in the countryside (Nabian et al., 2008). *D. raskemensis* was studied by Dhanda et al. in 1971 in India and Pakistan (Filippova, 1983). Hoogstraal has reported *D. raskemensis* from the protected area of Khosh-Yeylagh from Alborz herds (Hoogstraal, 1980). Nabian has reported this tick from the provinces of Semnan, Khorasan, Kurdistan, and Eastern Azerbaijan. (Nabian et al., 2008). *D. raskemensis* was isolated from the sheep in the present study in the majority of cases of late summer.

D. marginatus is able to transfer various pathogens, such as *Rickettsia slovaca* that has been reported by Sanogo et al., (Sanogo et al., 2003). Also this tick is able to transfer pathogens such as *Francisella tularensis*, *Coccinella brunetti*, tick-borne encephalitis virus, and rocky mountain spotted fever caused by Rickettsia (Rehacek, 1987; Radulovic et al., 1994; Tokhov, et al., 2001). According to the information available, there are no reports on pathogen transfer by *D. raskemensis*. In laboratory condition, *H. m. marginatum* tick is able to transfer *Theileria annulata* (Estrada-Pena et al., 2004). In a study done by Razmi on sheep affected by *Theileria lestoquardi*, he could not diagnose *T. lestoquardi* in the *H. m. marginatum* that isolated from the sheep (Razmi et al., 2003). This tick is the main carrier of the virus that causes Crimean-Congo haemorrhagic fever (CCHF) in Europe (Estrada-Pena et al., 2004). The virus of CCHF has also been detected in *H. m. marginatum* in Darrehshahr of Ilam Province (Sharifinia et al., 2014).

There is some information regarding the distribution of ticks on the sheep showing the preferred infestation sites, so-called predilection sites, which might contribute to control measures such as mechanical removal and acaricide treatment. The most common assumption regarding the behavior of ticks looking for a place to feed is that they wander around searching for thin and soft skin in sheltered places on the host after being wiped off the vegetation. The study on distribution of ticks on the sheep showed that it was attached in summer pasture just around the ears and perineal areas and in countryside only in the sternum and the neck. In a study in Kermanshah, the highest accumulation of hard ticks was on the ears of the sheep (Sohrabi et al., 2013). In another study that was conducted in villages around Oshnavieh, perineal region and udder were reported as the most important attached site of ticks (Yakhchali & Hajihasanzadehzarza, 2004). Maximum tick infection on the perineal region and hip area of the sheep has been reported in Torbatejam (Yakhchali & Ranjbargarmabolia, 2008) and also in Urmia City (Yakhchali & Hosseine, 2006). Taib has reported the highest number of ticks in from ear's sheep (Taib et al., 2007).

In early summer, the sheep herd was treated using Cypermethrin.Cypermethrin was first employed as an ectoparasiticide dip in 1987 and has been widely used since then for such control. The advantage of Cypermethrin is its long lasting nature for several weeks due to its adhesion to animal wool and hair (O'Brien et al., 1997). During sampling, carried out the day after deeping the sheep, all isolated ticks were dried and killed. However, 2 weeks after deeping, of the 53 animals examined, 12 (22.6%) were infected to ticks, and totally 64 ticks were removed. Tick prevalence is considerably less, compared to the months before and after administration of cypermethrin in the same year. In preliminary studies in 1997, the effect of cypermethrin was observed up to 4 weeks after treatment (O'Brien et al., 1997).

Nonetheless, studies by Khaladj, to evaluate the effects of acaricide on ticks, showed that the effectiveness rate of the acaricide was 94.7% one day after treatment, which would be reduced to 49% and 25.3% trend in the fourteenth and twenty-first days after treatment, which led to the acceptable effect of acaricide until the 14th day (Khaladj, 2007). In another study, it was shown that the use of Cypermethrin acaricide at concentrations recommended was not able to kill larvae Boophilus with rate of 99% (Khaladj, 2007). Due to a decrease in the prevalence and intensity of infection in the calculation of annual incidence and severity of infection, the data obtained on the first day and 2 weeks after deeping were not considered. In the monthly sampling done about 4 weeks after deeping, the prevalence of infestion was 50% (Table 1). Tick resistance to Cypermethrin has been reported in various studies (Abbas et al., 2014; Kaladj, 2007).

There are several methods to treat external parasites of domestic animals. However, regardless of the different methods of treatment, farmers should become familiar with the proper use of these acaricide. In addition, the regular examination of ticks in animals for resistance to various acaricide should be placed on the agenda of veterinary organization and research centers (FAO, 2002).

In this study, the mean intensity of ticks removed from the adult animals (ewe) was significantly ($p < 0.01$) less than that of lambs. It appears that feeding of tick on the host causes some immunological responses in the host that finally results in the reduction of the population of ticks in ewe compared to lamb. It is noteworthy that the reduction in the number of ticks in ewe as compared to the lamb was due to the reduction of the male population, and the difference observed in female ticks was not significant in ewe and lamb. However, studies on questing ticks in the open space attached to the host have shown that the number of ticks that are divided into male and female ones is the same (Bowman & Nuttall, 2008; Estrada-Pena et al., 2004; Sonenshine, 1991). Also, reports have indicated that metasetriata male ticks remain on the host longer than the female ticks. The male ticks attach to the host in the proximity of the female ticks for mating; then, they are separated and start blood feeding and get ready for remating (Bowman & Nuttall, 2008; Stich et al., 2008). In the current study, there was an equal ratio between the male and female ticks only in the first month of their activities; however, in the remaining months, the male ticks were always more than the female ones. This is due to the start of the activities of the ticks in April when the number of male and female ticks was equal; after a while, the blood-fed female ticks got separated and male ticks remained on the host, and therefore the number of male ticks increased. Despite the high number of male ticks in each host in comparison with the female ones, the total number of male ticks removed from ewe was significantly less than the lamb. The difference were observed in the male tick population is statistically significant ($p < 0.01$).

Suggestions: 1. Regarding the high number of female ticks as opposed to male ones in the ewe compared to lamb, and the possible relationship with secretion of some proteins by the male ticks in *D. marginatus*, *D. raskemensis* and *H. marginatum*, it is suggested that in future studies these proteins get separated and examined and their possible role in immunity be investigated.

2. According to the study done, it is recommended that spraying the animal in the countryside in the chest area be administered monthly. In the winter, due to higher risk of affecting more areas of the body, deeping the animal with the amounts mentioned is recommended. In addition, it is recommended not to save materials and replace the use of acaricide at the proper time.

Acknowledgments

The author appreciates the support of parasitology department of faculty of veterinary medicine, Tehran University in conducting the study. I would like to thank Dr salaimi Bejestani & Mr Darvishi for their contribution in preparing the article & lab work. This project was financially supported by research council of Semnan University.

References

1. Abbas, R.Z., Zaman, M.A., Colwell, D.D., Gilleard, J., Iqbal, Z. (2014) Acaricide resistance in cattle ticks and approaches to its management: the state of play. Vet Parasitol. 203: 6-20.
2. Bowman, A.S., Nuttall, P.A. (2008) Ticks Biology, Disease and Control. (1st ed.) Cambridge University Press. London, UK.
3. Estrada-Pena, A., Eastrada-Pena, R. (1991) Notes on Dermacentor Ticks: redescription of *D. marginatus* with the synonymies of *D. niveus* and *D. daghestanicus* (Acari: Ixodidae). J Med Entomol. 28:

2-15.
4. Estrada-Pena, A., Bouattour, A., Camicas, J.L., Walker, A.R. (2004) Ticks of Domestic Animals in the Mediterranean Region. (1st ed.) University of Zaragoza. Zaragoza, Spain.
5. FAO (2002) Guidelines for resistance management and integrated parasite control in ruminants.
6. Filippova, N.A. (1983) Redescription of *Dermacentor raskemensis* pomerantzev, 1946 (Ixodidae) - a representative of the mountain fauna of the southern regions of the USSR and adjacent territories, Parasitologiia. 17: 283-92.
7. HeidarpourBami, M., Khazraiinia, P., Haddadzadeh, H.R., Kazemi, B. (2010) Identification of *Theileria* species in sheep in the eastern half of Iran using nested PCR-RFLP and microscopic techniques. Iran J Vet Res, Shiraz University. 11: 262-266.
8. Hoogstraal, H. (1980) Ticks (Ixodoidea) from wild sheep and goats in Iran and medical and veterinary implications. Fieldiana Zool new series. 6: 1-16.
9. Jongejan, F., Uilenberg, G. (1994) Ticks and control methods. Rev Sci Tech Oie. 13: 1201-1226.
10. Kettle, D.C. (1995) Medical & Veterinary Entomology. (2nd ed.) CAB International. Wallingford, Oxon, UK.
11. Khaladj, M., Rahbari, S., Nabian, S., Laddonni, H., Atarod, V., Sadeghian, G.A., Samani, A.A.S. (2007) Evaluation of some acaricide against hard ticks. J Vet Res. 62: 53-56.
12. Nabian, S., Rahbari, S., Shayan, P., Haddadzadeh, H.R. (2008) Identification of tick species of *Dermacentor* in some localities of Iran. J Vet Res. 63: 123-126.
13. O'Brien, D.J., Morgan, J.P., Lane, M.F., O'Reilly, P.F., O'Neill, S.J. (1997) Treatment and prophylaxis of psoroptic mange of sheep by a 10% w/w dip formulation of high CIS-cypermethrin. Vet parasitol. 69: 125- 131.
14. Radulovic, S., Feng, H.M., Crocquet-Valdes, P., Morovic, M., Dzelalija, B., Walker, D.H. (1994) Antigen-capture enzyme immunoassay: a comparison with other methods for the detection of spotted fever group Rickettsia in ticks. Am J Trop Med Hyg. 50: 359-64.
15. Razmi, G.R., Hosseini, M., Aslani, M.R. (2003) Identification of tick vectors of ovine theileriosis in an endemic region of Iran. Vet Parasitol. 116: 1-6.
16. Rehacek, J. (1987) Epidemiology and significance of Q fever in Czechoslovakia. Zbl Bakt-Int J Med M, Series A. 267: 16-9.
17. Sanogo, Y.O., Davoust, B., Parola, P., Camicas, J.L., Brouqui, P., Raoult D. (2003) Prevalence of Rickettsia spp. In *Dermacentor marginatus* ticks removed from game pigs (*Sus scrofa*) in southern France. Ann Ny Acad Sci. 9: 191-195.
18. Sharifinia, N., Rafinejad, J., Hanafi-Bojd, A.A., Chinikar, S., Piazak , N., Baniardalan, M., Biglarian, A., Sharifinia, F. (2014) Hard ticks (Ixodidae) and Crimen-Congo hemorrhagic fever virus in South West of Iran. Acta Med Iranica, Article in Press.
19. Sohrabi, Sh., Yakhchali, M., Ghashghai, O. (2013) Hard ticks (Acarina: Ixodidae) diversity in the natural habitat of Iranian domestic ruminants: A provincial study in Kermanshah. J Vet Res. 68:39-46.
20. Sonenshine, D.E. (1991) Biology of Ticks, vol. 1. Oxford University Press. New York, USA.
21. Stich, R.W., Schaefer, J.J., Bermer, W.G., Needham, G.R., Jittapalapong, S. (2008) Host surveys, ixodid tick biology and transmission scenarios as related to the tick-borne pathogen, *Ehrlichia canis*. Vet. Parasitol. 158: 267-273.
22. Taib, O.L., Kadir, M.A.A., Seitzer, U., Ahmed, J.S.(2007) A survey of ticks (Acari: Ixodidae) on cattle, sheep and goats in the Dohuk Governorate, Iraq. Parasitol Res. 101: 189-194.
23. Thrusfield, M. (1995) Veterinary Epidemiology. (2nd ed.) Black Wellscience Ltd. Oxford, UK.
24. Tokhov, IuM., Sysoliatina, G.V., Chumakova, I.V., Popova, E.V. (2001) Specific features of the parasitic system of Crimean haemorrhagic fever in Stavropol'region during epidemic season of 2000, Zh Mikrob Epid Immun. (6Suppl): 98-99.
25. Yakhchali, M., Hajihasanzadehzarza, S.H. (2004) Study on some ecological aspects and prevalence ofdifferent species of hard ticks (Acarina: Ixodidae) oncattle, buffalo and sheep in Oshnavieh suburb. Pajuhesh Va Sazandegi. (In Persian). 63: 31-35.
26. Yakhchali, M., Hosseine, A. (2006) Prevalence and ectoparasites fauna of sheep and goats flocks in Urmia suburb, Iran. Vet Arhiv. 76: 441-450.
27. Yakhchali, M., Ranjbargarmabolia, B. (2008) A studyon ixodid ticks fauna in sheep and goats of Salehabadin Torbatjam, Iran. Pajuhesh Va Sazandegi. (In Persian). 80: 27-32.

The photoperiod and heat stress effects on histometrical structure of rat prostate gland

Erfani Majd, N.[*]**, Sehab Negah, S., Fatemi Tabatabaei, S.R.**

Department of Basic Sciences, Faculty of Veterinary Medicine, Shahid Chamran University of Ahvaz, Ahvaz, Iran

Key words:
heat stress, histometrical, photoperiod, rat prostate

Correspondence
Erfani Majd, N.
Department of Basic Sciences,
Faculty of Veterinary Medicine,
Shahid Chamran University of
Ahvaz, Ahvaz, Iran

Email: naeemalbo@yahoo.com

Abstract:

BACKGROUND: There is not enough information about the effects of heat stress and photoperiod on different lobes structure. **OBJECTIVES:** The present study aims at determining the histological changes and the rate of changes in each lobes of rat prostate, affected by photoperiod changes and heat stress. **METHODS:** To this end, 15 adult male wistar rats were divided to three groups: 1. the control group in which the rats were kept in 12L: 12D and 25°C temperature condition, 2. the heat stress group in which the rats were kept in 12L: 12D and 42+1 °C temperature condition for 4 to 5 hours per day, and 3. the photoperiod group in which the rats were kept in 16L: 8D and 25°C temperature condition. After 30 days, samples were taken from different lobes and sections with 5 to 6μ thickness were made and stained by H&E and PAS. **RESULTS:** The microscopic results showed that histomorphometrical structure and histochemical reactions of the different lobs of normal prostate of the rats are different. The proportion of parenchyma to stroma decreased by heat stress; however, it increased by photoperiod. The maximum changes were seen in ventral lobe. The epithelial thickness, lumen diameter, and number of secretory units also increased by photoperiod (16L:8D), but it decreased by heat stress. The number of secretory cells were increased by heat stress because the cell size decreased; however, they decreased by long photoperiod regime. The number of folded secretory units increased by photoperiod, while heat stress has an adverse effect ($p<0.001$). The serum testosterone increased by long photoperiod and decreased by heat stress ($p<0.01$). **CONCLUSIONS:** This study shows that long photoperiod has important effects on increasing the rat prostate parenchyma and its activity.

Introduction

The prostate gland is the largest accessory sex gland in mammals. This gland surrounds the urinary bladder neck and urethra opening. Its secretion is important for sperm fertility (Guyton and Hall, 2010). Thomson (2001) reported that the earliest signs of prostate formation were observed in 17 or 18 days and approximately 9 to 10 weeks of embryonic development in mice, rats, and human, respectively. Androgens are essential factors for the survival of prostate epithelial cells. Although there are other androgen formation in ducts, channels, and having to be involved in the differentiation of epithelial tissue, the main androgen is testosterone (Donjacour and Cunha, 1998).

In the male, there is a period of growth in which the prostate is fully functional and it will be alternate with a period of regression in which the prostate parenchyma is changed. During this regression period, a dramatic decreasing will occur in the weight and function of the prostate. These changes are regulated by environmental cues; the major ones are photoperiod and heat stress (Bronson and Heideman, 1994; Bronson, 1985). It has been shown that the photoperiod length has a major effect on the morphology and function of the mature testes of male hamsters (Breckon and Cawood, 1985; Darrow et al., 1980) and juvenile ones (Gunduz and Stetson, 1994). Moreover, the epididymis luminal diameter decreases in a short-day light regime. The aim of this study was to identify some details of the changes induced by long-day light regime (16:8h. light: dark) and induced heat stress on the different lobes of rat prostate.

Materials and Methods

Animals were prepared from laboratory animal center of Jondy Shapour university of medical sciences of Ahwaz. For this study, 15 adult male wistar rats were divided into three groups (5 rats in each group): 1. The control group (G1) in which the rats were kept in 12L: 12D and 25°C temperature condition, 2. The heat stress group (G3) in which the rats were kept in 12L:12D and 42 +1°C temperature condition for 4 to 5 hours per day, 3. The photoperiod group (G2) in which the rats were kept in 16L:8D and 25°C temperature condition. The rats were fed with standard diet. After 30 days, the rats were easy drawing with chloroform, and blood samples were taken from heart; in addition, then the level of testosterone was measured by the Elisa (Power work Biotek X52). Abdominal cavity was explored and samples were taken from different lobes of rat's prostate gland. Sections with 5 to 6μ thickness were made by paraffin embedding method and were stained by H&E and PAS (Bancroft and Gamble, 2003). The PAS staining was used to show the glycoprotein secretion in each lobe. The histomorphotrical studies were done using digital Dino-Lite lens and Dino-capture1 software. Secretory cells were counted in 50 micrometer length of the alveolus wall in magnification of 40.

Statistical Analyses: Data are expressed as mean ± standard variation. One-way analysis of variance (ANOVA) was performed on the data. Differences between groups were considered to be significant at $p < 0.05$.

Table 1. Epithelial thickness of secretory units in different lobes of rat prostate (μm). Letters in superscript means significant difference ($p<0.05$).

Groups / Lobes	Control (G1)	Photoperiod (G2)	Heat stress (G3)
Ventral	24±1.07	26±2.97	23±3.2
Dorsal	18±2.40	21±3.52	20±3.71
Anterior	22±2.56	24±2/43 ^{C}	18±2.35 ^{B}
Lateral 1	19±1.26	21±1.34	16±1.26 ^{AB}
Lateral 2	21±2.30	17±1.59	17±2.37

Table 2. Lumen diameter of secretory units in different rat prostate lobes (μm).

Groups / Lobes	Control (G1)	Photoperiod (G2)	Heat stress (G3)
Ventral	298±60.80	299±61.86	226±59.47
Dorsal	175±71.21	195±14.49	184±78.02
Anterior	202±40	405±79.38 ^{AC}	281±44.46
Lateral 1	280±68.92	525±156.7 ^{AC}	250±24.73
Lateral 2	211±46.06	247±53.28 ^{C}	166±37.41 ^{B}

Table 3. The number of secretory cells in 50 μ length of secretary unit wall in different rat prostate lobes. Letters in superscript means significant difference ($p<0.05$).

Groups / Lobes	Control (G1)	Photoperiod (G2)	Heat stress (G3)
Ventral	9±1.30	10±1.22	10±0.83
Dorsal	9±1.4 B ^{C}	8±0.54 ^{AC}	10±1.3 ^{AB}
Anterior	8±1.58	9±1.41	9±1.92
Lateral 1	8±0.83	8±0.79	9±0.54 ^{AB}
Lateral 2	8±1	9±0.83 ^{C}	10±1 ^{B}

Table 4. The proportion of parenchyma to stroma in different lobes of rat prostate. Letters in superscript means significant difference ($p<0.05$).

Groups / Lobes	Control (G1)	Photoperiod (G2)	Heat stress (G3)
Ventral	79±1.92 ^{C}	75±1.86	68±6.85 ^{A}
Dorsal	72±2.80	55±7.61	59±9.50
Anterior	62±5.11	58±3.87	57±9.5
Lateral 1	69±12.56	68±8.41	56±6.68 ^{AB}
Lateral 2	79±8.22 ^{BC}	61±8.34 ^{AC}	44±8.03 ^{AB}

Results

Microscopic results revealed that histomorpho-

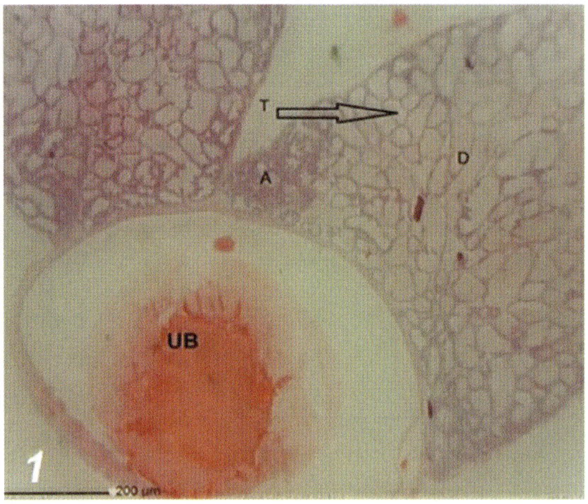

Figure 1. The ventral lobe of rat prostate gland in control group (X4, H&E). The folded secretory units in peripheral area (A), tubular units (T), and ducts (D).

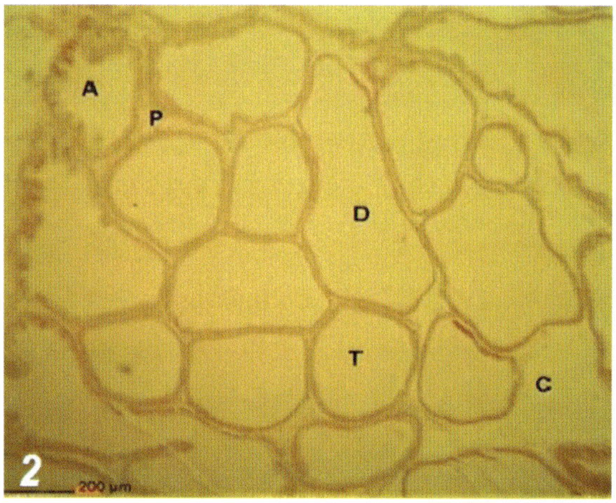

Figure 2. The ventral lobe of rat prostate gland, the control group (X4, H&E). The folded secretory units in peripheral area (P), alveolar (A), tubular units (T), ducts (D), and the central area of lobe (C).

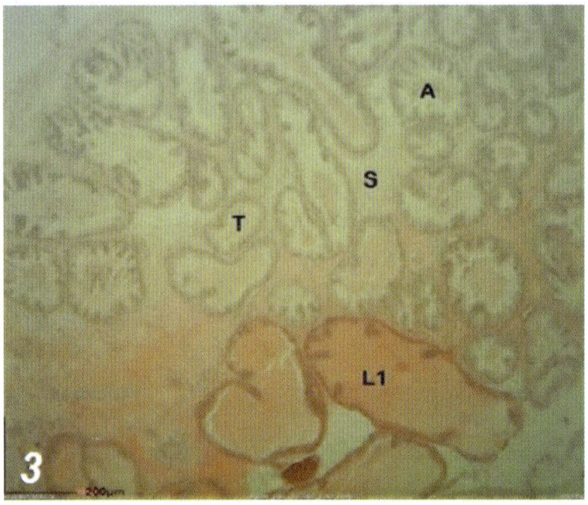

Figure 3. The dorsal lobe of rat prostate gland in control group (X4, H&E). The folded secretory units (A) dispersed in the entire lobe.

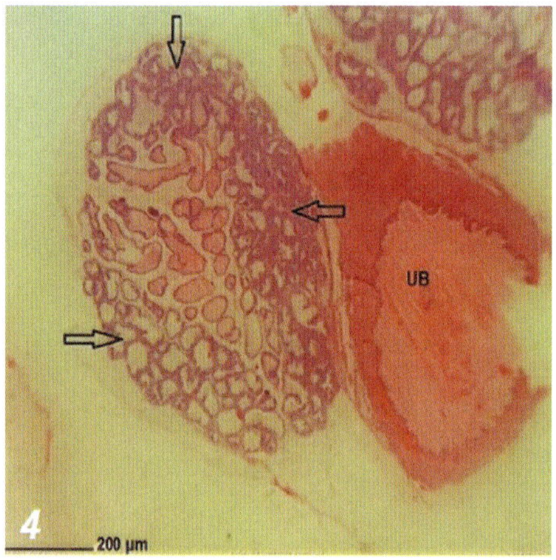

Figure 4. The ventral lobe of rat prostate gland in photoperiod group (X4, H&E). The increasing of peripheral folded secretory units in long-photoperiod group (arrows) is considerable.

metrical and histochemical reactions of different lobs of normal rat prostate are different. The ventral and dorsal have more parenchyma than other lobes, and the folded secretory units were concentrated peripherally in ventral lobe (Figure 1 & 2) while they were diffuse in dorsal lobe (Figure 3). Folded secretory units in long photoperiod group increased but decreased in heat stress group. These changes were more visible in the ventral lobe (Figure 4). Histological results showed that the proportion of parenchyma to stroma has changed in different groups. This proportion decreased by heat stress (Figure 5); however, it increased by long-photoperiod regime (Figure 6). These changes were more visible in the lateral lobes.

PAS Reaction: PAS staining showed that all secretory cells in different prostate lobes have positive PAS reaction in normal rat prostate; however, the staining intensity were maximum and minimum in ventral and anterior lobes, respectively. The tubular secretory units have more reaction to PAS staining than alveolar units. The results also indicated that PAS reaction increased by long-photoperiod regime; however, it decreased by heat stress.

Micrometrical Results: The micrometrical results showed that the epithelial thickness of secretory units were changed in different groups. It increased in long-photoperiod group (G2), while it decreased in heat stress group (G3). The most significant changes were seen in lateral lobe type 2 (Table 1).

The lumen diameter of secretory units increased

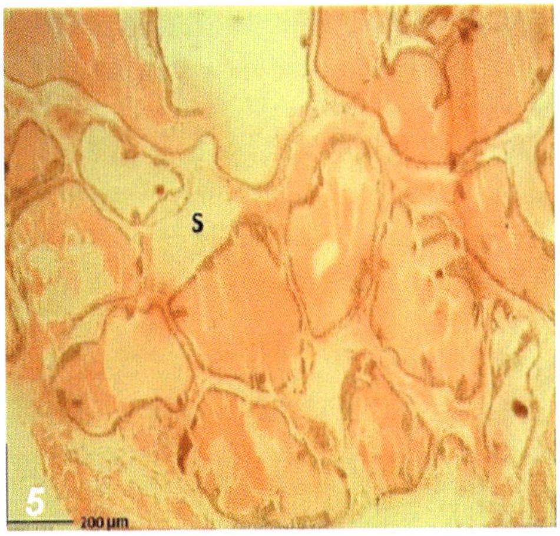

Figure 5. The lateral lobe 1 of rat prostate gland in heat stress group (X4, H&E). The decreasing of parenchyma (secretory units) and epithelium thickness and increasing of stroma (S) are considerable.

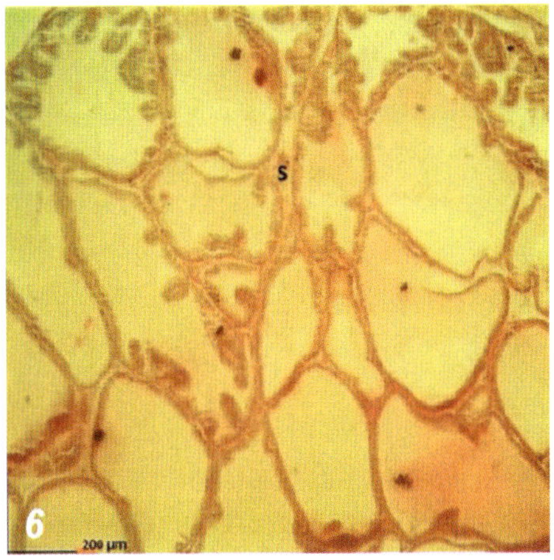

Figure 6. The lateral lobe 1 of rat prostate gland in photoperiod group (X4, H&E). The increasing of parenchyma (folded secretory units) and epithelium thickness and decreasing of stroma (S) are considerable.

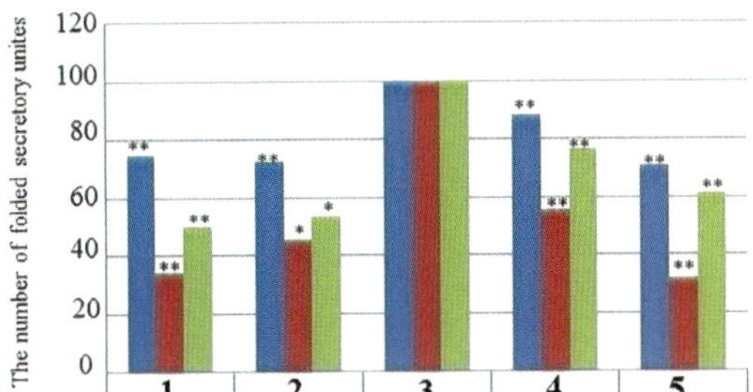

	1	2	3	4	5
Photoperiod G.	74.8	72.8	100	88.2	70.8
Heat Stress G.	34.2	45.4	100	55.6	32.2
Control G.	49.8	53.3	100	76.2	61.4

Figure 7. The number of folded secretory units in different lobes and groups (mean+SD). Ventral lobe (1), dorsal lobe (2), cranial lobe (3), lateral lobe (type1) (4), lateral lobe (type2) (5). (*) Indicate a significant difference ($p<0.01$). (**) Indicate a significant difference ($p<0.001$).

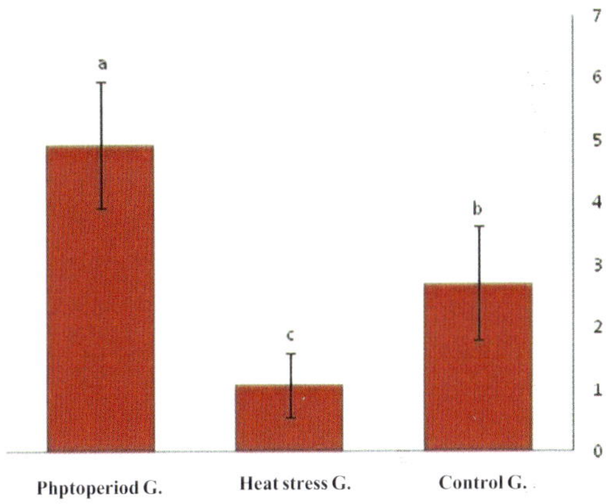

Figure 8. The serum testosterone (n/mg) in different groups. Different letters (a-c) indicate a significant difference ($p<0.01$).

in long-photoperiod group (G2) compared to heat stress group (G3) and control group (G1). The most significant changes were observed in lateral lobes (Table 2).

The number of secretory cells increased in heat stress group (G3), while they decreased in long-photoperiod group (G2), because cell size was increased. The most significant changes were observed in dorsal and lateral lobe type 1 (Table 3).

The proportion of parenchyma to stroma changed in different groups. It increased in long-photoperiod group (G2), while it decreased in heat stress group (G3) (Table 4).

The number of folded secretory units increased by long-photoperiod regime, whereas heat stress had an adverse effect (Figure 7).

Testosterone: The serum testosterone level increased by long-photoperiod regime and it decreased by heat stress (Figure 8).

Discussion

Androgen plays an essential role in embryonic development and in adult prostate (Bartsch et al., 2002; Schroder, 1994; Thomson, 2001). Androgens promote the growth and differentiation of prostate cells through ligand activation of the androgen receptor (AR) (Zhu and Kyprianou, 2008). Prostate secretory cells have androgen receptor and they are continuously stimulated by androgen in order to survive and function (Chatterjee, 2003), so that after castration which androgen cease, the apoptosis will occur in rat prostate epithelial cells (Kyprianou and Isaacs, 1988; Schroder, 1994). The photoperiod and temperature are important factors which affect the androgen levels (Carballada, 2006). Photoperiod is also an important factor for regulating the reproductive activity (Anne Grocock, 1981; Shimizu, 2003). Reproductive activity in long-day animals can be stimulated by a long light period (e.g. 16h) and followed by a shorter dark period (e.g. 8h). Carballada et al. (2006) reported that the percentage of apoptotic cells increased in animals which were maintained for 6, 8, or 12 weeks in a short photoperiod. This study shows that photoperiod has an important effect on increasing rat prostate parenchyma and its secretory activity. The results of the present study showed that prostate parenchyma was affected by a long-photoperiod (16h light and 8h dark) which has conformity with increasing of serum testosterone. The number of secretory cells in 50m length of secretory units wall decreased in the photoperiod group because the secretory cells size increased. The dorsal lobe of the prostate Golden hamster has more response to long-photoperiod regime than ventral lobe (8h dark, 16h light) (Carballada, 2006). It has also been shown that the ventral lobe of castrated rat prostate undergoes more changes than the dorsal lobe (Banerjee et al., 1995). The results of the present study showed that ventral lobe of rat prostate has more changes to long-photoperiod regime than dorsal lobe, which is consistent with Carballada (2006) in Golden hamsters and Banerjee et al. (1995) in rats. The finding of present study showed that the cranial lobes of rat prostate is an active lobe, while most researchers suggested that cranial lobe is an inactive lobe and it is not considered as a part of rat prostate (Jesik et al., 1982; Wylot et al., 2004 Hernandes, et al., 2006).

Heat Stress: It has been shown that cancer cells are relatively sensitive to heat stress. It has been reported that heat treatment (43oC) increased the expression of heat shock protein 70 (hsp70), and it increased apoptosis. Hsp70 is a protein that protects cells against heat damage (Nakanoma et al., 2001). It has been shown that increasing the temperature caused apoptosis in rat epididymis (Jara et al., 2002). The apoptosis in rat epididymis and ventral prostate lobes increased with age (Jara et al., 2004). The results of the present study showed that serum testosterone levels reduced with heat stress and subsequent prostate tissue also underwent changes, so that, the thickness of the epithelium and ratio of parenchyma to the stroma decreased. The number of secretory cells in 50m length of secretory units wall increased because the cell size decreased. Heat stress has often caused apoptosis which was inconsistent with the present results. It should be noted that in most studies cell culture is used for showing heat stress effects (Nakanoma et al., 1998). The maximum lumen diameter of tubular secretory units were seen in long-photoperiod regime group that it is consistent with the statements of Fink et al. (2005); they reported that the lumen diameter of secretory units increased with increasing of prostate activity.

The results of the present study showed that long-photoperiod increased prostate parenchyma and activity, while heat stress has inverse effects.

Acknowledgments

The authors wish to express their gratitude to the Research Council of Shahid Chamran University of Ahvaz for their financial supports.

References

1. Banerjee, P.P., Banjeree, S., Tilly, K.I., Tilly, J.L., Brown, T.R., Zirkin, B.R. (1995) Lobe-specific apoptotice cell death in rat prostate after androgen ablation by castration. Endocrinology. 136: 4368-76.
2. Bartsch, G., Rittmaster, R.S., Klocker, H. (2002) Dihydrotestestrone and the concept of 5 alpha reductase inhibitions in human benign prostatic hyperplasia. World J Urol. 19: 413-425.
3. Breckon, G., Cawood, A.H. (1985) Photoperiodic control of meiosis in the male Syrian hamster (*Mesocricetus auratus*). J Reprod Fertil. 75: 177-181.
4. Bronson, F.H., Heideman, P.D. (1994) Seasonal regulation of reproduction in mammals. In: Knobil and Neill's Physiology of Reproduction. Knobil E., Neil E. J. (eds.). Raven Press, New York, USA. p. 541-583.
5. Bronson, F.H. (1985) Mammalian reproduction: an ecological perspective. Biol Reprod. 32: 1-26.

6. Carballada, R., Jara, M., Esponda, P. (2006) Photoperiod-induced apoptosis in the male genital tract epithelia of the golden hamster. Int J Androl. 30: 73-79.
7. Chatterjee, B. (2003) The role of the androgen receptor in the development of prostatic hyperplasia and prostate cancer. Mol Cell Biochem. 253: 89-110.
8. Darrow, J.M., Davis, F.C., Elliott, J.A., Stetson, M.H., Turek, F.W., Menaker, M. (1980) Influence of photoperiod on reproductive development in the golden hamster. Biol Reprod. 22: 443-450.
9. Donjacour, A.A., Cunha, G.R. (1998) The effect of androgen deprivation on branching morphogenesis in the mouse prostate. Dev Biol. 128:1 14.
10. Fink, J.W., Bernie, J., Mcleod-Stephen, J., Assinder-Laura, J., Parry-Helen, D., Nicholoson, H.D. (2005) Seasonal change in Mesotocin and localization of its receptor in the prostate of the brushtail possum (*Trichosurus vulpecula*). Biol Reprod. 72: 470- 478.
11. Grocock, A. (1981) Effect of different photoperiods on testicular weight changes in the vole, *Microtus agrestis*. J Reprod Fertil. 62: 25-32.
12. Gunduz, B., Stetson, M.H. (1994) Effects of photoperiod, pinealectomy, and melatonin implants on testicular development in juvenile Siberian hamsters (*Phodopus sungorus*). Biol Reprod. 51: 1181-87.
13. Guyton, A.C., Hall, J.E. (2010) Texbook of Medical Physiology. (10th ed.) W.B. Saunders Company. Philadelphia, USA.
14. Hernandes, M.E., Abraham, S.C., Fausto, R., Luz, I.P., Gonzalo, E., Aranda-Abreu, R.T., Luis, I.G., Andres, Q.S., Jorge, M. (2006) Prostate response to prolactin in sexualy active male rats. Reprod Biol Endocrinol. 4: 28, doi: 10.1186/1477-7827-4-28.
15. Jara, M., Carballada, R., Esponda, P. (2004) Age-induced apoptosis in the male genital tract of the mouse. Reproduction. 127: 359-366.
16. Jara, M., Esponda, P., Carballada, R. (2002) Abdominal temperature induces region specific p53-indipendent apoptosis in the cauda epididymis of the mouse. Biol Reprod. Vol.67, No.2,1189-96.
17. Jesik, C.J., Holand, J.M., Lee, C. (1982) An anatomic and histologic study of the rat prostate. The Prost. 3: 81-97.
18. Bancroft, J.D., Gamble, M. (2003) Theory and Practice of Histological Techniques. (5th ed.). Churchil Livingstone, Edinburgh, UK.
19. Kyprianou, N., Isaacs, J.T. (1988) Expression of transforming growth factor-β in the rat ventral prostate during castration induced programmed cell death. Mol Endocrinol. 3: 1515-22.
20. Nakanoma, T., Ueno, M., Iida, M., Hirata, R., Deguchi, N. (2001) Effects of quercetin on the heat-induced cytotoxicity of prostate cancer cells. Int J Urol. 8: 623-30.
21. Nakanoma, T., Ueno, M., Ohigashi, T., Nonaka, S., Iida, M., Hirata, R., Suzuki, M., Murai, M., Deguchi, N. (1998) Anti-proliferative effects of heating on the human prostatic carcinoma cells in culture. Humen Cell. 11: 167-74.
22. Schroder, F.H. (1994) Medical treatment of benign prostatic hyperplasia: the effect of surgical or medical castration. Prog Clin Biol Res. 386: 191-196.
23. Shimizu, A. (2003) Effect of photoperiod and temperature on gonadal activity and plasma steroid levels in a reared strain of the mummichog (*Fundulus heteroclitus*) during different phases of its annual reproductive cycle. Gen Comp Endocrinol. 131: 310-324.
24. Thomson, A.A. (2001) Role of androgens and fibroblast growth factors in prostatic development. Reproduction. 121: 187-195.
25. Wylot, M., Laszczynska, M., Stuczanowska-Glaboska, P.M. (2004) Aging process of epithelial cells of the rat prostate lateral lobe in experimental hyperolactinemia induced by haloperidol. Rocz Akad Med Bialymst. 49: 111-113.
26. Zhu, M.L., Kyprianou, N. (2008) Androgen receptor and growth factor signaling cross-talk in prostate cancer cells. Endocr Relat Cancer. 15: 841-849.

Development of antibody-based microarray assay for quantitative detection of aflatoxin B_1

Beizaei, A., Kamkar, A.*, Misaghi, A.

Department of Food Hygiene and Quality Control, Faculty of Veterinary Medicine, University of Tehran, Tehran, Iran

Key words:
aflatoxin B_1, dot blot, immunoassay, microarray, optimization

Correspondence
Kamkar, A.
Department of Food Hygiene and Quality Control, Faculty of Veterinary Medicine, University of Tehran, Tehran, Iran

Email: akamkar@ut.ac.ir

Abstract:

BACKGROUND: Aflatoxin B1 (AFB1) is a toxic metabolite produced by *Aspergillus* species that contaminates a wide range of agricultural products. **OBJECTIVES:** This study was designed to develop a rapid and highly sensitive immunoassay method in microarray format for quantitative detection of AFB1 to evaluate the potential of microarray platform for high-throughput screening, which can be beneficial in food and feed industry. **METHODS:** Following successful optimization, using an indirect competitive immunoassay in dot blot format, AFB1-bovine serum albumin (AFB1-BSA) conjugate was contact-printed onto 16 isolated sub-arrays on multi-pad nitrocellulose coated slides; subsequently used in competitive binding assays. **RESULTS:** Using the aforementioned assay, AFB1 was determined from 15 pg/g to 3.04 ng/g working range with detection limit (LOD) of 1 pg/g. To evaluate assay performance in real food matrices, the authors spiked wheat samples with different concentration of AFB1. After extraction, working ranges of 0.11-4.15 ng/g with detection limit of 30pg/g was determined. Good recoveries (94±9%) were obtained, demonstrating accurate detection of AFB1 concentrations in wheat samples. Assay procedure completed in 3 hours. **CONCLUSIONS:** The results indicated that the proposed developed assay in microarray format could be used for rapid and sensitive detection of AFB1in wheat samples.

Introduction

Aflatoxin B_1 (AFB_1) is a toxic metabolite produced mainly by *Aspergillus flavus* and *A. parasiticus*. AFB_1 was listed as a Group I carcinogen by the International Agency for Research on Cancer (IARC) (IARC, 2002). It is a potent carcinogen, teratogen, and mutagen (Speijers and Speijers, 2004). Aflatoxins can affect a wide range of vegetable commodities such as cereals, nuts, peanuts, fruits, oilseeds, and dried fruits both in the field and during storage (Doradimos et al., 2000). The most common aflatoxin exposure is consumption of grains contaminated by aflatoxin-producing fungal strains during growth, harvest, or storage (Bakirci, 2001; Lopez et al., 2001).

European Community legislation has established a maximum level of 2 μg/kg (2ppb) of AFB_1 in foodstuffs (Anklam et al., 2002); Levels above that result in toxic manifestations, which in turn leads to liver cancer (hepatocellular carcinoma), which is the fifth most commonly occurring cancer throughout the world and the third greatest cause of cancer mortality (Parkin et al., 2001).

Aflatoxin production occurs in a wide range of foods and because of its harmful effects on humans and animals, several methods and techniques have been developed for Aflatoxin determination over the last few years. There are well-established methodologies for analyzing aflatoxins in many different foodstuffs; e.g., thin-layer chromatography (TLC), high-performance liquid chromatography (HPLC), overpressure-layer chromatography (OPLC), immune affinity chromatography (IAC), and near infrared spectroscopy (NIR) (Li et al., 2009).

These methods typically require skilled operators, extensive sample pretreatment, and expensive equipments (Stroka and Anklam, 2002; Papp et al., 2002).

The goal of more recent studies has been to simplify and expedite the method of detection while attempting to maintain or improve sensitivity.

Immunological techniques have been used for a long time for the detection and identification of Aflatoxin in different assays. Antibody based detection methods for AFB_1 include standard immunoassays coupled to colorimetric (Garden and Strachan, 2001; Delmulle et al., 2005; Xiulan et al., 2005), electrochemical (Ammida et al., 2004) or surface plasmon resonance (Daly et al., 2000; Dunne et al., 2005) detection, as well as enhanced immunoassays such as the enzyme-linked immunosorbent assay (ELISA) (Bhattacharya et al., 1999; Pal and Dhar, 2004; Lee et al., 2004). Dot blot is a simple technique to detect proteins. It is a quick assay in which sample proteins are spotted on a membrane and hybridized with an antibody that acts as a probe. Dot blot results give semi-quantitative measurements of the spotted proteins. Therefore, in this study, a dot blot technique has been used for initial optimization towards development of sensitive microarray format for detection of AFB_1. To achieve microarray optimization, an immunoassay was applied on the spotted polyvinylidene difluoride (PVDF) membrane. A simple dot blot technique offers significant savings in time and can be used for designing the layout of microarray. Thus, using these findings, a toxin microarray has been developed for rapid and sensitive detection of AFB_1. The efficacy of this microarray assay was evaluated in food samples using spiked wheat flour as a model of real matrices.

Materials and Methods

16-pad nitrocellulose coated slides and incubation chambers were purchased from Whatman Int. Ltd. AFB_1 standard solution (2μg/mL) in acetonitrile was purchased from Sigma. AFB_1-bovine serum albumin (AFB_1-BSA), monoclonal anti- AFB1 antibody (Mab), sheep anti mouse IgG -Cy3 (Ab2-Cy3), and goat anti mouse IgG- Alkaline phosphatase (Ab2-AP) were obtained from Sigma-Aldrich. Alexa Fluor® 647 Goat Anti-Mouse IgG was purchased from Invitrogen. All other chemicals were of analytical grade (A.R.) and purchased from Sigma-Aldrich.

Assay optimization using dot blot: One volume of AFB1-BSA (400-10 μg/mL), phosphate buffered saline (PBS) (as the negative control), monoclonal, and secondary antibodies (as internal control) were spotted on pre- activated PVDF membrane to optimize microarray layout according to the schemes in the Figure 1, 2 and 3. The spotted membranes were stored at 4°C overnight for further application.

A simple indirect immunoassay procedure was performed on the spotted membranes. After blocking for 1h in 5% (w/v) low-fat milk prepared in tris-buffered saline -T (150mM NaCl, 10 mM Tris-HCL pH 7.5, 0.05% v/v Tween 20), membranes were washed three times with TBS-T for 5 min. Then, Mab was applied in different dilutions; 1:10000, 1:20000, and 1:30 000 (from 33 mg/mL concentration) and incubated for 1 h. Following 3 washes, two different detection methods were applied by using two secondary antibodies. Ab2-AP was tested in dilution series of 1:1000, 1:5000, and 1:10 000 (1mg/mL). Ab2-Cy3 was tested in dilution series of 1:500, 1:5000, and 1:10 000 (1mg/mL). The secondary antibodies were incubated for 45 min. Additional steps were applied for those Ab2-APs that were used in the detection method. The membrane was equilibrated in AttoPhos® buffer (100mM Tris-HCL pH 9.5, 1mM MgCl2) for 10 mins, then transferred to a 1:40 dilution of AttoPhos® substrate in its buffer and incubated in the dark for 5 mins. In the detection step, all the membranes were scanned using LAS3000 Fuji imager (Figure 1 and 2) or G: BOX (SYNGENE) (Figure 3).

Contact printing and immobilization of toxin microarray: Q-Array System (Genetix) was used to generate microarrays. 16-pad nitrocellulose coated FAST slides were used as reacting chips (Figure 4). An image of each identical subarray is shown in Figure 1A. The identical layout of sub-arrays is shown in Figure 1B. The printing design of each sub array consisted of 32 replicates of AFB1-BSA, 8 replicates of mouse Ab2-Cy3 (printing control), 4 replicates of monoclonal anti- AFB_1 antibody (internal control), and 4 replicates of BSA 2% in PBS (negative control). After printing, the microarray slides were stored in a slide box at 4°C for at least 24 h before use.

Microarray assay: The spotting chambers were fixed on each slide and an indirect competitive immunoassay was performed on each sub array. First, the chips were blocked with BSA 2% in PBS (100μL per sub array) to minimize the nonspecific binding of the AFB_1 to the chips. They were then incubated at room temperature for 1 h. Subsequently, the chips were washed thoroughly (100μL per sub array) two times with PBST. Standard solutions of AFB_1 at different concentrations were prepared in BSA 1% PBS 0.01% (v/v) Tween 20, mixed with monoclonal anti-AFB1 (0.19μg/mL, diluted in BSA 1% PBS 0.01% (v/v) Tween 20) and then pre-incubated at 37°C for 20 min, before application to each sub array (50 μL per sub array). The chips were incubated at 37°C for 30 min. After incubation, the chips were washed (100μL per sub array) three times with PBST (each wash for 3 min).

The secondary antibody, Alexa Fluor® 647 anti-mouse IgG (I mg/mL) was diluted 1:5000 (v/v) in BSA 1%- PBS- 0.01 % (v/v) Tween and added to the subarrays (50 μL per sub array). The chips were incubated at 37°C for 45. After three washes, the chips were centrifuged at 3000rpm for 3 min at 4°C and scanned using confocal microarray reader (Genepix 4000B) at a wavelength of 635 nm. The total assay procedure was completed in 3 hours.

Food Sample preparation: Wheat flour samples were artificially contaminated by adding 100 μL of AFB_1 standard solutions (0, 0.1, 1 and 10 μg/mL) to 5 g of sample. The extraction method used was a modification of the method used by Strachan and Garden (Garden and Strachan, 2001). To this end, 15 ml methanol-water (80: 20) was added to 5 g of sample. The suspension was vortexed for 1 min and then centrifuged at 4000g for 15 min. The aqueous layer was diluted 1 in 10 for the assays. The concentration of AFB1 in diluted sample extracts was measured by reference to a calibration curve and was used to estimate the concentration in the original sample.

Data extraction and analysis: Quantitative data was extracted using Genepix Pro 5.1 software (Axon Instruments), generating the value "mean foreground minus mean background" intensity for each spot, applied for analysis. Finally, calibration graphs were handled with Origin 6.0. Standard curves generated from one chip in parallel and were repeated two times.

Results

Dot blot optimization: Each microarray has a layout that should be set up and designed properly. Therefore, AFB_1-BSA, PBS (as negative control), and a primary and two secondary antibodies (as internal controls) were spotted to establish the optimum design for future use on a microarray platform. The concentration of 100μg/mL was selected as the optimal concentration for AFB_1-BSA, as it was the lowest concentration that was detectable using the dilution of both primary and secondary abs. (Figure 1, 2 and 3). The dilution of 1:5000 of Mab was the only dilution that could be detected by Ab2-AP and nothing was detected by Ab2-Cy3 (Figure 1). Although all dilutions of spotted secondary antibodies have been detected with imager, using Ab2-AP as the detection method the signals were stronger. With regard to the final result of spotting dilutions, a 1:100 dilution of both Mab (330μg/mL) and secondary antibodies (10μg/mL) was chosen for the positive controls (Figure 1).

Antibodies titrations: Antibody detection always plays an important role in an indirect immunoassay system; therefore, the conditions for using two different secondary Abs, Ab2-AP, and Ab2-Cy3 were optimized (Figure 2). As It was expected, Ab2-AP was more sensitive than Ab2-Cy3, as the dilution of 1:10 000 (v/v) for Cy3 has made a weak signal but was strong enough for Ab2-AP. Thus, the dilution of 1:5000 (0.2 μg /mL) was established as the optimal detection dilution for use in final format of microarray design.

Different dilutions of Mab were applied on the final figure of designed chip. Although the Ab2-AP was more sensitive, further optimization was carried out using Ab2-Cy3 as detection method because the final microarrays format adapts to the florescent detection. The images showed that the dilution of 1:30 000 (1.1 μg/mL) can still detect AFB_1 and can be used as a starting point for further optimization on expensive microarray surfaces (Figure 3).

Utilizing the dot blot technique, the concentrations of 100 μg/mL of AFB1-BSA, 330μg/mL of Mab and 10μg/mL of secondary antibodies (as positive controls) were chosen for designing the final

Table 1. Estimation of LOD for AFB1 detection using antibody-based microarray assay.

Matrix	Standard curve	LOD (ng/g)	Working range (ng/g)
Buffer	y=2.1386+ 1.2023/(1+(x/0.3708^2.1386))-1.2023,R2=0.98	0.001	0.015 - 3.04
Wheat	y=4.0836+ 0.3898/(1+(x/1.0089^0.7033))-0.3898,R2=1	0.03	0.11- 4.15

Table 2. Measurements of AFB1 in wheat samples by antibody-based microarray assay . Each extraction value was represented the average value of 16 measurements on each sub-array. Each sub-array measurement was repeated two times.

Sample(ng/g)	AFB1 spiked	AFB1 measured after extraction (ng/g)		(Mean ± SD)	R.S.D. (%)	Recovery (%)
		First extraction	Second extraction			
Wheat	2	2.01	1.79	1.9±0.15	7.87	95.3
	20	16.02	17.99	17.01±1.39	8.19	85.06
	200	206.28	199.8	203.04±4.58	2.25	101.52

feature of microarrays on suitable surface. For developing the immunoassay, the dilution of 1:30 000(v/v) of Mab can be used as a starting point for further optimization. The dilution of 1:5000(v/v) of secondary antibodies was established as the optimum.

Optimization on microarray: To establish the working range in the microarrays format, further titration starting from 1.1 μg/mL concentration of Mab antibody was performed. The four final optimized concentrations of monoclonal antibody on the sub arrays performance were evaluated by generating standard competition curves for AFB_1 (Figure 3). All the experimental data were fitted using non-linear four-parameter logistic calibration plot. The four-parameter logistic (Fare et al., 1996) is given by the equation:

$$f(x) = a-d/1+(x/c)^b+d$$

in which and are the asymptotic maximum and minimum values, the value of at the inflection point (IC50), and the slope. Comparison of the calibration curves generated using the toxin microarray indicated that the dilution of 1: 170 000 (v/v) (0.19 μg/mL) is optimal for quantitative detection of AFB1. Several microarrays were screened without competitors in order to evaluate the experimental variation in spot intensities among each array. Relative standard deviation no higher than 10 % was observed. The variation across the slide was affected by the distance of the slide from microtitre plate and the exact location on the slide. Therefore, a non-contact form of printing the variation should be overcome.

Calibration curves: In Table 1, the result of calibration curves, the equations for estimation of limit of detection (LOD) values (equivalent to IC10) and working ranges are shown. Each concentration of AFB_1 had 32 replicates in a sub array and each sub array value representing two time measurements. The logistic correlation coefficient (R2), which was above 0.98, indicated the excellent analytical performance of this optimized toxin microarray assay method. The results reveal that this microarray assay can detect the pure toxin at a level of 1 pg/mL. It should be pointed out that the sensitivity of assay in wheat samples was 30 pg/mL, i.e. near 30 fold higher. The reduction of sensitivity for AFB1 detection in real samples is explainable due to food matrix effect; nonetheless, this assay achieves adequate sensitivity for applications in food samples.

Recovery in food samples: The recovery analysis of artificially contaminated wheat flour samples has been shown in Table 2. Good recoveries (94±9%), demonstrating the suitability of the proposed assay for accurate determination of AFB1 concentration in wheat samples was obtained. Each extraction value indicated the average of 16 measurements. The recovery values were represented the mean value of two extraction procedure repeated on two different days. The precision was estimated by calculating the relative standard deviation (% R.S.D) for replicate measurements.

Discussion

In recent years, the development of array-based biosensors and microarray technology has offered using them in various applications, including the study of disease, drug discovery, genetic screening, clinical diagnostic, and food screening. Antibody-based microarrays provide a powerful tool that can be used to generate rapid and detailed expression profiles of a defined set of analytes in complex samples, and they are potentially useful for generating rapid immunological assays of food contamin-

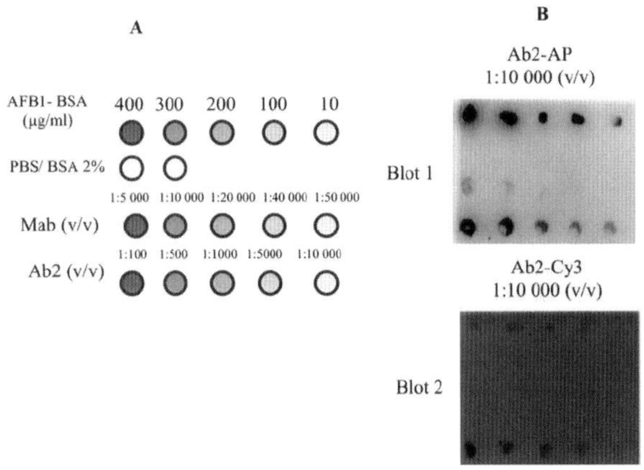

Figure 1. Optimization of microarray feature using dot blot. (A)The illustration of the spotted elements and related concentrations; AFB1-BSA, BSA 2% in PBS, Mab and Ab2 on each blot has been shown in cartoons. (B) Corresponding image of spotted blots. A 1:10 000 (v/v) dilution of Mab and Ab2-AP or Ab2-Cy3 has been applied for immunoassay detection.

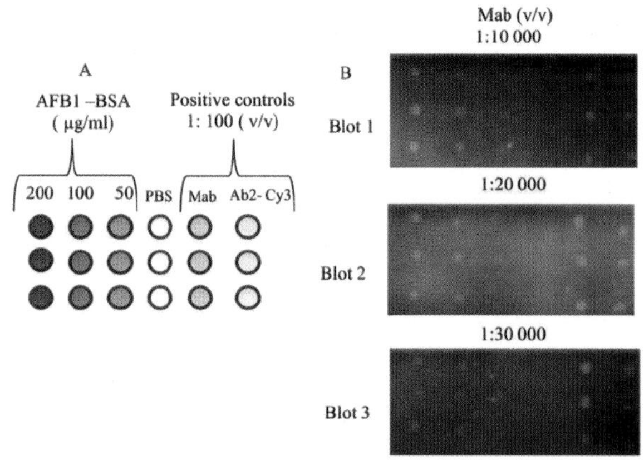

Figure 2. Secondary antibodies titration using dot blot. (A) The illustration of the spotted elements on each blot in cartoons. (B) Corresponding image of spotted blots. From left to the right, Ab2-AP and Ab2-Cy3 were applied in three different dilutions on each blot for immunoassay detection.

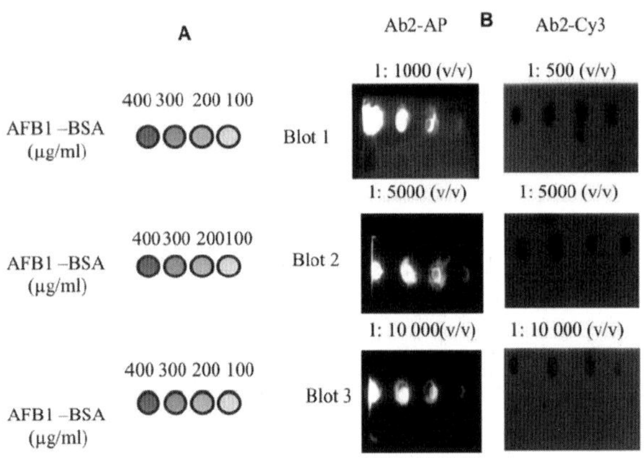

Figure 3. Primary antibody titration using dot blot. (A) The illustration of the spotted feature on each blot has been shown in cartoons. (B) Corresponding image of spotted blots. Three different dilutions of Mab were applied on each blot for immunoassay detection.

ants.

There are different issues that should be addressed for optimal microarray performance, e.g., the type of antibody molecules, solid supports and binding chemistries, detection system, blocking reagents, stability of printed antibodies, sensitivity and labeling strategies, specificity and cross-reactivity, immunoassay format, analysis of microarray data, and normalization (Parro, 2010). Considering all these factors looks challengeable and has made this technology complicated. Most of the microarray reagents and equipments (e.g., buffers, solid Supports, etc.) are expensive; therefore, the need to use an inexpensive method for initial optimizations prior to the actual microarray platform seems to be crucial. Dot blot is a simple technique to detect proteins. Thus, in an attempt to develop an antibody-based assay for detection of AFB_1 in microarray format, dot blot technique was applied for primary optimization. Different concentrations of AFB_1-BSA, monoclonal and secondary antibodies, sheep anti-mouse IgG-Cy3 conjugated (Ab2-Cy3), or goat anti mouse IgG-Alkaline phosphatase conjugate (Ab2-AP) (as internal control) were spotted in series of dilution to establish the optimum conditions for microarray layout. The concentration of 100μg/mL was selected as the optimal concentration for AFB_1-BSA, as it was the lowest concentration that was detectable using the optimized immunoassay. For positive internal controls, a 1:100 dilution of Mab (330μg/mL) and secondary antibodies (10μg/mL), was determined as optimal (Figure 1 and 3).

The type of antibody molecules (polyclonal-monoclonal, phage-display, Fab, affybodies, etc.) and detection systems, label-dependent (e.g. fluorescence, chemoluminiscence, enzymatic, etc.) or label free, always plays an important role for optimal antibody microarrays function. (Parro, 2010). Minimum antibody titers of 1:30 000 (1.1 μg/mL) of Mab and 1:5000 (0.2 μg/mL) for secondary antibodies were established as suitable dilutions for immunoassay. Ab2-AP was more sensitive than Ab2-Cy3 as 1:10 000 (0.1 μg /mL) of Ab2-Cy3 has made a

A

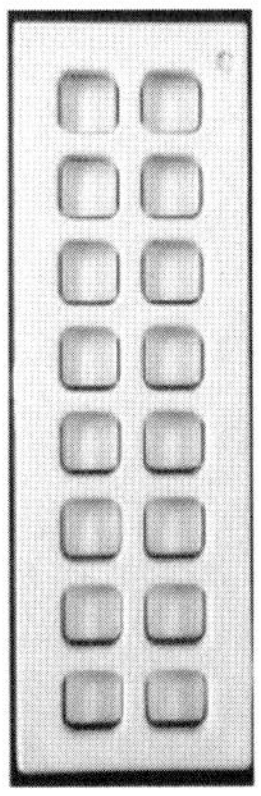

B

Anti-AFB1 Mab	Anti-AFB1 Mab	AFB1-BSA	AFB1-BSA	AFB1-BSA	AFB1-BSA
IgG-Cy3	IgG-Cy3	AFB1-BSA	AFB1-BSA	AFB1-BSA	AFB1-BSA
BSA 2%	BSA 2%	AFB1-BSA	AFB1-BSA	AFB1-BSA	AFB1-BSA
IgG-Cy3	IgG-Cy3	AFB1-BSA	AFB1-BSA	AFB1-BSA	AFB1-BSA

Figure 4. Image of a microarray chip. (A) An image of a Nitrocellulose coated slide containing 16 physically isolated subarrays assembled with reaction chamber has been shown. (B) A representing order of the layout of each subarray has been shown in table. Every subarray was consisted of two replicates of this printing layout.

weak signal but was strong enough for Ab2-AP. (Figure 2). For the final titration of monoclonal antibody, only Ab2-Cy3 was used because of the advantage of one step detection.

In all of the studies designed to detect mycotoxins, the LOD, which reflects sensitivity, is an important parameter e.g., the LOD of AFB_1 was 3.00 ng/ml using surface plasmon resonance (Daly et al., 2000), 12.5 ng/g by ELISA in food stuffs (Saha et al., 2007), 0.16 ng/mL by HPLC (Ghali et al., 2009) and 1.00 ng/mL using LC/APPI-MS/MS (Capriotti et al., 2010); 1 ng/mL by novel selective immunochromatographic assay (Zhang et al, 2011); and 1 mg/kg by lateral flow immunoassay (Anfossi et al., 2011).

In comparison with the current published methods for aflatoxin detection, the LOD of our developed method was 1 pg/mL, indicating the high sensitivity of developed assay, which is more sensitive than the currently available commercial methods. Total assay time was 3h, which indicates the rapid detection ability of the proposed method. The performance of the microarray assay in commodities was evaluated using spiked wheat flour samples. The sensitivity of this method was determined as 30 pg/g. The reduction of sensitivity in actual food samples is explainable by the effect of food matrices. Therefore, further investigation needs to be carried out to address this issue. A good recovery (98±11%) indicates the accuracy of the proposed assay for AFB1 detection in real food samples. In conclusion, microarray technology has the potential to be used as a screening tool for monitoring food samples on a large scale. Using this method, small quantities of reagents and samples are required. In addition, parallel assays can be performed for multiple analyses. Dot blot is a simple and inexpensive technique which confirms the presence or absence of a biomolecule. A successful dot blot optimization can be considered as a significant cost benefit step toward designing an effective microarray. Future work can focus on larger scale application of this method in commercial foodstuffs. In addition, this method could be extended to detect other foodborne hazards (such as food borne pathogens, bacterial toxins, chemicals, antibiotics residues, etc.) on a single chip format.

Acknowledgments

This study was supported by the Ministry of Science, Research, and Technology of Iran, the Research Council of University of Tehran and the facilities of Conway Institute of Biomedical and Bimolecular Research, University College Dublin, Dublin, Ireland.

References

1. Ammida, N.H.S., Micheli, L., Palleschi, G. (2004) Electrochemical immunosensor for determination of aflatoxin B_1 in barley. Anal Chim Acta. 520: 159-164.
2. Anfossi, L., D'Arco, G., Calderara, M., Baggiani, C., Giovannoli, C., Giraudi, G. (2011) Development of a quantitative lateral flow immunoassay for the

detection of aflatoxins in maize. Food Addit Contam. 28: 226-234.

3. Anklam E., Saroka J., Boenke A. (2002) Acceptance of analytical methods for implementation of EU legislation with a focus on mycotoxins. Food Control. 13: 173-183.
4. Bakirci, I. (2001) A study on the occurrence of aflatoxin M1 in milk and milk products produced in van province of Turkey. Food Control. 12: 47-51.
5. Bhattacharya, D., Bhattacharya, R., Dhar, T.K. (1999) A novel signal amplification technology for ELISA based on catalyzed reporter deposition. Demonstration of its applicability for measuring aflatoxin B1. J Immunol Methods. 230: 71-86.
6. Capriotti, A.L., Foglia, P., Gubbiotti, R., Roccia, C., Samperi, R., Lagana, A. (2010) Development and validation of a liquid chromatography/atmospheric pressure photoionization-tandem mass spectrometric method for the analysis of mycotoxins subjected to commission regulation (EC) No. 1881/2006 in cereals. J Chromatogr A. 1217: 6044-6051.
7. Daly, S.J., Keating, G.J., Dillon, P.P., Manning, B.M., O'Kennedy, R., Lee, H.A., Morgan, M.R.A. (2000) Development of surface Plasmon resonance-based immunoassay for aflatoxin B_1. J Agric Food Chem. 48: 5097-5104.
8. Daradimos, E., Marcaki, P., Koupparis, M. (2000) Evaluation and validation of two fluorometric HPLC methods for the determination of aflatoxin B1 in olive oil. Food Addit Contam. 17: 65-73.
9. Delmulle, B.S., De Saeger, S.M.D.G., Sibanda, L., Barna-Vetro, I., Van Peteghem, C.H. (2005) Development of an immunoassay-based lateral flow dipstick for the rapid detection of aflatoxin B_1 in pig feed. J Agric Food Chem. 53: 3364-3368.
10. Dunne, L., Daly, S., Baxter, A., Haughey, S., O'Kennedy, R. (2005) Surface plasmon resonance-based immunoassay for the detection of aflatoxin B1 using single-chain antibody fragments. Spectrosc Lett. 38: 229- 245.
11. Fare, T.L., Sandberg, R.G., Herzoge, D.P. (1996) Environmental Immunochemical Methods. Perspectives and Applications, American Chemical Society. Vanehmon, J.H., Gerlach, G.L. (eds.). Washington DC, USA.
12. Feldstein, M.J., Golden, J.P., Rowe, C.A. MacCraith, B.D., Ligler, F.S. (1999) Array biosensor: optical and fluidics systems. J Biomed Microdev. 1: 139-153.
13. Ghali, R., Belouaer, I., Hdiri, S., Ghorbel, H., Maaroufi, K., Hedilli, A. (2009) Simultaneous HPLC determination of aflatoxins B_1, B_2, G1 and G2 in Tunisian sorghum and pistachios. J Food Compos Anal. 22: 751-755.
14. Garden, S.R., Strachan, N.J.C. (2001) Novel colorimetric immunoassay for the detection of aflatoxin B_1. Anal Chim Acta. 444: 187-191.
15. International Agency for Research on Cancer (IARC). (2002) Aflatoxins in some naturally occurring substances: Food items and constituents, heterocyclic aromatic amines and mycotoxins. Mono-graphs on the evaluation of carcinogenic risk to humans, IARC, Lyon, France. p. 245-395.
16. Lamberti, I., Tanzarella, C., Solinas, I., Padula, C., Mosiello, L. (2009) An antibody-based microarray assay for simultaneous detection of aflatoxin B_1 and Fumonisin B_1. J Mycotox Res. 25: 193-200.
17. Lee, N.A., Wang, S., Allan, R.D., Kennedy, I.R. (2004) A rapid aflatoxin B_1 ELISA: development and validation with reduced matrix effects for peanuts, corn, pistachio and soybeans. J Agric Food Chem. 52: 2746-2755.
18. Li, P., Zhang, Q., Zhang, W., Zhang, J., Chen, X., Jiang, J., Xie, L., Zhang D. (2009) Development of a class-specific monoclonal antibody-based ELISA for aflatoxins in peanut. J Food Chem. 115: 313- 317.
19. Lopez, C., Ramos, L., Ramadan, S., Bulacio, L., Perez, J. (2001) Distribution of aflatoxin M1 in cheese obtained from milk artificially contaminated. Int J Food Microbiol. 64: 211-215.
20. Ngundi, M.M., Shriver-Lake, L.C., Moore, M.H., Lassman, M.E., Ligler, F.S., Taitt, C.R. (2005) Array biosensor for detection of ochratoxin A in cereals and beverages. Anal Chem. 77: 148-154.
21. Pal, A., Dhar, T.K. (2004) An analytical device for on-site immunoassay. Demonstration of its applicability in semiquantitative detection of aflatoxin B1 in a batch of samples with ultrahigh sensitivity. J Anal Chem. 76: 98-104.
22. Papp, E., H-Otta, K., Z´aray, G., Mincsovics, E. (2002) Liquid chromatographic determination of aflatoxins. Microchem J. 73: 39-46.
23. Parro, V. (2010) Antibody microarrays for environmental monitoring. In: Handbook of Hydracarbon and Lipid Microbiology. Timmis K.N. (ed). Springer-Verlag Berlin Heidelberg, Germany. p. 2700-2705.
24. Parkin, D.M., Bray, F., Ferlay, J., Pisani, P. (2001)

Estimating the world cancer burden: Globocan 2000. Int J Cancer. 94: 153-156.

25. Saha, D., Acharya, D., Roy, D., Dhar, T.K. (2007) Filtration-based tyramide amplification technique-a new simple approach for rapid detection of aflatoxin B_1. Anal Bioanal Chem. 387: 1121-1130.
26. Sapsford, K.E., Taitt, C.R., Loo, N., Ligler, F.S. (2005) Biosensor detection of Botulinum A toxoid and staphylococcal enterotoxin B in food. Appl Environ Microbiol. 71: 5590-5592.
27. Shriver-Lake, L.C., Shubin, Y.S., Ligler, F.S. (2003) Detection of staphylococcal enterotoxin B in spiked food samples. J Food Prot. 66: 1851-1856.
28. Shriver-Lake, L.C., Taitt, C.R., Ligler, F.S. (2004) Applications of array biosensor for detection of food allergens. JAOAC Int. 87: 1498-1502.
29. Speijers, G., Speijers, M. (2004) Combined toxic effects of mycotoxins. J Toxicol Lett. 153: 91-98.
30. Stroka, J., Anklam, E. (2002) New strategies for the screening and determination of aflatoxins and the detection of aflatoxin-producing moulds in foods and feed. Trends Anal Chem. 21: 90-95.
31. Sweeney, M.J., Dobson, A.D.W. (1998) Mycotoxin production by Aspergillus, Fusarium and Penicillium species. Int J Food Microbiol. 43: 141-158.
32. Taitt, C.R., Shubin, Y.S., Angel, R., Ligler, F.S. (2004a) Detection of *Salmonella enterica* serovar Typhimurium by using a rapid, array-based immunosensor. Appl Environ Microbiol. 70: 152-158.
33. Taitt, C.R., Golden, J.P., Shubin, Y.S., Shriver-Lake, L.C., Sapsford, K.E., Rasooly, A., Ligler, F.S. (2004b) A portable array biosensor for detecting multiple analytes in complex samples. Microbiol Ecol. 47: 175- 185.
34. Xiulan, S., Xiaolian, Z., Jian, T., Zhou, J., Chu, F.S. (2005) Preparation of gold-labeled antibody probe and its use in mmunochromatography assay for detection of aflatoxin B1. Int J Food Microbiol. 99: 185- 194.
35. Zhang, D., Li, P., Yang, Y., Zhang, Q., Zhang, W., Xiao, Z., Ding, X. (2011a) High selective immunochromatographic assay for rapid detection of aflatoxin B_1. Talanta. 85: 736-742.

Pneumonic pasteurellosis in a goat

Jesse Abdullah, F.F.[1,3*], Tijjani, A.[2,4], Adamu, L.[1,4], Teik Chung, E.L.[1], Abba, Y.[2,4], Mohammed, K.[1,4], Saharee, A.A.[1], Haron, A.W.[1,3], Sadiq, M.A.[2], Mohd, A.M.L.[2]

[1]*Department of Veterinary Clinical Studies, Faculty of Veterinary Medicine, Universiti Putra Malaysia, Serdang, Selangor, Malaysia*

[2]*Department of Veterinary Pathology and Microbiology, Faculty of Veterinary Medicine, Universiti Putra Malaysia, Serdang, Selangor, Malaysia*

[3]*Research Centre for Ruminant Disease, Faculty of Veterinary Medicine, Universiti Putra Malaysia, Serdang, Selangor, Malaysia*

[4]*Faculty of Veterinary Medicine, University of Maiduguri, Borno State, Nigeria*

Key words:
goat, *Pasteurella multocida*, pneumonic Pasteurellosis

Correspondence
Jesse Abdullah, F.F.
Department of Veterinary Clinical Studies, Faculty of Veterinary Medicine, Universiti Putra Malaysia, 43400 UPM Serdang, Selangor, Malaysia

Email: jesseariasamy@gmail.com

Abstract:

A 3-year-old goat weighing 40 kg was presented to the Large Animal Unit, University Veterinary Hospital, Universiti Putra Malaysia with complains of in appetence, lateral recumbency, and weakness. Physical examination findings were pyrexia, tachycardia, tachypnea, and pale mucous membrane. Harsh and crackles lung sound was noticed upon auscultation. The case was tentatively diagnosed as pneumonic pasteurellosis, and the goat was treated with broad spectrum antibiotic, non-steroidal anti-inflammatory drug (NSAID), and fluid therapy. The prognosis of this case was guarded and the goat died on day after hospitalization and post mortem examination was carried out. Samples were taken from the lungs, heart, and pericardial fluid for bacterial isolation and identification. The post mortem findings were consolidations of the left and right craniolateral lung lobes, frothy exudates along the trachea, bronchi and the cut surface of the lungs and presence of straw-colored pericardial fluid. The bacterial culture yielded *Pasteurella multocida* growth from all the samples. Based on the clinical signs, post mortem findings, and bacteriology result, this case was finally diagnosed as pneumonic pasteurellosis.

Case History

Pneumonic pasteurellosis is one of the most important economically infectious diseases of ruminants with a wide prevalence throughout the continents. The disease is characterized by an acute febrile course with severe fibrinous or fibrino-purulent bronchopneumonia, fibrinous pleurisy, and septicaemia (Mohammed and Abdelsalam, 2008). *M. haemolytica*, *P. trehalosi*, and *P. multocida* are common commensal organisms of the tonsils and nasopharynx of healthy sheep and goats. They are non-motile gram-negative rods that cause cranioventral bronchopneumonia affecting sheep and goats of all ages worldwide (Cynthia and Scott, 2012). Infections from these pathogens are associated with poor management practices and occur as a secondary infection or as a consequence of severe stress. Transportation stress, viral infections, overcrowded pens, poor housing conditions, sudden environmental changes, and other stressful conditions increase goats' susceptibility to *P. multocida* and *M. haemolytica* pneumonias (Maria, 2007).

Drugs such as penicillin, ampicillin, tetracycline, oxytetracycline, tylosin, florfenicol, and ceftiofur have been reported to be effective in the treatment of pneumonia in goats (Maria, 2007). Vaccination is the best form of control of the disease. Effective vaccine such as alum precipitated and oil adjuvant vaccines have been developed (Chandrasekaran et al., 1994; Myint and Jones 2007). Recently, recombinant DNA vaccines that confer significant protection and antibody response in goat have been reported (Ina-Salwany, 2011; Sabri et al., 2013).

Clinical presentations

A 3-year-old male Jamnapari goat weighing 40 kg was managed semi-intensively and was presented to the University Veterinary Hospital, Universiti Putra Malaysia with complaints of inappetence and weakness. The goat was on lateral recumbency as at the time of presentation. The owner reported to have noticed the condition for the past three days and presented the case to the hospital when he realized the condition of the goat was deteriorating.

Physical examination findings were pyrexia, tachycardia, and tachypnea. The mucous membrane was pale with capillary refill time and skin tenting of more than 2 seconds. The goat was having abdominal breathing with harsh and crackles lung sound upon auscultation.

Post mortem findings for this goat were consolidations of the left and right craniolateral lung lobes (Figure 2). In addition, we noticed froth along the trachea, bronchi, and cut surface of the lung (Figure 3). Also, the presence of straw-colored pericardial fluid was observed (Figure 4). Based on the clinical signs, post mortem findings, and bacteriology result, this case was finally diagnosed as pneumonic Pasteurellosis.

Diagnostic Testing

Swab samples of the lungs, heart, and pericardial fluid were aseptically collected and sent to the bacteriology laboratory of the Faculty of Veterinary Medicine, Universiti Putra Malaysia for bacteriological isolation and identification. The samples were cultured on 5% horse blood agar and McConkey agar at 37°C for 24 hours. Bacterial identification was done using gram staining and biochemical characterization according to the methods of Carter (1990). Oxidase, urea broth, Sulphur Indole Motility (SIM), Triple Sugar Iron (TSI), and citrate test were performed. *Pasteurella multocida* was isolated from all the samples submitted to the laboratory.

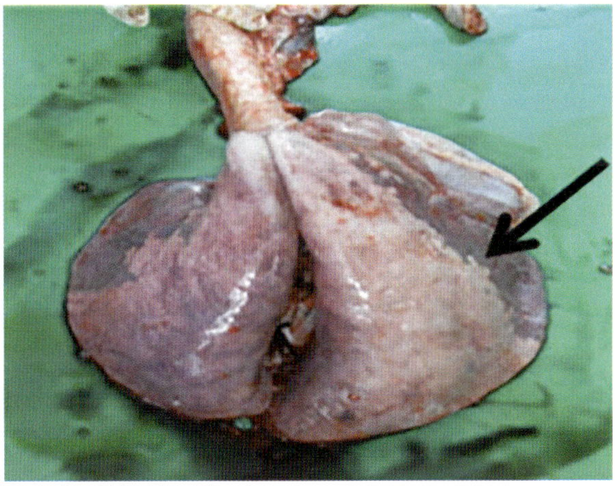

Figure 1. Showed consolidation of the Left and Right craniolateral lung lobes.

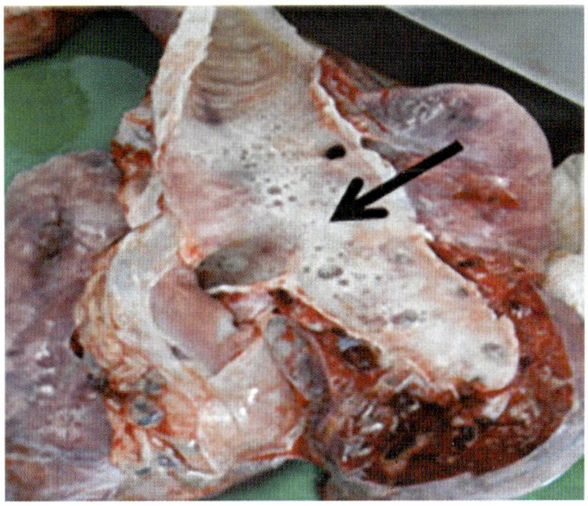

Figure 2. Showed froth along the trachea, bronchi, and cut surface of the lungs.

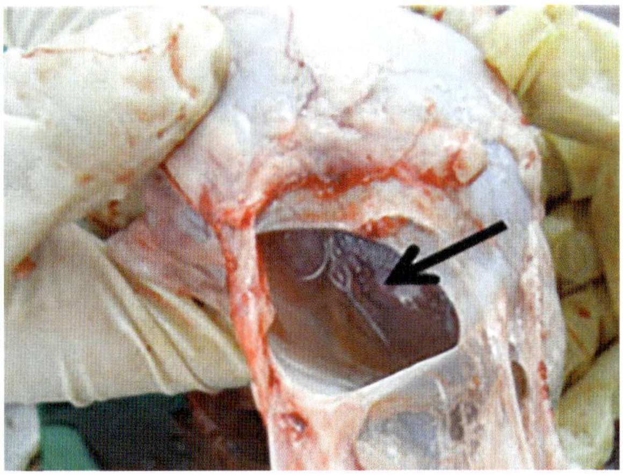

Figure 3. Showed the presence of straw-color pericardial fluid in pericardium.

Swab samples of the lungs, heart, and pericardial fluid were aseptically collected and sent to the bacteriology laboratory of the Faculty of Veterinary Medicine, Universiti Putra Malaysia for bacteriological isolation and identification. The samples were cultured on 5% horse blood agar and McConkey agar at 37 ^{o}C for 24 hours. Bacterial identification was done using gram staining and biochemical characterization according to the methods of Carter (1990). Oxidase, urea broth, Sulphur Indole Motility (SIM), Triple Sugar Iron (TSI), and citrate test were performed. *Pasteurella multocida* was isolated from all the samples submitted to the laboratory (This paragraph is a repetition of the paragraph above).

The prognosis of this case was guarded, and the goat died one day after hospitalization and post mortem examination was carried out.

Based on the clinical presentation and physical examination findings, the case was tentatively diagnosed as pneumonic pasteurellosis. The treatment plan for this goat were Norodine 24 (Trimethoprim 2.5g and sulfadiazine 12.5g) (1 mL/ 16 kg) injection intravenously (I/V) for 3 days as broad spectrum antibiotic, Flunixine meglumine (2.2 mg/kg), intravenously (I/V) for 2 days as anti-inflammatory and analgesic, coupled 0.9% sodium chloride fluid therapy intravenously to replenish the dehydration status of the goat.

Assessments

The present case was diagnosed as pneumonic pasteurellosis based on the clinical presentations, post mortem results, and bacterial culture findings. The clinical signs of inappetence, weakness, pyrexia, and harsh and crackles lung sound corroborates the reports of Zamri et al. (1994) who reported similar clinical signs in an experimental infection of goats with *Mannheimia haemolytica* A2. The present case can be said to be an acute form of the disease as it has been reported that the disease in goats can manifest in acute, sub-acute, or chronic form (Zamri et al., 1996). The post mortem findings of consolidation of the lung lobes, frothy exudates in the trachea, bronchi, and lung surfaces coupled with straw-colored pericardial fluids depict the postmortem case definition of pneumonic Pasteurellosis by the FAO (2010). The reports of isolation of *Pasteurella multocida* in the lungs from cases of pneumonic Pasteurellosis in the abattoir and in outbreaks of the disease (Momin et al., 2011; Sadhukan et al., 2011, Salaheden and Hanan, 2012; Marru et al., 2013) affirms the isolation of the same organism from the lungs, heart, and pericardial fluids in the present case. The bacteria have been reported to be a normal flora of the nasopharynx in healthy sheep and goats (Cynthia and Scott, 2012). Stress factors such as transportation, concurrent infections, overcrowding, poor housing, and sudden environmental changes increase goats susceptibility to pneumonic pasteurellosis (Maria, 2007). The administration of Norodine in the present case is in line with that of Maria (2007) who reported that antibiotics such as penicillin, ampicillin, tetracycline, oxytetracycline, tylosin, florfenicol, and ceftiofur were effective in the treatment of pneumonia in goats. Vaccines have been developed for the control of pneumonic pasteurellosis. These include alum precipitated and oil adjuvant vaccines (Chandrasekaran et al., 1994; Myint and Jones 2007). Recently, recombinant vaccine for Mannheimiosis have been developed which was reported to substantially reduce incidence of the disease in Malaysia (Sabri et al., 2013).

In conclusion, pneumonic pasteurellosis is one of the important and devastating diseases in sheep and goats. The disease is caused either by *Mannheimia haemolytica* or *Pasteurella multocida*, and it causes great economic losses to small ruminant industry worldwide. Prevention via vaccination and control of stress factors are the best ways to prevent this disease.

Acknowledgements

The authors wish to offer their gratitude to En Nazim Razali Kanini, En Mohd Jefri and Mr. Velloo of University Veterinary Hospital (UVH), and Faculty of Veterinary Medicine Universiti Putra Malaysia for their technical assistance.

References

1. Carter, R.G. (1990) Isolation and Identification of bacteria from clinical specimens. In: Diagnostic Procedures in Veterinary Bacteriology and Mycology. Carter, G.R., Cole, J.R. (eds.). (5th ed.) Academic press Inc., San Diego, California, USA.
2. Chandrasekaran, S., Kennett, L., Yeap, P.C., Muniandy, N., Rani, B., Mukkur, T.K.S. (1994)

Characterization of immune response andduration of protection in buffaloes immunized with haemorrhagic septicaemia vaccine. Vet Microbiol. 41: 213-219.

3. Cynthia, M.K., Scott, L. (2012) Pasteurellosis of sheep and goats. In: Merck Veterinary Manual, Merck Sharp & Dohme Corp. Whitehouse Station, N.J., USA.
4. FAO. (2010) Case definition of livestock diseases. In: Report of the Food and Agriculture Organization (FAO) of the United Nations, Disaster Response and Rehabilitation Unit (DRRU) Addis Ababa, Ethiopia, accessed 26/1/2014: www.fao.org/world/ethiopia.
5. Ina-Salwany, M.Y., Sabri, M.Y., Zamri-Saad, M., Effendy, A.W.M. (2011) Efficacy of an inactivated recombinant vaccine encoding a fimbrial protein of PasteurellamultocidaB: 2 against hemorrhagic septicemia in goats. Trop Anim Health Prod. 43: 179-187.
6. Maria, L. (2007) Bacterial Pneumonia in Goats. In: Alabama Cooperative Extension System online publication. www.aces.edu/urban. accessed 26/1/2014.
7. Marru, H.D., Anijajo, T.T., Hassen, A.A. (2013) A study on Ovine pneumonic pasteurellosis: Isolation and Identification of Pasteurellae and their antibiogram susceptibility pattern in Haramaya District, Eastern Hararghe, Ethiopia. BMC (Biomed Central) Vet Res. 9: 239.
8. Mohammed, R.A., Abdelsalam, E.B. (2008) A review on pneumonic pasteurellosis (respiratory mannheimiosis) with emphasis on pathogens virulence mechanisms and predisposing factors. Bulg J Vet Med. 11: 139-160.
9. Momin, M.A., Islam, M.A., Khatun, M.M., Rahman, M.M., Islam, M.A. (2011). Characterization of Bacteria Associated with Pneumonia in Black BengalGoats. Bangl J Vet Med. 9: 67 - 71
10. Myint, A., Jones, T.O. (2007) Efficacy of haemorrhagicsepticaemiaalum precipitated vaccine, Vet Rec. 160: 172.
11. Sabri, M.Y., Shahrom-Salisi, M., Emikpe, B.O. (2013) Comparison prior and post vaccination of inactivated recombinant vaccine against mannheimiosis in Boer Goats Farm in Sabah. J Vaccines Vaccin. 4:1.
12. Sadhukhan, T.K., Dutta, T.K. (2010) Investigation of an outbreak of pneumonic pasteurellosis in water buffaloes in West Bengal associated with fimbriated *Pasteurella multocida*. Indian J Comp Microbiol Immunol Infect Dis. 31: 37-40.
13. Salaheddin, O.H., Hanan, M.E. (2012) Pneumonia in Goats in Sudan. Int J Anim Vet Adv. 4: 144-145.
14. Sirous, S., Mohammed, R.M.D., Gholam, A.K., Taghi, T.B., Abbas, T. (2011) *Pasteurella multocida* pneumonic infection in goat: Hematological, biochemical, clinical and pathological studies. Small Rum Res. 100: 189-194.
15. Zamri-Saad, M., Azri, A., Nurida, A.B., Sheikh-Omar, A.R. (1994) Experimental Respiratory Infection of Goats with *Mycoplasma arginini* and *Pasteurella haemolytica* A2. J Trop Agric Sci. 17: 239-242.
16. Zamri-Saad, M., Effendy, W.M., Maswati, M.A., Salim, N., Sheikh-Omar, A.R. (1996) The goat as a model for studies of pneumonic pasteurellosis caused by *Pasteurella multocida*. Br Vet J. 152: 453-458.

The efficacy of a poultry commercial anticoccidial vaccine in experimental challenge with *Eimeria* field isolates

Arabkhazaeli, F.[1], Nabian, S.[1*], Modirsanei, M.[2], Madani, S.A.[3]

[1] *Department of Parasitology, Faculty of Veterinary Medicine, University of Tehran, Tehran, Iran*

[2] *Department of Animal and Poultry Health and Nutrition, Faculty of Veterinary Medicine, University of Tehran, Tehran, Iran*

[3] *Department of Avian Diseases, Faculty of Veterinary Medicine, University of Tehran, Tehran, Iran*

Key words:
anticoccidial vaccine, coccidiosis, efficacy, poultry *Eimeria*

Correspondence
Nabian, S.
Department of Parasitology, Faculty of Veterinary Medicine, University of Tehran, Tehran, Iran

Email: nabian@ut.ac.ir

Abstract:

BACKGROUND: The control of coccidiosis in poultry industry is dominated by prophylactic chemotherapy; however, drug resistance is a serious problem. Alternative control methods such as vaccination have been accepted as a practical method for controlling coccidiosis in chickens. Considering the immunological variation of *Eimeria* strains, the efficacy of live coccidiosis vaccines may be compromised. **OBJECTIVES:** To evaluate the efficacy of a commercial anticoccidial vaccine in poultry, vaccination was followed by experimental challenge with 3 *Eimeria* field isolates. **METHODS:** The efficacy of Livacox® Q anticoccidial vaccine was evaluated on male broiler chicks, reared in battery cages. Different factors including weight gain, FCR, OPG (oocysts per gram of feces) and intestinal lesion scores were assessed. **RESULTS:** Vaccinated challenged groups (VC) gained less weight than the un-vaccinated un-challenged (UVUC) birds ($p \leq 0.05$). Fourteen days post-challenge, the weight gain of VC groups challenged with isolate 2 differed significantly from its un-vaccinated challenged (UVC) counterpart; however, there were no significant differences in weight gain of groups challenged by isolates 1 and 3 with their respective UVC groups. Lesion score and FCR were significantly improved in VC groups comparing with their associated UVC groups ($p \leq 0.05$). Lesion score and FCR were significantly improved in VC groups comparing with their UVC counterparts ($p \leq 0.05$). **CONCLUSIONS:** The present study suggests that the use of live anticoccidial vaccine has the potential for improving live weight gains and FCR; nonetheless, immunity to local *Eimeria* species should be evaluated separately and in trial designs it should be more approximate to the actual field condition.

Introduction

Avian coccidiosis, caused by the substantial replication of seven species of coccidian parasites belonging to the genus *Eimeria*, is a major parasitic disease within the intensively reared poultry (Shirley & Bedrnik 1997; Allen & Fetterer 2002). Coccidiosis is considered as one of the commonest pernicious diseases of poultry and costs the world's commercial chicken producers at least US$ 1.5 billion every year (Yadav & Gupta 2001). The intensive use of anti-coccidial drugs which has led to the development of resistance and the public concern of chemical residues in poultry products and pollution of the environment has stimulated research for alternative control methods such as applying a vaccine early in life or development of new drugs (Barriga 1994; Chapman 1997; Li et al., 2004; De Pablos et al., 2010; Yim et al., 2010). The first commercial anticoccidial vaccine, CocciVac®, which is a live vaccine comprising several wild-type strains of *E. tenella* (*E. t*) oocysts, was introduced to the US market in 1952 (Shirley & Bedrnik 1997). Attenuated vaccines are produced mainly by either passaging through embryonated eggs, such as *E. t* in Livacox® vaccines, or by selection for precocity, such as the other species of Livacox vaccines and the Paracox® vaccines (Rami & Lillehoj 2006). Live vaccines comprising attenuated or virulent oocysts of various *Eimeria* species have offered a practical alternative to anticoccidial drugs for the sustainable control of coccidiosis in chickens, and in fact several such vaccines have been commercially available in the world market. However, *Eimeria* sp. induces solid immunity to homologous challenge and immune variation, as documented in *Eimeria maxima* (*E. ma*), may provide the basis for the lack of cross protective immunity among geographically isolated strains (Williams 1998; Chapman et al., 2002; Allen et al., 2005; McDonald & Shirley 2009). The degree of heterologous protection by a given vaccine may be addressed by obtaining local samples from where the vaccine is intended for use, and carrying out cross protection studies with the candidate vaccine lines. The aim of this study was to assess the efficacy of a commercial live attenuated vaccine available and widely used in poultry industry in Iran in terms of weight gain, feed conversion ratio, oocyst per gram of feces, and lesion score in experimentally infected chickens with three representative local mixed *Eimeria* field isolates.

Materials and Methods

Calculation of infectious dose. Three mixed isolates with a known biopathogenecity (Arabkhazaeli et al., 2011) were used as domestic poultry *Eimeria* isolates briefly containing 12% *E. acervulina* (*E. a*), 16% *E. brunetti* (*E. b*), 44% *E. ma*, 12% *E. mitis* (*E. mi*), 12% *E. t* and 4% *E. necatrix* (*E. n*) in isolate 1, 24% *E. a*, 6% *E. b*, 34% *E. ma*, 16% *E.* mi, 18% *E. t* and 2% *E. n* in isolate 2 and for isolate 3 containing 40% *E. a*, 15% *E. b*, 25% *E. ma*, 8% *E. mi*, 6% *E. t* and 6% *E. n*.

Based on observations during propagation, the challenge dose of the three selected farm isolates were estimated as following: for isolates 1 and 2, originating from Mazandaran province, 300000 sporulated oocyst per bird and for isolate 3, from Hamedan province, 250000 sporulated oocyst per bird.

Animals and husbandry. Two hundred and forty male one-day-old Ross308 broiler chicks were assigned by a randomized procedure to 8 groups of approximately equalized initial weights. Each group contained 30 chicks, comprising of three replicates of 10 and kept in battery cages. The birds were leg tagged so that individual data could be recorded. They were provided with a diet based on corn and soybean meal, which has been formulated to meet or exceed all required nutrients for the birds (NRC, 1994), and food and water were provided ad-libitum throughout the experimental period.

Vaccination and Challenge inocula. One hundred and twenty birds were orally inoculated with Livacox Q® (Biopharm, Research Institute of Biopharmacy and Veterinary Drugs, Czech Republic) at 3rd day of age, according to the manufacturer's recommendation. The control group received PBS orally. The infectious dose was given orally on the 14th day of age (10 days post-vaccination) to one hundred and eighty birds. A group of 30 chicks was allocated as uninfected unvaccinated negative control (Table 1).

Evaluation of the vaccine efficacy. Data regarding weight gain (WG), feed intake (FI), lesion score (LS), oocysts index (OI), and mortality were recorded in a 7-day period after inoculation of the infectious dose. Feed conversion ratio (FCR) was calculated (Daugschies et al., 1998; Conway et al., 2007; Arabkhazaeli et al., 2011).

On the 7th day post-inoculation, 9 birds from each group were selected for post-mortem examination and intestinal lesion score for a mixed infection, according to Conway and McKenzie (2007). Faecal examination was conducted daily up to 10 days post-challenge, and number of oocyst per gram of droppings was calculated by using the McMaster counting technique (Ryley et al., 1976).

Statistical analysis. All data were subjected to

ANOVA and two way t-test to see whether the differences between groups are significant. Differences among means were considered significant at $p<0.05$.

Results

There were significant differences in weight gain between unvaccinated-challenged (UVC) and unvaccinated- unchallenged (UVUC) groups for each isolates. These results confirm that the challenge dose was sufficient. The results are summarized in table 1. The vaccinated unchallenged (VUC) birds' weight gain, lesion score, and FCR were not significantly different ($p\leq0.05$) from those of the control group (UVUC). Expectedly vaccinated challenged (VC) groups gained less weight than the UVUC birds ($p\leq0.05$). Seven days post-challenge weight gain of the VC groups challenged with isolates 1 and 2 were significantly more than their respective unvaccinated challenged (UVC) counterparts. In VC groups challenged with isolate 3, weight gain was not significant caompared to the related UVC group ($p\leq0.05$). Fourteen days post-challenge, the weight gain of VC groups challenged with isolates 1 and 3 did not differ significantly from their UVC counterparts. However, there was significant difference in weight gain of groups challenged by isolate 2 ($p\leq0.05$).

FCR were significantly improved in VC groups comparing with their respective UVC groups ($p<0.05$). The best FCR was calculated for UVUC group which was not significantly different from the FCR of the VUC group ($p\leq0.05$).

The VUC group showed the lowest lesion score and VC groups had lower lesion scores comparing to their related UVC cgroups ($p\leq0.05$).

OPG results were inconclusive (Fig. 1). Although numerically the UVC groups had higher OPG, there were no significant differences among the groups ($p\leq0.05$).

No mortality was observed during the experiment. Our results about growth factors showed a coordination with apparent clinical sings in three UVC groups challenged with three different isolates. Accordingly, clinical signs as morbidity, emaciation, and diarroeha were more severe in UVC challenged with isolate 3.

Table 1. Effect of immunization† and subsequent‡ challenge with local *Eimeria* field isolates on the performance of birds kept in battery cages. A VC1, VC2 & VC3: Vaccinated and Challenged by isolate 1, 2 & 3, respectively; UVC1, UVC2 & UVC3: Unvaccinated and Challenged by isolate 1, 2 & 3, respectively; UVUC: Unvaccinated and Un-Challenged; FCR: Food conversion Ratio (Mean food consumption/Mean weight); SEM: Standard Error of Means; a-h: Means followed by different letters are significantly different ($p<0.05$). B Mean weight gain (7 days post-challenge). C Mean weight gain (14 days post-challenge). † Male broiler chicks orally inoculated with Livacox Q® at 3rd day of age. ‡ The infectious dose (3.0×10^5 oocyst/bird for isolates 1 &2 and 2.5×10^5 oocyst/bird for isolate 3) was given orally to the challenged birds on 14th day of age.

Group	Treatment A	mean weight gain ± (g) (mean±SEM)		FCR	Lesion score
		7B	14C		
1	VC1	268.7 ± 7.6^{b}	719.0 ± 17.4^{bc}	1.8^{bc}	1^{b}
2	VC2	246.0 ± 9.7^{bc}	758.4 ± 46.8^{ab}	1.9^{d}	0.7^{b}
3	VC3	151.9 ± 8.9^{e}	610.3 ± 25.7^{d}	2.5^{f}	1.7^{c}
4	VUC	340.0 ± 7.9^{a}	789.3 ± 24.5^{ab}	1.7^{ab}	0.2^{a}
5	UVC1	237.0 ± 9.8^{c}	648.5 ± 25.5^{cd}	2.0^{e}	1.8^{c}
6	UVC2	205.6 ± 8.0^{d}	669.0 ± 27.1^{cd}	2.0^{e}	1.5^{c}
7	UVC3	145.3 ± 8.9^{e}	612.0 ± 20.2^{d}	2.7^{g}	2.3^{d}
8	UVUC	349.6 ± 10.9^{a}	816.2 ± 28.5^{a}	1.6^{a}	0^{a}

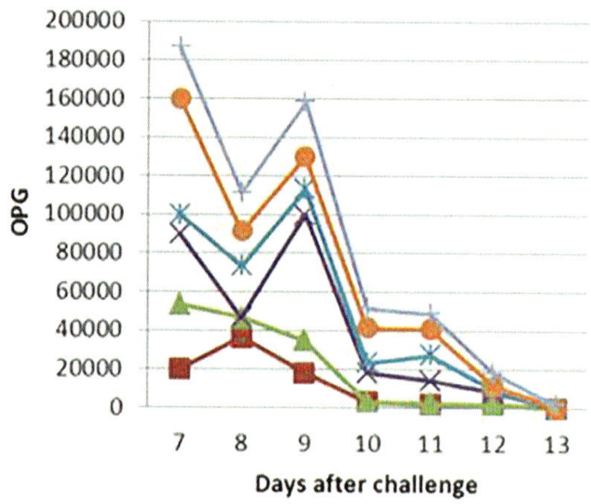

Figure 1. Effect of immunization and subsequent challenge with local *Eimeria* field isolates on oocyst per gram of feces (OPG) of birds vaccinated with Livacox®. VC1, VC2 & VC3: Vaccinated and Challenged by isolate 1, 2 & 3, respectively; UVC1, UVC2 & UVC3: Unvaccinated and Challenged by isolate 1, 2 & 3, respectively. — UVC3 —●— UVC2 —✱— UVC1 —✕— VC3 —▲— VC2 —■— VC1

Discussion

Many laboratory and experimental studies have demonstrated that a live multivalent vaccine induces a strong immunity to challenge with virulent homologous or heterologous *Eimeria* strains in chickens (Martin et al., 1997; Li et al., 2004). Immune-variation in five strains of *E. ma* taken from different geographical areas of North America indicated that vaccination with a given suspension of oocysts may not be effective in protecting against field strains in different geographical locations (Danforth 1998). To assess the degree of heterologous protection by a vaccine line, researchers should test local samples in cross protection studies (Chapman et al., 2005).

In this research, the efficacy of a live multivalent anticoccidial vaccine was tested on performance of broilers (male Ross308) reared in battery cages in response to challenge with three local *Eimeria* field isolates. The present study suggests that the use of live attenuated anticoccidial vaccines has the partial potential to relatively improve live weight gains and FCR; although none of the immunized birds had significantly higher average weight gains than the UVUC group for the entire experiment, VC group challenged by isolate 2 had a significant higher weight gain than the analogous UVC group and comparable weight gain to the UVUC group showing that the vaccinated birds were immune to the virulent challenge (Table 1).

On the subject of criteria for evaluating vaccine efficacy, it has been previously reported that unlike lesion score, the criterion of weight gain during seven days following challenge with virulent coccidia strains and the numerical results of FCR calculations can provide definitive evidence for the degree of the bird immunity (Williams & Catchpole 2000). Whilst the absence of lesions following virulent challenge of a vaccinated bird may be taken as evidence for protection against coccidiosis in parasitological terms, the presence of lesions does not necessarily indicate a lack of protection (Williams & Catchpole 2000). As seen with our results, the lesion scores of all VC groups were significantly different from their related UVC counterparts which may be inferred as protection efficacy of the vaccination; however, weight gains of the unvaccinated groups challenged with isolates 1 and 3, 14 days post-challenge shows compromised vaccine efficacy.

Based on oocyst count, no conclusion could be inferred. Although the absolute numbers varied among the groups, the pattern of oocyst production remained consistent overall. Oocyst production is affected by various factors including the inherent potential of each species to reproduce; the 'crowding' factor; competition with other species of coccidia or other infectious agents; nutrition of the host and genetic differences in strains of parasites (Fayer 1980; Chapman et al., 2002), hence oocyst counting alone for assessing immunity in chicks, whilst proving to be a sensitive method of detecting maternally transferred antibodies, is inappropriate for demonstrating protection against clinical coccidiosis (Williams & Catchpole 2000).

Livacox® Q is a quadrivalent live attenuated coccidiosis vaccine containing the economically important *Eimeria* species, namely: *Eimeria acervulina*, *E. ma*, *E. tenella* and *E. n* all of which were identified in domestic isolates used in this study (Arabkhazaeli et al., 2011). According to the manufacturer, the vaccine is applicable to layer and breeder chickens raised both on litter and in cages; however, birds must have access to the droppings as a reservoir of attenuated coccidian oocysts as booster antigen. Apparently, birds reared in cages with wire-mesh floors have limited exposure to fecal material, little opportunity for auto-reinfection and do not develop full immunity (Chapman et al., 2005). Despite this fact, based on FCR, the vaccine prevented adverse effects of challenge with the three tested isolates; however, based on weight gain, it was not fully effective against isolates 1 and 3 which may be due to immune variation of vaccine strains and challenge isolates. Since immunized chickens were challenged with multiple *Eimeria* species as a mixture, it was impossible to determine which one or more of the species, included in the challenge dose, adversely affected vaccine efficiency. Such experiences provide good reason for assessing immunity to each *Eimeria* species separately (Williams & Catchpole 2000).

Drug resistance and a relatively short life span (40-45 days) in raising broiler chickens has forced certain withdrawal periods for the safety of consumers. Such concerns have made vaccination an applicable practice in poultry industry. However, the degree of heterologous protection by a given vaccine should be evaluated in a given geographical region. The present study suggests that the use of live attenuated anticoccidial vaccine has the potential to partially improve live weight gains and FCR; nevertheless, immunity to local *Eimeria* species should be evaluated separately and in trial design more approximate to the actual field condition.

Acknowledgements

The authors would like to thank the faculty of Veterinary Medicine, University of Tehran, for funding the project number 7506009/6/8 and thank Dr. Rahbari for his valuable comments.

References

1. Allen, P.C., Fetterer, R.H. (2002) Recent advances in biology and immunobiology of *Eimeria* species and in diagnosis and control of infection with these coccidian parasites of poultry. Clin Microbiol Rev. 15: 58-65.
2. Allen, P.C., Jenkins, M.C., Misjka, K.B. (2005) Cross protection studies with *Eimeria maxima* strains. Parasitol Res. 97: 179-185.
3. Arabkhazaeli, F., Nabian, S., Modirsaneii, M., Mansoori, B., Rahbari, S. (2011) Biopathologic characterization of three mixed poultry *Eimeria* spp. isolates. Iran J Parasitol. 6: 23-32.
4. Barriga, O.O. (1994) A review on vaccination against protozoa and arthropoda of veterinary importance, Vet Parasitol. 55: 29-55.
5. Chapman, H.D. (1997) Biochemical, genetic and applied aspects of drug resistance in *Eimeria* parasites of the fowl, Avian pathol. 26: 221-244.
6. Chapman, H.D., Cherry, T.E., Danforth, H.D., Richards, G., Shirley, M.W., Williams, R.B. (2002) Sustainable coccidiosis control in poultry production: the role of live vaccines. Int J Parasitol. 32: 617-629.
7. Chapman, H.D., Roberts, B., Shirley, M.W., Williams, R.B. (2005) Guidelines for evaluating the efficacy and safety of live anticoccidial vaccines, and obtaining approval for their use in chickens and turkeys, Avian Pathol. 34: 279-290.
8. Conway, D.P., McKenzie, M.E. (2007) Poultry Coccidiosis Diagnosis and Testing Procedures. (3rd ed.) Blackwell publishing, Iowa, USA.
9. Danforth, H.D. (1998) Use of live oocyst vaccines in the control of avian coccidiosis experimental studies and field trials, Int J Parasitol. 28: 1099-1109.
10. Daugschies, A., Gässlein, U., Rommel, M. (1998) Comparative efficacy of anticoccidials under the conditions of commercial broiler production and in battery trials. Vet Parasitol. 76: 163-171.
11. De Pablos, L.M., dos Sontos, M.F., Montero, E., Garcia-Garnados, A., Parra, A., Osuna, A. (2010) Anticoccidial activity of maslinic acid against infection with *Eimeria* tenella in chickens, Parasitol Res. 107: 601-604.
12. Fayer, R. (1980) Epidemiology of protozoan infections: the coccidian. Vet Parasitol. 6: 75-103.
13. Li, G.Q., Kanu, S., Xiang, F.Y., Xiao, S.M., Zhang, L., Chen, H.W., Ye, H.J. (2004) Isolation and selection of ionophore-tolerant *Eimeria* precocious lines: *E.tenella*, *E.maxima*, and *E.acervulina*. Vet Parasitol. 119: 261-276.
14. Martin, A.G., Danforth, H.D., Barta, J.R., Fernando, M.A. (1997) Analysis of immunological cross-protection and sensitivities to anticoccidial drugs among five geographical and temporal strains of *Eimeria maxima*. Int J Parasitol. 27: 523-534.
15. McDonald, V., Shirley, M.W. (2009) Past and future: vaccination against *Eimeria*. J Parasitol. 136: 1477-1489, DOI: 10.1017/S0031182009006349.
16. Nutrient Requirements of Poultry (1994) National Academy Press. (9th ed.) Washington DC, USA.
17. Dalloul, R.A., Lillehoj, H.S. (2006) Poultry coccidiosis: recent advances in control measures and vaccine development, Expert Rev Vaccines. 5: 143-163.
18. Shirley, M.W., Bedrník, P. (1997) Live attenuated vaccines against avian coccidiosis: Success with precocious and egg-adapted lines of *Eimeria*, Parasitol Today. 13: 481-484.
19. Williams, R.B., Catchpole, J. (2000) A new protocol for a challenge test to assess the efficacy of live anticoccidial vaccines for chickens, Vaccine. 18: 1178-1185.
20. Williams, R.B. (1998) Epidemiological aspects of the use of live anticoccidial vaccines for chickens. Int J Parasitol. 28: 1089-1098.
21. Yadav, A., Gupta, S.K. (2001) Study of resistance against some ionophores in *Eimeria tenella* field isolates. Vet Parasitol. 102: 69-75.
22. Yim, D., Kang, S.S., Kim, D.W., Kim, S.H., Lillehoj, H.S., Min, W. (2011) Protective effects of Aloe vera-based diets in *Eimeria maxima*-infected broiler chickens, Exp Parasitol. 127: 322-325.

A case of perosomus elumbis concurrent with visceral abnormalities in a Holstein calf

Eslami, M.[1], Gharagozloo, F.[2*], Rahimi Feyli, P.[3], Vojgani, M.[2], Soroori, S.[4]

[1]Department of Theriogenology and Poultry, Faculty of Veterinary Medicine, University of Urmia, Urmia, Iran

[2]Department of Theriogenology, Faculty of Veterinary Medicine, University of Tehran, Tehran, Iran

[3]Department of Clinical Sciences, Faculty of Veterinary Medicine, Razi University, Kermanshah, Iran

[4]Department of Surgery and Radiology, Faculty of Veterinary Medicine, University of Tehran, Tehran, Iran

Key words:
congenital abnormality, Holstein calf, perosomus elumbis, vertebral column

Correspondence
Gharagozloo, F.
Department of Theriogenology,
Faculty of Veterinary Medicine,
University of Tehran, Tehran, Iran

Email: faramarz@ut.ac.ir

Abstract:

Perosomus elumbis is an occasional congenital anomaly of cattle, swine, sheep, and dogs with unknown etiology. This congenital abnormality occurs in both sexes. A dead Holstein calf characterized by musculoskeletal and external genitalia abnormalities was referred to the large animal hospital of University of Tehran. Radiographic evaluation and subsequent dissection revealed that the vertebral column was truncated at the level of first lumbar vertebra (L1). Moreover, L2-L5, sacrum and coccygeal vertebrae were absent. The dorsum of the lumbosacral region contained only soft tissues. Urogenital tract was incomplete, and it contained agenesis of the ovaries, uterine tubes, cervix, and vulva concurrent with unilateral umbilical artery agenesis. Small and large intestine contained blind-ended sacs. No testes, scrotum, and penis were found. The intact ureter was attached to a thin-walled fluid fill sac. The laboratory finding showed that the pH of the fluid was 6 and contained hemoglobin, white blood cells, bacteria, a few red blood cells, oxalate crystalline, and epithelial cells. It was concluded that the collected fluid was urine. This is the first report of perosomus elumbis in a Holstein calf having a lot of visceral abnormalities in Iran.

Case History

Perosomus elumbis, which occurs in ruminants and swines, is characterized by hypoplasia or aplasia of the spinal cord, which ends in the thoracic region. The regions of the body including the hindlimbs, which are normally supplied by the lumbar and sacral nerves, exhibit muscular atrophy, and joint movement does not develop. The rigidity of the posterior limbs may then cause dystocia (Noakes et al, 2009). This abnormality is a fairly common congenital defect in cattle (Roberts, 1986). It usually includes arthrogryposis of the hind limbs, characterized by ankylosis of the joints, with associated malformations of the musculature (Roberts, 1986). This abnormality occurs in both sexes (Jones, 1999). Perosomus elumbis in a calf was first reported in the veterinary literature in 1832 by Ernst Gurlt, and since then cases have been reported (Jones, 1999). Congenital abnormalities may cause obstetrical problems and economic losses; hence, reporting more of these cases accompanied with other defects may help us to identify the exact etiology and prevent this complication in the future.

Perosomus elumbis with visceral abnormalities is less reported worldwide. This paper describes the clinical, necropsy, and radiographic evaluation of perosomus elumbis concurrent with a lot of visceral abnormalities in a Holstein calf.

Clinical Presentation

A dead Holstein calf characterized by angular hind limb and lumbar deformities, atresia of anus, rectum, vulva, and tail, and distended abdomen was referred to the animal hospital of University of Tehran (Figure 1). The calf was born alive but died after 2 days. The calf's birth weight was 27.3 kg.

Diagnostic Testing

Radiographic analysis and subsequent necropsy revealed that the vertebral column was truncated at the first lumbar (L1) level (Figure 2) with attached iliac wings, narrowed pelvic canal, and agenesis of the L2-L5, sacral and coccygeal vertebrae (Figure 3). The femurs were malformed. Spinal cord continued until L1. Thoracic vertebrae and ribs were normal. The back of the lumbosacral region was composed of only soft tissues.

Abdominal dissection showed a plenty of abnormalities. Agenesis of the ovaries, uterine tubes, cervix, and vulva concurrent with unilateral agenesis of renal and adrenal gland, ureter and umbilical artery were observed (Figure 4). No testes, scrotum, and penis were found. The intact ureter was attached to a thin-walled sac. The sac was instead of the urinary bladder and was passed by a vestibule like structure through the narrowed pelvic canal then fused to perianal region to excrete the urine. The fluid inside the sac was evacuated to analyze its component. The laboratory finding showed that the pH of the fluid was 6 and contained hemoglobin, white blood cells (WBC), bacteria, a few red blood cells (RBC), oxalate crystalline, and epithelial cells. As a result, the collected fluid was considered urine, as was expected.

The spiral and distal colon composed of moderately distended thin-walled blind-ending sacs. The blind sacs fused with narrow connective tissue to each other and filled with brown-yellow materials. The distal portion of the distal colon was dead-ended and the calf showed anal and rectal atresia.

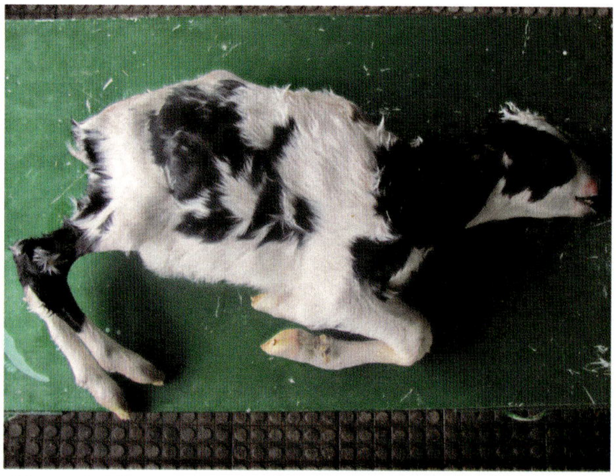

Figure 1. A Perosomus Elumbis calf with angular hind limb and lumbar deformities.

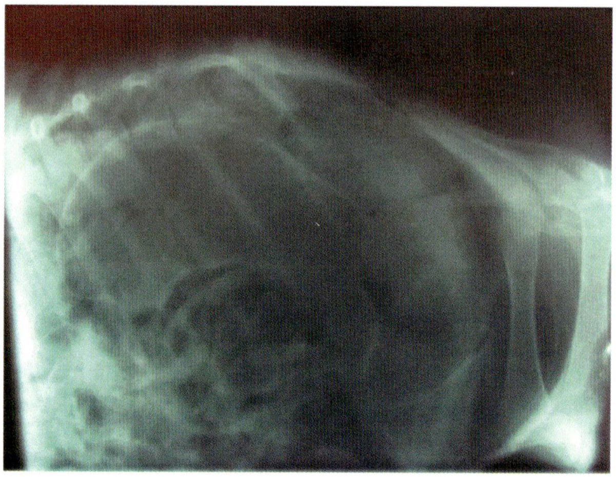

Figure 2. Radiographic region of vertebrae indicating the lack of L2-L5 lumbar vertebras.

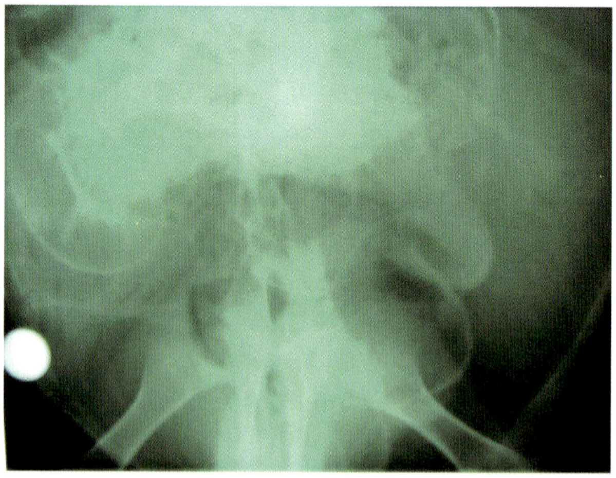

Figure 3. Ventrodorsal radiograph showing narrowed pelvic canal with attached iliac wings.

Assessments

Congenital defects can result from disruptive events at one or more stages during the complex transitions of embryonic and fetal development (Greene, 1973). Bovine inbreeding has increased the percentage of congenital defects in this species

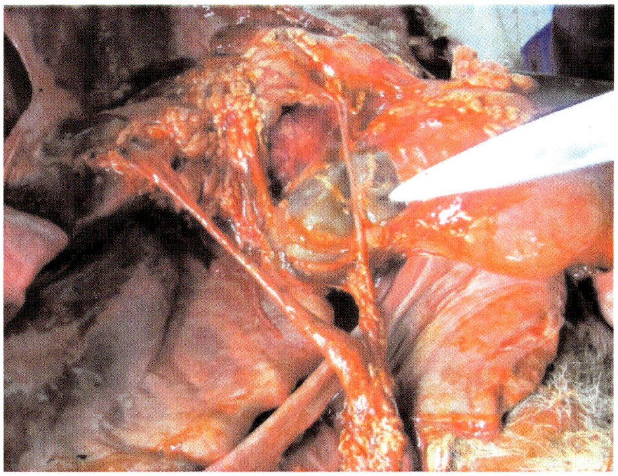

Figure 4. Unilateral aplasia of kidney, ureter and umbilical artery.

compared to the others. Although heredity has been shown to contribute to a number of well documented defects, environmentally induced defects can and do occur in any genotype (Jones, 1999).

Malformation or improper migration of the neural tube during the tail-bud stage, accompanied by partial agenesis of the caudal spinal cord, appears to be the cause of this abnormality (Gentile, 2006). Abnormal development usually occurs when a threshold of genetic and environmental insults is attained and the fetal compensatory mechanisms are overcome. Thus, purely genetic defects can originate from the dam, the sire or both, and environmental teratogens are usually numerous, as are nutritional imbalances, chemicals, drugs, and biotoxins (Rousseaux and Ribble, 1998). However, the accurate etiology of purely genetic defects is still unknown.

The laboratory finding showed that the pH of fluid evacuated from the sac (instead of the bladder) was 6 and contained hemoglobin, WBC, bacteria, a few RBC, oxalate crystalline, and epithelial cells. The collected fluid was found to be urine contaminated with blood and/or the presence of ascending infection in the incomplete urinary system after birth.

To the authors' best knowledge, anal atresia, Cryptorchidism, testicular agenesis (Williams, 1931), unilateral, intestinal malformation, vaginal and uterine malformation (Hirago, 1983), and bilateral renal agenesis (Gurlt, 1832) have been reported in perosomus elumbis cases; however, unilateral umbilical artery agenesis concurrent with all of these abnormalities has not been reported yet.

Acknowledgement

The authors would like to express their sincere gratitude to Mr. Noshahri for his kind assistance.

References

1. Gentile, A., Testoni, S. (2006) Inherited disorders of cattle: A selected review. Slov Vet Res. 43: 17-29.
2. Greene, H.J., Leipold, H.W., Huston, K., Noordsy, J.L., Dennis, S.M. (1973) Congenital defects in cattle. Iran Vet J. 27: 37-45.
3. Gurlt, E.F. (1832) Lehrbuch der pathogischen Anatomie der Haus-Sa¨ugethiere, 2. Teil, Atlas. plate IV, no. 1. G. Reimer, Berlin, Germany. p. 88-91.
4. Hirago, T., Abe, M. (1983) A case of perosomus elumbis in a calf. J Jap Vet Med Assoc. 36: 277-279.
5. Jones, C.J. (1999) Perosomus elumbis (vertebral agenesis and arthrogryposis) in a stillborn Holstein calf. Vet Pathol. 36: 64-70.
6. Noakes, D.E., Parkinson, T.J., England, G.C.W. (2009) Veterinary Reproduction and Abstetrics. (9th ed.) Elsevier, Saunders. Edinburg, London, UK.
7. Roberts, S.J. (1986) Veterinary Obstetrics and Genital Diseases (Theriogenology). Roberts, S.J. (ed.). (3rd ed.) Woodstock, Vermont. USA.
8. Rousseaux, C.G., Ribble, C.S. (1998) Developmental anomalies in farm animals. II. Defining etiology. Can Vet J. 29: 30-40.
9. Williams, W.L. (1931) Studies in teratology. Cornell Vet. 21: 25-53.

PERMISSIONS

All chapters in this book were first published in IJVM, by Faculty of Veterinary Medicine of University of Tehran; hereby published with permission under the Creative Commons Attribution License or equivalent. Every chapter published in this book has been scrutinized by our experts. Their significance has been extensively debated. The topics covered herein carry significant findings which will fuel the growth of the discipline. They may even be implemented as practical applications or may be referred to as a beginning point for another development.

The contributors of this book come from diverse backgrounds, making this book a truly international effort. This book will bring forth new frontiers with its revolutionizing research information and detailed analysis of the nascent developments around the world.

We would like to thank all the contributing authors for lending their expertise to make the book truly unique. They have played a crucial role in the development of this book. Without their invaluable contributions this book wouldn't have been possible. They have made vital efforts to compile up to date information on the varied aspects of this subject to make this book a valuable addition to the collection of many professionals and students.

This book was conceptualized with the vision of imparting up-to-date information and advanced data in this field. To ensure the same, a matchless editorial board was set up. Every individual on the board went through rigorous rounds of assessment to prove their worth. After which they invested a large part of their time researching and compiling the most relevant data for our readers.

The editorial board has been involved in producing this book since its inception. They have spent rigorous hours researching and exploring the diverse topics which have resulted in the successful publishing of this book. They have passed on their knowledge of decades through this book. To expedite this challenging task, the publisher supported the team at every step. A small team of assistant editors was also appointed to further simplify the editing procedure and attain best results for the readers.

Apart from the editorial board, the designing team has also invested a significant amount of their time in understanding the subject and creating the most relevant covers. They scrutinized every image to scout for the most suitable representation of the subject and create an appropriate cover for the book.

The publishing team has been an ardent support to the editorial, designing and production team. Their endless efforts to recruit the best for this project, has resulted in the accomplishment of this book. They are a veteran in the field of academics and their pool of knowledge is as vast as their experience in printing. Their expertise and guidance has proved useful at every step. Their uncompromising quality standards have made this book an exceptional effort. Their encouragement from time to time has been an inspiration for everyone.

The publisher and the editorial board hope that this book will prove to be a valuable piece of knowledge for researchers, students, practitioners and scholars across the globe.

LIST OF CONTRIBUTORS

Salari, S., Zahraei Salehi, T. and Nayeri Fasaei, B.
Department of Microbiology, Faculty of Veterinary Medicine, University of Tehran, Tehran, Iran

Karimi, V.
Department of Poultry Diseases, Faculty of Veterinary Medicine, University of Tehran, Tehran, Iran

Davoudi, Y.
Islamic Azad University, Sarab Branch, Sarab, Iran

Nourmohammadzadeh, F. and Abdollahpour, G.
Department of Internal Medicine, Faculty of Veterinary Medicine, University of Tehran, Tehran, Iran

Nouri, A.
Razi Vaccine and Serum Research Institute, Karaj, Iran

Nowrouzian, I.
Department of Surgery,Faculty of Veterinary Medicine,University of Tehran,Tehran, Iran

Seidabadi, M.
Graduated from the Faculty of Veterinary Medicine, Ferdowsi University of Mashhad, Mashhad, Iran

Razmi, Gh. R. and Naghibi, A.
Department of Pathobiology, Faculty of Veterinary Medicine, Ferdowsi University of Mashhad, Mashhad, Iran

Najizadeh, M.H., Pourjafar, M., Chalmeh, A., Badiei, Kh., Nazifi, S. and Naghib, M.
Department of Clinical Sciences, School of Veterinary Medicine, Shiraz University, Shiraz, Iran

Ghalyanchi Langroudi, A. and Madadgar, O.
Department of Microbiology and Immunology, Faculty of Veterinary Medicine, University of Tehran, Tehran, Iran

Hosseini, H.
Department of Clinical Sciences, Faculty of Veterinary Medicine, Islamic Azad University, Karaj Branch, Karaj, Iran

Karimi, V.
Department of Poultry Diseases, Faculty of Veterinary Medicine, University of Tehran, Tehran, Iran

Hashemzadeh, M.
Department of Research & Production of Veterinary and Poultry Vaccines, Razi Vaccine and Serum Research Institute, Karaj, Iran

Ghafouri, S. A.
Department of Poultry Health and Diseases, Iranian Veterinary Organization, Tehran, Iran

Bagheri Ghadikolaei, S. S. and Vahedi, S. M.
Students' Scientific Association of Microbiology, Faculty of Veterinary Medicine, University of Tehran, Tehran, Iran

Khanzadi, S. and Jamshidi, A.
Department of Food Hygiene and Aquaculture, Faculty of Veterinary Medicine, Ferdowsi University of Mashhad, Mashhad, Iran

Razmyar, J.
Department of Clinical Sciences, Faculty of Veterinary Medicine, Ferdowsi University of Mashhad, Mashhad, Iran

Borji, Sh.
Graduated from the Faculty of Veterinary Medicine, Ferdowsi University of Mashhad, Mashhad, Iran

Alirezaei, M.
Division of Biochemistry, School of Veterinary Medicine, Lorestan University, Khorram Abad, Iran

Arabkhazaeli, F.
Department of Parasitology, Faculty of Veterinary Medicine, University of Tehran, Tehran, Iran

Madani, S. A.
Department of Avian Diseases, Faculty of Veterinary Medicine, University of Tehran, Tehran, Iran

Jafari Dehkordi, A.
Department of Large Animal Internal Medicine, Veterinary Faculty of Shahrekord University, Shahrekord, Iran

Mohebbi, A. N.
Department of Veterinary Clinical Pathology, Veterinary Faculty of Shahrekord University, Shahrekord, Iran

Balali Dehkordi, Sh.
Graduated from the Faculty of Veterinary Medicine, Shahrekord University, Shahrekord, Iran

Akhtardanesh, B.
Department of Clinical Sciences, Faculty of Veterinary Medicine, Shahid-Bahonar University of Kerman, Kerman, Iran

Sharifi, H.
Department of Food Hygiene, Faculty of Veterinary Medicine, Shahid-Bahonar University of Kerman, Kerman, Iran

Rasooli, R. and Aghazamani, M.
Graduated from the Faculty of Veterinary Medicine, Shahid Bahonar University of Kerman, Kerman, Iran

Pourjafar, H. and Noori, N.
Department of Food Hygiene and Quality Control, Faculty of Veterinary Medicine, University of Tehran, Tehran , Iran

Ghasemnejad, R.
Department of Food Hygiene and Quality Control, Science and Research Campus, Islamic Azad University, Tehran, Iran

Mohammadi, Kh.
Department of Food Hygiene and Quality Control, Faculty of Veterinary Medicine, Tabriz Branch, Islamic Azad

Kheradmand, A.
Department of Clinical Sciences, School of Veterinary Medicine, Lorestan University, Khorram Abad, Iran

Kamali Sangani, A.
Graduated from the Faculty of Agriculture, University of Tarbiat Modares, Tehran, Iran

Masoudi, A. A.
Department of Animal Sciences, University of Tarbiat Modares, Tehran, Iran

Hosseini, S. A.
Department of Animal and Poultry Nutrition, Animal Sciences Research Institute, Karaj, Iran

Masoudifard, M., Vajhi, A. R. and Molazem, M.
Department of Surgery and Radiology, Faculty of Veterinary Medicine, University of Tehran, Tehran, Iran

Mansouri, Sh.
Private Veterinary Practitioner, Tehran, Iran

Bahonar, A. R.
Department of Food Hygiene and Quality Control, Faculty of Veterinary Medicine, University of Tehran, Tehran, Iran

Zehtabvar, O.
Department of Basic Sciences, Faculty of Veterinary Medicine, University of Tehran, Tehran, Iran

Pirali Kheirabadi, Kh.
Department of Pathobiology, Faculty of Veterinary Medicine, Shahrekord University, Shahrekord, Iran

Fallah, A.
Department of Food Hygiene and Quality Control, Faculty of Veterinary Medicine, Shahrekord University, Shahrekord, Iran

Abolghasemi, A.
Graduated from the Faculty of Veterinary Medicine, Shahrekord University, Shahrekord, Iran

Mokhtari, A. and Mahzounieh, M. R.
Department of Pathobiology, Faculty of Veterinary Medicine, University of Shahrekord, Shahrekord, Iran

Rassouli, A., Amani, Z., Shams, Gh. and Abdolmaleki, Z.
Department of Pharmacology, Faculty of Veterinary Medicine, University of Tehran, Tehran, Iran

Bahonar, A.
Department of Food Hygiene and Quality Control, Faculty of Veterinary Medicine, University of Tehran, Tehran, Iran

Ebrahimzadeh, E., Pazhoom, F., Nabian, S., Shayan and P., Bakhshani, A.
Department of Parasitology and Tick and Tick Born Diseases Center, Faculty of Veterinary Medicine, University of Tehran, Tehran, Iran

Omidi, A.
Department of Animal Health Management, School of Veterinary Medicine, Shiraz University, Shiraz, Iran

Sajedi, Zh. and Montazer Torbati, M. B.
Department of Animal Sciences, Agriculture Faculty, Birjand University, Birjand, Iran

Mostafai, M.
Research Centre for Agriculture and Natural Resources, Ardabil, Iran

Mahmoodi Afsah, T., Vojgani, M. and Gharagozlou, F.
Department of Theriogenology, Faculty of Veterinary Medicine, University of Tehran, Tehran, Iran

Akbarinejad, V.
Young Researchers and Elites Club, North Tehran Branch, Islamic Azad University, Tehran, Iran

Nazem, M. N.
Department of Basic Sciences, Faculty of Veterinary Medicine, Shahid Bahonar University of Kerman, Kerman, Iran

Sami, M.
Department of Food Hygiene and Public Health, Faculty of Veterinary Medicine, Shahid Bahonar University of Kerman, Kerman, Iran

Askari, N.
School of Veterinary Medicine, Shahid Bahonar University of Kerman, Kerman, Iran

Alishahi, M.
Department of Clinical Sciences, Faculty of Veterinary Medicine, Shahid Chamran University of Ahvaz, Ahvaz, Iran

Esmaeili Rad, A.
Graduated Student from the Faculty of Veterinary Medicine, Shahid Chamran University of Ahvaz, Ahvaz, Iran

Ghorbanpour, M.
Department of Pathobiology, Faculty of Veterinary Medicine, Shahid Chamran University, Ahvaz, Iran

Zarei, M.
Department of Food Hygiene, Faculty of Veterinary Medicine, Shahid Chamran University of Ahvaz, Ahvaz, Iran

Mansoori, F. and Roshani, H.
Department of Basic Sciences, School of Veterinary Medicine, Shahid Bahonar University of Kerman, Kerman, Iran

Shemshadi, B. and Ranjbar-Bahadori, Sh.
Department of Parasitology, Faculty of Veterinary Medicine, Garmsar Branch, Islamic Azad University, Garmsar, Iran

Faghihzadeh-Gorji, S.
Graduated from the Faculty of Veterinary Medicine, Garmsar Branch, Islamic Azad University, Garmsar, Iran

Changizi, E.
Deparment of Pathobiology, Faculty of Veterinary Medicine, Semnan University, Semnan, Iran

Erfani Majd, N., Sehab Negah, S. and Fatemi Tabatabaei, S. R.
Department of Basic Sciences, Faculty of Veterinary Medicine, Shahid Chamran University of Ahvaz, Ahvaz, Iran

Beizaei, A., Kamkar, A. and Misaghi, A.
Department of Food Hygiene and Quality Control, Faculty of Veterinary Medicine, University of Tehran, Tehran, Iran

Teik Chung, E. L. and Saharee, A. A.
Department of Veterinary Clinical Studies, Faculty of Veterinary Medicine, Universiti Putra Malaysia, Serdang, Selangor, Malaysia

Jesse Abdullah, F. F. and Haron, A. W.
Department of Veterinary Clinical Studies, Faculty of Veterinary Medicine, Universiti Putra Malaysia, Serdang, Selangor, Malaysia
Research Centre for Ruminant Disease, Faculty of Veterinary Medicine, Universiti Putra Malaysia, Serdang, Selangor, Malaysia

Sadiq, M. A. and Mohd, A. M. L.
Department of Veterinary Pathology and Microbiology, Faculty of Veterinary Medicine, Universiti Putra Malaysia, Serdang, Selangor, Malaysia

Tijjani, A. and Abba, Y.
Department of Veterinary Pathology and Microbiology, Faculty of Veterinary Medicine, Universiti Putra Malaysia, Serdang, Selangor, Malaysia
Faculty of Veterinary Medicine, University of Maiduguri, Borno State, Nigeria

Adamu, L. and Mohammed, K.
Department of Veterinary Clinical Studies, Faculty of Veterinary Medicine, Universiti Putra Malaysia, Serdang, Selangor, Malaysia
Faculty of Veterinary Medicine, University of Maiduguri, Borno State, Nigeria

Arabkhazaeli, F. and Nabian, S.
Department of Parasitology, Faculty of Veterinary Medicine, University of Tehran, Tehran, Iran

Modirsanei, M.
Department of Animal and Poultry Health and Nutrition, Faculty of Veterinary Medicine, University of Tehran, Tehran, Iran

Madani, S. A.
Department of Avian Diseases, Faculty of Veterinary Medicine, University of Tehran, Tehran, Iran

Eslami, M.
Department of Theriogenology and Poultry, Faculty of Veterinary Medicine, University of Urmia, Urmia, Iran

Gharagozloo, F. and Vojgani, M.
Department of Theriogenology, Faculty of Veterinary Medicine, University of Tehran, Tehran, Iran

Rahimi Feyli, P.
Department of Clinical Sciences, Faculty of Veterinary Medicine, Razi University, Kermanshah, Iran

Soroori, S.
Department of Surgery and Radiology, Faculty of Veterinary Medicine, University of Tehran, Tehran, Iran

Index